FENG SHUI
AND HEALTH

THE ANATOMY OF A HOME

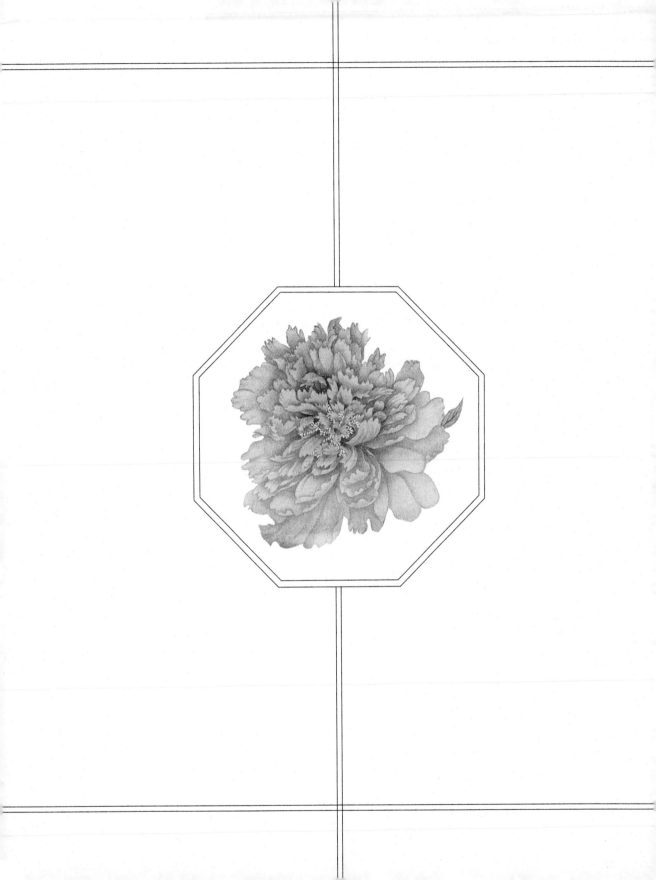

FENG SHUI
AND HEALTH

THE ANATOMY OF A HOME

Using Feng Shui to Disarm Illness,
Accelerate Recovery, and Create Optimal Health

NANCY SANTOPIETRO

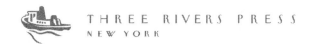
THREE RIVERS PRESS
NEW YORK

Published by Three Rivers Press, New York, New York.
Member of the Crown Publishing Group, a division of Random House, Inc.

www.randomhouse.com

THREE RIVERS PRESS and the Tugboat design are registered trademarks
of Random House, Inc.

Printed in the United States of America

DESIGN BY LYNNE AMFT

Illustrations by Cindy Booth

Library of Congress Cataloging-in-Publication Data
SantoPietro, Nancy.
Feng shui and health: the anatomy of a home: using Feng Shui to disarm illness,
accelerate recovery, and create optimal health / Nancy SantoPietro.—1st ed.
1. Feng shui—Health aspects.   2. Alternative medicine.   3. Mind and body.
4. Self-care, Health.   5. Interior design and health.   6. Interior design and illness.
7. Chakra Energy System and health.   8. Chakra Energy System and illness.
9. Chakra Energy System and Feng Shui Design.   10. Color, Feng Shui, Chakras, and health.
I. Title.

RZ999 .S325 2001
613—dc21   2001034067

ISBN 0-609-80661-0
10 9 8 7 6 5 4

TO MY FIVE THUNDERS:

Susan Olsen

Robin Spiegel

Greer Jonas

Lisa Braun

H. H. Professor Thomas Lin Yun Rinpoche . . .

for continued love and support,

and for walking beside me,

lifetime after lifetime.

To each one of you, thank you—108 times over. . . .

Acknowledgments

AS WITH ALL CREATIVE ENDEAVORS, many tangible and intangible factors need to come together to help birth the final project. Many wonderful individuals have participated, some knowingly and some unknowingly, in the birthing of this book. I thank the following people for their love, generosity, and heartfelt contributions: Lisa Aldisert; Irene Prokop; Doveen Schecter; Julie Anna Alverez; Petra Sacco; Silvana Occhialini and Márcia Silva De Luca, my Brazilian angels; Durga Das Patello; Pat Coliene; Judy Wicker; Jenny Parra; Ma Baghavati; Nurit Schwarzbaum; Carolyn Rangel; Marina Lighthouse; Janine Sneider; Crystal Chu; Dr. Lien Nguyen; Mary Hsu; Lin-Lin Cheng; the Yun Lin Temple and Monastery staff; Jeneane Willyard; Melissa Willyard; Erik Willyard; Marie Alvino; Jazan Higgins; Faye Lane; Jill Higgins; Mary Zimmerman; Susan Sollinger; Eddie Sollinger; Julia Sollinger; Florence Kapovich; the Hayslip family; Howard Jaffe; Irene Jaffe; Katherine Cohen; Jerry Cohen; Benjamin Cohen; Audrey Levy; Carole Katz; Patricia Belfanti; Gabriella Messina; Gigi Estabrook; Dr. Serafina Corsella; Dr. Howard Bezoza; Dr. Richard Ash; Michel J. Landron; my Black Hat Sect family and colleagues; R. D. Chin; Melanie Lewendowski; Sarah Rossbach; Lillian Garnier; Robin Lennon; Mary Cordaro; Carol Adrienne; Gregg Braden; Ruby Holladay; my mother, Matilda Amendolare; my sisters, Cathy

SantoPietro and Rita Harrison; my aunt, Virginia Siniscalco; Susan Failla; Phillip Reinhardt; Aralys Estevez; Rev. Charmaine Colon; all my Feng Shui Consultation and Therapy clients; the students, lightworkers, and graduates of my Feng Shui Consultant Training Program, The Accelerated Path™; all the volunteers, merchants, and Feng Shui consultants who have contributed their time, expertise, and monies to the Feng Shui Across America and Feng Shui Around the World Projects; a big thanks and appreciation to Shelly Sparks and the Gang in L.A. for continuing to Light the Way . . .

SPECIAL THANKS TO . . .

Denise Linn for her love and friendship, and her spiritual example of what true "heart-based" leadership really is; Katherine Metz for her commitment to excellence and for eloquently preserving the Black Hat Lineage and H. H. Professor Thomas Lin Yun Rinpoche's teachings; Dr. Heather Anne Harder for her cutting-edge work and for bringing my understanding of the bigger picture of life to a whole new dimension; Nancy Rosanoff for continued brilliance, fifteen years of mentoring, guidance, and a treasured friendship—her teachings on the Chakras and intuition continue to have the most powerful influence on my work and my life today; Deepak Chopra for his generous blessings and his embodiment of "limitless possibilities"; my Chinese mother, Dr. Catherine Yi-yu Cho Woo, for teaching me the things I didn't know I needed to learn—with love from Little Dog to Big Dog; Cindy Booth for her wonderful illustrations and constant serenity; Candice Fuhrman, my agent; Agnes Krup, my foreign-rights agent; my editorial team, Patty Gift, Carrie Thornton, Stephanie Gunning, Jazan Higgins, Robin Spiegel, and Susan Olsen; Nora Adela Montoya for her gift of healing the manuscript, so it could heal others; Diane Hoffmann for her heartfelt assistance, editing, and ongoing support; Sarah Spataro, whose support and years of loyalty helped shape the beginnings of my work, my business, and the manuscript of this book . . . thank you, thank you, old friend. And to . . . Hey, *What's An Angel Doing Here?* With "flower candy kisses" I thank you for your love, kindness, and incredible support! And to all of you readers who have struggled in the face of a chronic illness, never give up hope that a healing is not only possible, but expected!

AND TO MY FIVE THUNDERS . . .

Robin Spiegel for a bonding and a friendship that always was and slways will be; Greer Jonas for love without conditions; Lisa Braun for spiritual guidance and compassionate, wise counsel; Susan Olsen, whose continued love, friendship, humor, camaraderie, and assistance carried me, once again, past the finish line of this manuscript, thank you for everything; and a special acknowledgment of thanks and gratitude to H. H. Professor Thomas Lin Yun Rinpoche, who single-handedly, with much grace and humility, changed the world for the better, and me along with it . . .

A VERY SPECIAL THANK-YOU TO . . .

My late stepdad, Dominick Amendolare, for his love and support that has emanated from the Yang life, and continues to flow through the Yin life . . . you are always in my heart.

AND IN MEMORY OF . . .

My friend the late Holly Huang of the Yun Lin Monastery. Thank you for all your years of dedication, service, and quiet acts of kindness. You will be greatly missed.

Contents

CONTENTS

CONTENTS

xiv

Foreword

By H. H. Grandmaster Professor Thomas Lin Yun
Rinpoche, Head Master and Spiritual Leader of the Third
and Fourth Stages of the Black Hat Sect School of
Tibetan Tantric Buddhism

NANCY SANTOPIETRO'S NEW BOOK, *Feng Shui and Health: The Anatomy of a Home,* promises to be a masterpiece that will help people in need and bring great benefits to the world. This is a unique and unparalleled new book that accelerates the process of regaining our health. The author's main goal is to break through traditional medical treatment theories, perspectives, and methods to extinguish illnesses speedily, so that people can recover their physical health as soon as possible. These brand-new and amazing diagnostic methods are really rare and very hard to come by. In addition to paying respect to traditional physiological, psychological, pathological, emotional, medical, pharmacological, and Western-based healing methods, the author clearly outlines how to use Feng Shui Design, spiritual cultivation, and the Chakra Energy System to accelerate the recovery of our health. The reader should not overlook the "Vibrational Medicine" healing methods that Ms. SantoPietro introduces in this book. These methods analyze our bodies' internal vibrational patterns to illuminate the spiritual cultivation, past lives, dispositions, religious beliefs, personalities, body shapes, and body weights that are formed as a result of our different physical bodies, emotions, and frequencies. This book also teaches us about the "Nine Hallmarks" of the spiritual revolution that are unfolding in this new millennium, and their impact on our health. She repeatedly explains the various types and patterns of energy and how they have a close relationship to the emotional, spiritual, and physiological ESPs of our illnesses.

Ms. SantoPietro, who is wise as well as benevolent, has the remarkable foresight to let her readers know that Feng Shui is the complement and "added boost" to traditional medicine in the next millennium. Feng Shui will bring unimaginable changes to our lives, life spans, and health. Therefore, the author created another chapter to teach us numerous ways to assess our own health through the Feng Shui design of our space. Once we are aware of our own health condition, in addition to continuing mundane treatment methods, the author also sincerely introduces nine transcendental treatment methods, which are rare to find even in our historical folklore cultures. These cures are the "accelerated ch'i and illness adjustment methods" according to Black Sect Tantric Buddhism. Of course, it is only by determining how and when to do these transcendental methods that we will achieve the best and most obvious results. Ms. SantoPietro also explains that the bedroom is the most sacred place to best adjust our physical and emotional health issues and what specifics are needed to create ideal Feng Shui in that room. The author also tirelessly points out architectural layouts that will bring negative effects to our bodies, and teaches us how to align our personal ch'i with Feng Shui Design and the power of visualization so that we can accurately receive the most benefits for healing. At the end of the book, the author even presents the most treasured Black Sect Tantric Buddhist Transcendental Solutions for health, which are of the highest order of secrecy and not usually taught publicly. These transcendental solutions are some of the best spiritual medicines available to solve all problems, miseries, and health conditions. They are the "Six Tone, Six Ch'i Meditation Method" and the "Healing Medicine Buddha Prayer." These are very rare and very sacred. "Color Healing Methods" are also included for adjusting the ch'i of the body and the home through the use of the colors of the Chakras and the many colors of the Feng Shui Bagua. These adjustments will enhance your happiness, well-being, and overall physical health.

In summary, the compassionate and munificent Ms. SantoPietro has utilized all of her mundane and transcendental knowledge, especially that of the Chakra Energy System, to employ multiple ways of dismantling many challenging but common illnesses. Finally, she has asked clients who have had past experiences in dealing with these illnesses to give personal testimonies to the actual effectiveness of the healing methods contained in this book. Therefore, when I said that this book is a masterpiece that will bring great benefits to the world, I definitely was not exaggerating!

It is always difficult to write the foreword for a book, but it is especially difficult for a book that is written by an expert. In addition to formally taking refuge with me and becoming my so-called disciple, this kindhearted author is also my good friend of many years. In addition to her bountiful mundane and transcendental knowledge, she often travels to hospitals all over the world to give aid and assistance to those people who are in need. Even though many know of her virtue and benevolence, it has not yet been widely recognized that her conduct and ideology have already reached the apex of the world. An ancient Chinese proverb says, "The indigo ink is bluer than the indigo plant from which it comes."★ Every time I read her books or hear that she is traveling around the world providing assistance to the needy, a deep sense of respect grows within me. I believe that through this book, all readers will receive the secrets to receiving good health and longevity. Even though the book itself may be easy to obtain, the methods provided in it are very difficult to find. The Chinese have another saying: "Opening a book will bring great benefits." Now that Ms. SantoPietro has provided both the book and the methods, I truly know that readers throughout the world will receive good health and great happiness. . . . I strongly believe that as long as you read the book seriously and follow the methods carefully, you will benefit from the author's dedication and efforts.

—LIN YUN, SEPTEMBER 10, 2000

★"The indigo ink is bluer than the indigo plant from which it comes" is a Chinese proverb that teachers often use to graciously praise the achievement of their students for having surpassed their own achievements.

—TRANSLATED FROM MANDARIN TO ENGLISH BY MARY HSU

THE STARFISH MAN

───

One morning at dawn, a young boy went for a walk on the beach. Up ahead, he noticed an old man stooping down to pick up starfish and fling them into the sea. Finally, catching up with the old man, the boy asked him what he was doing. The old man answered that the stranded starfish would die unless they were returned to the water. "But the beach goes on for miles, and there are millions of starfish," protested the boy. "How can what you're doing make any difference?" The old man looked at the starfish in his hand and then threw it to safety in the waves. "It makes a difference to this one," he said.

INTRODUCTION

*"Ms. SantoPietro, your test results are back
and all your blood work appears normal!"*

1990

MOST PEOPLE WHO are ill would breathe a sigh of relief or give their right arm to have those types of test results reported back to them. For me, it was just another part of my ongoing nightmare, for I was one year into an illness that baffled the medical profession and left me without a diagnosis or any hope. My test results continually came back normal, but my health was rapidly declining. With every new day, I was becoming more and more despondent and scared.

In 1989 I was thirty years old and had a promising career as a psychospiritual therapist. I lectured extensively on the Chakra Energy System, conducted a full-time psychotherapy practice in New York City, and in the midst of it all, my life fell apart.

What started out as an apparent stomach virus turned into a ten-year nightmare that left me sick with daily fevers and swollen glands. At times I was unable to eat, sleep, or concentrate very well. For the first few years, each doctor I went to gave me the same diagnosis, that nothing was medically wrong with me. Unable to identify what was really wrong with me, most recommended sleep and rest. Some suggested changing my profession, because "listening to other people's problems all day must be very depressing." My personal favorite was from a noted gastrointestinal specialist who said, "I think you should consider getting married. It must be hard for a young woman like yourself to be single and only have a career"!

Needless to say, I was scared and had no clue what was happening in my life. I was so preoccupied with my daily survival that often just getting through the day was all I could handle. For lack of a better plan, I continued my weekly psychotherapy sessions, pursued medical treatment from numerous traditional and nontraditional practitioners, joined a twelve-step fellowship, read spiritual growth books, and prayed a lot.

My illness was very loud and demanding. Initially my physical distress manifested as an allergic reaction to dust, molds, common foods, and household products. My first thought was "Wow, my higher power really doesn't want me to clean my own house!" As my condition worsened and became not so funny anymore, I found myself frequently out of breath, not sleeping, not eating, and with constant flulike symptoms. At one point my condition became so bad that I wasn't able to climb the subway steps in Brooklyn to take the train into Manhattan to my office. I felt as if I weighed three hundred pounds and had chronic emphysema.

I didn't know what was happening to me. In retrospect, I truly believe that if I hadn't had a spiritual framework to hold on to, I would probably have taken my own life—not because I didn't want to live anymore, but because I didn't know how to stop feeling so sick, and couldn't find a strong enough reason to go on living. I cried daily for most of those years, and lived every day with constant fear and worry. My illness was chipping away not only at my physical health but at my mental and emotional well-being. I was scared about everything—that I would never get well, that I'd run out of money, not be able to work, and eventually just go insane. My fear escalated as the reality set in of having an undiagnosed chronic illness that was not only destroying my life, but perplexing my doctors, as well.

Needless to say, I was not a very "good" sick person. I spent most of my time feeling overwhelmed and out of control and trying to conceal from most people (especially myself) the fact that I was so sick. It took me several more years to figure out why I felt so much shame about being sick, and why I felt somehow it was a personal reflection on me. I felt that these sorts of things happened to other people, and that they shouldn't happen to people who are good or spiritually evolved. This illness shook me at the very center of my being because now I was faced with a set of circumstances that no longer made sense in relation to my core spiritual beliefs. Suddenly I was praying to what I thought to be a benevolent God who no longer heard my prayers and my call for help.

In the midst of all the confusion, something profound began to take shape. Some very strange symptoms began to emerge that made no apparent medical or logical sense. I began to notice that not only was I having a difficult time sleeping at night, but also that I was constantly changing the position I was sleeping in. At first I thought it was because I was just trying to get comfortable, but no position seemed better than another. Over time it evolved to the point that I was no longer able to sleep in my bedroom at all.

As my illness progressed, I became increasingly sensitive to the energy in my environment, especially in my bedroom. I started to notice that some places in my home were more stressful to be in than others. For reasons that were not yet obvious to me, my home became a place I was no longer comfortable living in. In a desperate attempt to deal with this awareness, I decided to rearrange not only the furniture, but the rooms in my apartment as well.

I rounded up several skeptical friends, and within two days they moved my bedroom furniture into what was formerly my living room/psychotherapy office. As it turned out, I never got to sleep in my new bedroom. After walking into my home for the first time after the furniture was rearranged, I had a sudden realization that I could no longer live there. Crazy as it seemed, I knew intuitively that I had to move. Three weeks later I was living in another place.

All I knew was that something had changed drastically in my apartment when I moved my furniture around. At the time it didn't make any sense to me, but as fate would have it, several months later I was going to be introduced to a set of design principles that would change my life forever.

One evening while getting a weekly bodywork session at the home of one of my neighbors, I commented on the arrangement of the furniture in her living room. I knew that something felt different from the week before; the space seemed clearer and much more expansive to me. She confirmed my observation and said that she had recently moved some furniture around after reading an article on the Chinese art of placement and design called Feng Shui.

This was in 1989. Not only had I never heard of Feng Shui before, but I was having quite a time just trying to say it correctly *(Fung Shway)*. She told me that the art originated more than four thousand years ago in Asia.

Its basic premise is that invisible energy fields exist in our homes and work spaces, and that those energy fields are created by the way we place our furniture and design our homes. As I inquired further, I discovered that every environment has its own metabolism, with its own unique flow of energy. These energy fields also have a profound effect on shaping all aspects of our lives, including finances, relationships, *and health.*

I immediately knew Feng Shui had something to do with what was happening to my health, and that my former apartment had somehow contributed to my getting ill. My neighbor lent me the two books she had on Feng Shui, written by Sarah Rossbach. I read them voraciously, along with any other information I could find on the subject. Those two books changed not only my life but the direction of my life's work.

I soon realized that if this concept of environment influencing life and life situations was true, I needed to seriously explore it and somehow add it to my approach as a holistic therapist. If, in fact, environments significantly influenced life situations—and since my clients spent only fifty minutes a week in my office, but then went back to spend the rest of their time in their homes and offices—then I must somehow start incorporating Feng Shui principles into my treatment plan, in order to treat the whole client. Suddenly my current approach to healing seemed limited at best, and to be missing some very crucial pieces.

I asked my therapy clients to bring their floor plans into their sessions. We would break a few minutes early and I would review those plans, making suggestions on where to move certain pieces of furniture or where, for example, to hang a wind chime. They would go home, rearrange things, and report back to me the following week on how the changes felt.

Most of these clients had been seeing me for years and were very active in their own healing process, but like everyone else, they were at times stuck in their own issues. As I began to incorporate Feng Shui into their treatment process, I witnessed many clients who had been blocked in various situations begin to move forward and make substantial changes. Some left unhappy marriages, others changed careers, while still others who were unemployed found fulfilling work. Needless to say, the Feng Shui process really caught my attention!

I started to make more aggressive changes and add adjustments to my own home, and soon a very interesting turn of events occurred. The adjustments somehow contributed to exacerbating my illness; I actually became so ill that I eventually had to close my second office in Manhattan. My life was unraveling once again, and after putting up a good fight and realizing that there was nothing more I could do about it, I eventually surrendered to it.

Just for the record, let me state that I didn't go willingly. The universe had to pry my fingers off my "old" life. I had no clue that anything good lay ahead for me; all I knew was that something was happening to my life that felt scary and devastating, and that my world was falling apart and I didn't know what was happening or why.

That period represented a major turning point for my health, my work, and myself. Though I didn't realize it at the time, I had to become sicker before I could get better. What transpired during those very frightening months actually forced me to go see other doctors, and eventually I found one who was not only empathetic, but who had also been sick for a time with the same illness! He diagnosed me with chronic viral syndrome and immune system failure. My immune system, continually overworked and overstressed, had basically collapsed and I'd picked up a retrovirus that was causing havoc in my body. Because of that diagnosis, I was eventually able to get on disability and take some time off to heal without the major pressures of full-time employment.

During that time I began to search out ways to understand what was happening to me. Even with my newfound diagnosis, medical treatment, and continued psychotherapy sessions, I was still pretty sick. In many ways it was actually a blessing, for it forced me to deal not only with my body's physical needs, but with other aspects of my life that were contributing to my illness. Over time I began to piece together the emotional and spiritual underpinnings of my physical illness that were keeping me sick, and to find the things that really needed changing in my life. I had to revisit my dysfunctional childhood and once again process my physical, emotional, and sexual-abuse issues. I had to complete my grieving process over my grandmother's suicide and rework the various ways that I'd learned to cope with it all. As I began to look back again, I realized that although I had survived all those past traumas, my immune system, the part of my being that was cleverly hidden away from everyone, wasn't in fact immune to those childhood and life traumas and their aftereffects.

The breakdown of my body, and subsequently my life, set me on a journey to uncover what was happening to me, why and how to best address and deal with it all. My concept of God and my understanding of illness and the way I worked with other people's lives, health, and healing processes were forced to be reevaluated.

Although I was gradually getting better, it always seemed that I was just one set of symptoms away from feeling truly well. I worked so hard, for so many years, at getting my health back, often to no avail, that I knew that somewhere there was something else I was missing regarding my sickness and my healing process. In the mid-1990s, while speaking at a health expo in Seattle, I had the good fortune to have my booth placed next to that of Dr. Heather Anne Harder. Dr. Harder had written several very interesting "life after life" books. Two of those books in particular, *Many Were Called, Few Were Chosen* and *Perfect Power in Consciousness,* changed the way I understood life and awareness. Heather wrote about the different levels of consciousness on which we all function, and how each of those levels affects the way we see life and the way we function in the world. She also discussed a major change that we were in the process of experiencing on the planet, a change she called the Paradigm Shift. As I read more, I began to piece together a theory of what might be happening to me and to my health from the perspective of planetary changes and their effect on our lives, our emotions, and the way we see the world. I began to apply some of those principles to my own healing, and then to connect them to the current Western resurrection of Feng Shui Design and to my prior knowledge of the Chakra Energy System. Over time I developed an eclectic approach to my own healing process. These followed a long decade of profound insights, spiritual enlightenments, and theoretical realizations that changed the way I saw my illness, my treatment process, and my approach to assisting people who were ill.

Understanding about energy patterns and their interplay with Feng Shui and the Chakras led me to design an approach to working with and transmuting illness in a very progressive, cutting-edge way, through the use of "vibrational medicines."

I came to realize that all illnesses have a specific vibration or vibrational pattern with which they resonate and that those same patterns of illness can be re-created in our homes and in our daily surroundings. I found that when an individual has an illness or a predisposition to an illness, if that individual finds himself living or frequenting an environment that also vibrates with the same illness patterns, we create a set of energetic variables that can come together and can either exacerbate an existing illness or manifest one that is otherwise dormant. I've discovered that by working with the internal energy system (the Chakras) and the external energy system (Feng Shui), you can approach dismantling your illness vibrationally from both the inside and the outside vibrational forms in which it exists. This dual approach can alter and transmute an illness, making it more receptive to medicines, treatment processes, and prayer. I've come to understand that no single approach can heal illness completely. As you will learn in the forthcoming chapters, many different solutions, tangible and intangible, visible and invisible, factor into our health quotient. By addressing the ESPs of Illness™ (the emotional, spiritual, and physical underpinnings of why you became sick), and what some of their variables may be that are affecting your disease and treatment plan, you can work to disarm its impact and source of origin.

Feng Shui opened my eyes and mind to the impact that the environment can have on one's life and health. It opened doors for me, and became the foundation for the theories contained in this book. By combining my Chakra work with Feng Shui and with the use of color as a healing tool, I was able to piece together what was happening not only to my health but to my life as well. I came to understand empathetically that all illness is not just black-and-white or scientifically measurable; we must also take into account energy fields, vibrational patterns, and Earth frequencies. Some of these may at first seem very esoteric and at times even a bit "out there," but they exist. In my opinion, these new concepts regarding vibrational patterns are on the cutting edge of where true "complementary medicine" is going. Whenever something new is presented to us that at first we don't completely understand, it's a very common reaction to diminish and sometimes dismiss what we hear. It's very typical to respond to new information this way, because it is not always easy to incorporate new ideas and concepts into our thinking, especially ones that might force us to change the way we do and see things.

I was faced with this dilemma until I realized that although these concepts initially confused me, eventually they gave me an expansive frame of reference in which I could truly understand what was happening to my life. If I had not discovered many of the other factors that were contributing to my deteriorating health, I would probably have spent my whole life blaming my illness exclusively on myself, my difficult childhood, and my failing immune system.

The environmental, chemical, technological, and electromagnetic changes that are continuing to take place on the planet today are directly affecting our health and many of the chronic diseases we face daily. The more you understand that these illnesses and challenges are due in part to the many "vibrational shifts" that are creating energetic imbalances and emotional challenges, the more sense it will make to you that the remedy for these "vibrationally based illnesses" are "vibrationally based medicines" such as homeopathy, color and sound therapy, Chakra Psychology, Feng Shui, and the like. As I explored my own recovery process, I became more aware of how and why venerable healing arts such as Feng Shui and the Chakra Energy System were being resurrected now. We live in a time in which we need to include the best of *all* medicines—traditional, nontraditional, allopathic, naturopathic, and vibrational as well. These various modalities are beginning to resurface to assist us specifically through this time of transition and great healing. If a total transmutation, or healing, is going to occur, you have to process all the emotional issues that are stored at the core of your illness, examine the spiritual, bigger-picture reasons why your soul chose the particular illness you have, and—*very important*—get the medical attention of your choice to help address its physical manifestation in your body. All these things need to be worked on simultaneously so that a complementary approach to healing illness can occur.

As you begin to explore the concept of vibrational patterns, you will begin to see how these patterns can manifest within both yourself and your environment. These two forms of patterns can create imbalanced or unhealthy patterns of energy, or ch'i flow; left uncorrected, they can cause blocks in your career, difficulties with your finances, poor health, illness and disease, as well as dissatisfaction in your love life. By learning to assess and analyze vibrational patterns and the Feng Shui of your environment, you will be able to tap in to a new approach in how to understand, diagnose, and treat illness and attend to your own health.

Since 1990, I have had the great honor and privilege of studying under the tutelage of H. H. Professor Thomas Lin Yun Rinpoche, Head Master and Spiritual Leader of the Black Hat Tibetan Tantric Buddhism School of Feng Shui. His grace, wit, spiritual presence, and compassion for the human struggle slowly turned my life and my healing process around. His impact on my life and work goes far beyond the classroom; what he did for me was to restore my hope and my self-value and to remind me constantly of the importance of "one solitary life," mine. In helping me see what was invisible to most people, I then was able to see, truly and fully, many things that most people often look away from.

I had to take a long, hard, and at times painful look at my life and the string of events that led up to my illness. Honestly, I didn't want to do it, but time and experience have taught me that the "only way out of it is through it," and through it I went, though often not very gracefully. I never had a conscious intention of writing a book on healing. Frankly, after twelve years of being sick, seeing doctors, and experiencing ongoing health-related setbacks, the last thing I wanted to be involved with was an illness-related treatment approach! But they say that "we teach what we need to learn," and I desperately needed to learn how to get well and make the changes in my life that would keep me well. During my years of study and illness, I developed various theories concerning how and why people become ill, then combined those theories with my years of experience as a psychotherapist and my training in the Chakra Energy System, along with the principles of Feng Shui Design, and developed concepts and methods to help myself, my clients, and my students.

It took me many years of hard work, honest introspection, and healing to realize that my whole life was preparation for what I needed in order to write this book—my background as a special-education teacher, ten years working as a psychotherapist, fifteen years teaching the Chakra Energy System, ten years as a Feng Shui practitioner, and, yes, a whole decade of my life spent being ill, becoming undone, and learning to let go and surrender.

This book is autobiographical, but not in the usual way. It's autobio-

INTRODUCTION

9

graphical in the sense that whatever exists in these pages, theory and practice alike, I have lived, experienced, utilized, and applied to my own life, healing process, and clients. There is nothing in this book that hasn't somehow passed through my personal and professional life. I have poured out the contents of my experiences, and put on paper a lot of what I know regarding illness and healing through the use of Feng Shui Design and the Chakra Energy System. What you will get in every chapter is a slice of my life, including experiences, theories, methods, approaches, and views on health, disease, and dismantling illness. I wrote this book for you, and I wrote this book for me. I am very grateful that the universe gave me the opportunity to do something constructive with all that I learned and struggled with regarding the reality of having a long-term illness. This book is a synopsis of my work over the past eighteen years, and I am truly honored and pleased to be able to pass it on to you and, I hope, shed some light on your particular illness or struggle. This contribution of my work and theories to the greater whole keeps me humble and moving forward during my own setbacks.

A lot of my work will make immediate sense to you, and you will choose to utilize some of it right away; other parts may fascinate you; and still others may feel quite esoteric and not in alignment with your reality or truth. Please feel free to keep only the theories and methods that ring true to you and feel close to your heart. The rest you may discard, ignore, or put on a back burner for later review. Some of the information, especially in the first few chapters, many of you may find very new and cutting-edge. My only request to you is to read it with an open mind and an open heart, for it is in that place that you will be at your most receptive and able to absorb these teachings from a more expansive, intuitive perspective. It is in that "authentic" place that you can be truly open to deciding how you feel about these teachings, and to your excitement about receiving these cures and processes.

Although a lot of this information may appear new to you, please keep in mind that when my first book, *Feng Shui: Harmony by Design,* was published five years ago, relatively few people had heard about Feng Shui, while today it is widely practiced. What is often considered cutting-edge or avant-garde today quickly becomes integrated into our everyday life and our belief systems tomorrow.

This book is a synopsis of all the experiences and tools that I have learned and applied along the way. It was written for those of you who are scared by the things unfolding in your life that make no logical sense. It was written for those of you who are ready to look at life from another perspective and use this material as a way of preventing illness. But mostly it was written for those of you who want to understand the true nature of your illnesses from an emotional, spiritual, and psychological perspective, and to learn how to work with the invisible energy fields that contribute to shaping your health and your lives. These energy fields, Feng Shui and the Chakras, are gifts to us from the universe to help us transmute the lower energies of illnesses and decipher how the configurations of our homes and offices can contribute to creating illnesses or exacerbating those that already exist.

As you begin to work with Feng Shui concepts to improve your health, it is important to remember that the art of Feng Shui, so rich in metaphors, will mirror your health and life back to you as you subconsciously re-create it in your environment. It will manifest and reveal all the aspects of your health that you are not able to see objectively. Interpreted correctly, the Feng Shui of your environment will reflect back to you all the emotional, spiritual, physical, conscious, unconscious, and subconscious issues that are contributing to many aspects of your disease. It provides you with an objective but tangible way of exposing the hidden pieces of your illness as it exists in your home. Then, by making energy changes and corrections to your environment, you can dismantle the part of your illness that is being supported by unhealthy energy patterns and design layouts. Although many factors govern why and how an individual gets sick, working with the Feng Shui of a space can help create the necessary energetic foundation to support the process of health and healing.

Still today, at times, I am sick. This is as important for you to hear as it is for me to say. My intention in saying it is not to discredit Feng Shui or undermine my own work, but instead to give you a very realistic view of what Feng Shui is, and the true ways that it can help you in your healing process. Feng Shui is *not* a magic bullet, and I ask you please not to think of it as one. Making it a magical, esoteric healing tool diminishes what it was sent here today to help you do; that is, create a better and more abundant, healthy life. Maintaining the correct focus will keep you and others from succumbing to its misuse and rapidly growing commercialization. By approaching it from this level of honesty and truth etched in your heart, you personally help to preserve its integrity and its true reason for being here. If you can do that, then I know I've done my job and that my twelve years of living with chronic illness were not in vain.

My story is a very special one, but not because I was one of the "lucky" ones who happened to be blessed and miraculously got well, but because I worked very hard at it, made the changes that were needed, and painstakingly looked at a lot of aspects of myself and my life that were sometimes not very pretty. You may think that this sort of healing happens only to other people and not to you. I used to feel the same way, but the truth is, it happened to me, and I can show you how it can happen to you. *The condition that kills more people, more than heart attacks, cancers, and all other diseases combined, is complacency!* The lack of will or hope to rise above your situation, and at the very least make it a little better, is what will stop you dead in your tracks, time and again. If you have the will to be truly dedicated, to "show up" for yourself, the work you are here to do, and your healing process, your life will be transformed in ways that you cannot even imagine.

Please know that throughout your life you may be physically challenged at times, and at other times you may be emotionally weakened by your journey here, but in the end, if you choose to live your life awake, the process will forever spiritually strengthen you. I pass that knowledge on to you and remind you that deep down inside, you have the courage and strength needed to see your healing process through.

Professor Lin says that when two people or two events come together, and the information that is exchanged changes the course of one of those lives for the better, that is what is referred to as having "good karma." Even if it is just through the pages of this book, I honor each of our auspicious connections, and I am truly grateful for the opportunity to assist you. May this book serve as an infinite catalyst that connects you, me, and the good karma of your healing process that we now both share.

It takes five hundred years of prayer and meditation for two people to cross on the same boat.

— H. H. PROFESSOR THOMAS LIN YUN RINPOCHE

CHAPTER ONE

FENG SHUI DESIGN

A New Paradigm for Understanding Health

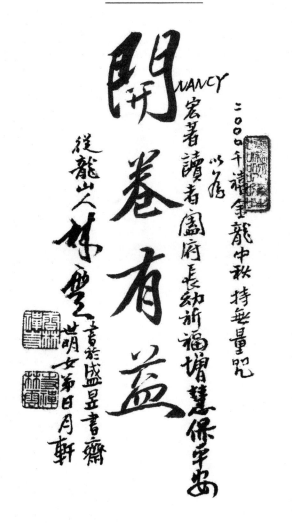

"Opening this book will bring great benefits."

CALLIGRAPHY BY H. H. PROFESSOR THOMAS LIN YUN RINPOCHE

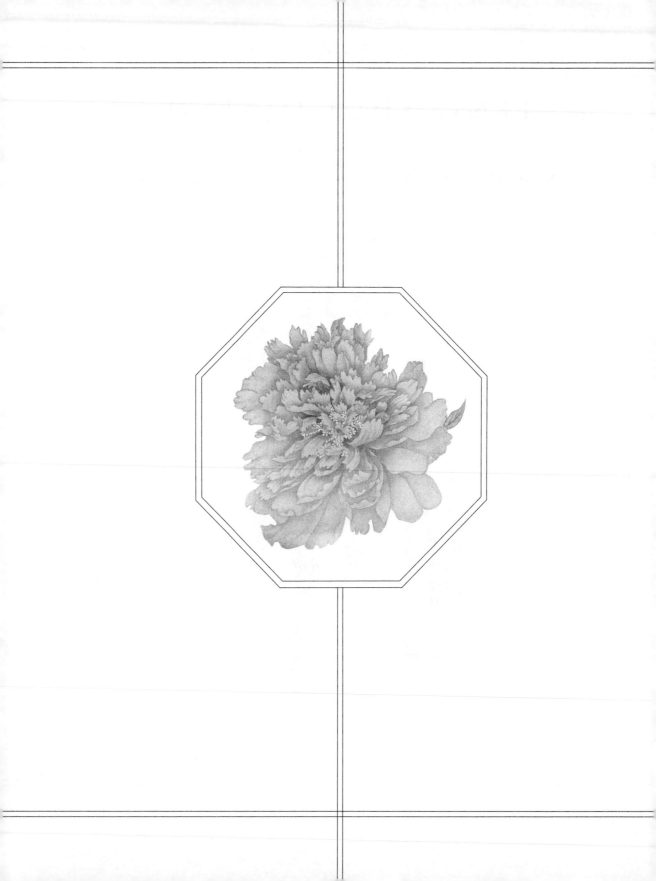

FENG SHUI IS A DESIGN SYSTEM based on the flow of energy (ch'i) through your home or environment. It differs from the principles of traditional interior design, which bases its concepts mainly on function, form, and aesthetics.

Although Feng Shui has been around for more than 4,000 years, Westerners first began to become aware of it in the mid-1980s, and it became popular in mainstream society in the 1990s. There are three main schools of thought in Feng Shui, but this book will exclusively address the nontraditional school of what is known as the Black Hat Sect. Unlike other schools, which utilize a compass (Lo' Pan), the Black Hat Sect uses entranceways and a mapping system called the Bagua to determine location and proper positioning.

But, no matter what the school of thought is, the primary objective of Feng Shui is always to create home and work environments that are in alignment with the healing forces of nature, thus creating spaces that naturally support and nurture the individuals who occupy them.

When these patterns of invisible energy are aligned, they produce environments that strengthen all the different circumstances an individual will encounter during his or her lifetime. Although the connection between Feng Shui and career opportunities, personal relationships, and finances is becoming better understood, until now, the connection to health has been less so.

As you further explore concepts of vibrational patterns, you will begin to see energy patterns both within an individual and within an environment.

Collectively, these two forms of patterns can create balanced and healthy energy patterns or unbalanced and unhealthy patterns of energy. Such patterns, when left uncorrected, can aggressively cause blocks in your career, poor health, illness and disease, dissatisfaction in your love life, and difficulties with your finances. By learning to assess and analyze vibrational patterns and the Feng Shui of your environment, you will be able to tap in to a new approach to understanding, diagnosing, and treating illness, and attending to your own health.

As you begin to work with Feng Shui concepts to improve your health, it is important to remember that the art of Feng Shui, so rich in metaphors, will mirror your health and life back to you as you subconsciously re-create them in your environment. It will manifest and reveal all the aspects of your health that you are not able to see objectively. Interpreted correctly, the Feng Shui of your environment will reflect back to you all the emotional, spiritual, physical, conscious, unconscious, and subconscious issues that are contributing to many aspects of your disease. It will provide you with an objective, tangible way to expose the hidden pieces of your illness as revealed in your home. Then, by making energy changes and corrections to your environment, you can dismantle the part of your illness that is being supported by unhealthy energy patterns and design layouts.

This book will gently invite you to look at your life, your home, and your health from a new perspective. It will challenge you to rethink illness from an understanding that our home and office environments have a direct impact on the quality and status of our health.

As you explore these principles, you might be surprised to find that there are *many* ways to assess the Feng Shui and health status of your home. Although many factors play into why and how an individual gets sick, working with the Feng Shui of a space can help create the necessary energetic foundation to support the process of health and healing. By learning to decipher the hidden health codes in our environment, we can furnish, decorate, and design our homes so that we unlock health issues that have plagued us for years. The principles of Feng Shui and health supply us with the understanding of how our environment affects our well-being from an invisible-energy perspective. By putting logical thought to one side for just a moment, you might see the other side of the invisible coin. By allowing yourself to abandon rational thinking momentarily, you may also discover a missing link to your own recovery process.

When we willingly get out of our own way and open ourselves to the higher wisdom that is available to us all, we move toward not only healing what ails us, but also toward transforming our whole lives along the way.

The information throughout this book is cutting-edge "spiritual technology" at its best. But keep in mind that although it is progressive and supportive, it represents only one component of why we get sick. Do not exchange good common sense for a quick Feng Shui fix. That would be a misuse of Feng Shui's many gifts. If you are sick or not feeling well, please remember to seek the appropriate medical help. *Feng Shui is a strong and powerful medicine, but only when used responsibly as an adjunct to other healing methods.* Different healing methods can strengthen and support one another. The more approaches we use to heal ourselves, the more we increase our chances of transforming that illness.

So pull out all the stops, call on the powers that be, and, above all, take action. "Your health is your wealth," and you deserve the best of all that is now being made available to you!

"If you are in the ocean and feel yourself beginning to drown, pray to God, but start swimming toward the shore, also!"

—PROVERB

GOOD HEALTH BEGINS WITH THE LAND

The more we understand the nature of illness and explore the impact of environment on disease, the more we can take responsibility for changing the aspects that we do have control over, with the environment being the main one.

At the beginning of the Feng Shui assessment process, most people know very little about the principles of Feng Shui. Often they have read books or articles on the subject containing conflicting information that only serves to confuse them.

The best and least overwhelming way to approach the Feng Shui assessment is to start with a thorough step-by-step process. By looking at all the variables and their impact on one another, you can start to create an "energetic profile" of your space and all its surroundings. In this way you can slowly start to discover areas of your home that are contributing to poor health and are in need of your love and attention.

The first thing you need to remember is that energy (or ch'i) is created through a process that involves many steps, on many levels. If you are going to work with it, assess it, and modify its constitution, it then becomes very important that you understand as best you can where it comes from and how it eventually arrives at your home affecting your life and subsequently your health.

ASSESSING THE CH'I OF THE LAND

Keep in mind that the closer the ch'i from the universe gets to the individual, the stronger becomes its effect on human ch'i. For instance, the ch'i that's around your bed will affect you more profoundly than will the ch'i that circulates throughout your country of origin. Conversely, human ch'i, as it extends outward, has a direct impact on the world and all the things in it.

The Circle of Life

The initial source of ch'i is the universe. The stars, the moon, the sun, and other celestial bodies radiate ch'i that filters down through Earth's atmosphere, eventually reaching the planet's surface. The ch'i then divides, and is distributed throughout the world. As it circulates through the various countries, it divides even further, funneling itself into states, cities, neighborhoods, communities, acres, and blocks. Finally it arrives at our apartment buildings and homes, making its way through the individual rooms, circulating around furniture and various objects, and eventually affecting the ch'i of all the occupants.

As the ch'i circulates throughout your home, it merges with the energy emitted by other elements in the environment, such as the color of the walls, the shapes of the rooms, and the positioning of the furniture, and the combinations create certain forms and invisible energy patterns. These patterns of energy then shape the ch'i that exists in our bodies and in our external energy system called The Chakras. The ch'i in our bodies transmits these energy patterns to the world, drawing to us, like a magnet, certain life situ-

Fig. 1. Circle of Life Chart

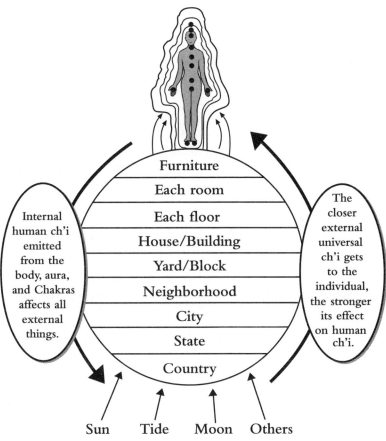

Internal human ch'i emitted from the body, aura, and Chakras affects all external things.

Furniture
Each room
Each floor
House/Building
Yard/Block
Neighborhood
City
State
Country

The closer external universal ch'i gets to the individual, the stronger its effect on human ch'i.

Sun   Tide   Moon   Others

All the Universal Elements of Nature Emit Ch'i

ations (relationships, jobs, health issues, etc.) that reflect those same energy patterns.

In turn, these different life situations also have very specific energy patterns of their own, which send ch'i back to our immediate environment, our neighborhoods, our communities, and eventually back to the universe. This energy exchange fuels and operates the "circle of life" (see Fig. 1).[1]

Learning how to detect the flow of ch'i throughout your house allows you to locate the areas where energy is blocked, stagnant, oppressive, or flowing too strongly. Any energy imbalance can trigger or lead to various ill-nesses. The assessment of ch'i in your home—its Feng Shui—will give you the information you need to make the proper adjustments to bring the ch'i back to its natural balance. Such adjustments may be as simple as moving your desk into a better energy position, adding extra light to a room, or sim-ply changing the color of your bedroom. By learning how to work with energy to design the interior of your home, you can ultimately shape and alter your health and the many different situations in your life.

Although ch'i emanates from a variety of universal sources such as the tide and the moon, just before it enters your home it is actually filtered down from the next higher level of energy, found on the land on and around your property. Before we begin to address the inside of your home, we first have to look at the Feng Shui of the surrounding area. The quality of that exte-rior energy and the uninterrupted flow of its ch'i has an immediate and pow-erful impact on the interior ch'i—how it flows through your home will determine how it affects your health and your life.

The environment around you is full of clues that can alert you to ener-getic problems. Your job is to decipher the clues and then begin to make the changes necessary to correct those conditions. Keep in mind that there are hundreds of such possible exterior factors, far too numerous to list here. If you know the right questions to ask yourself, and if you remain open to mak-ing discoveries of your own, you will be well on your way to doing a thor-ough health and Feng Shui assessment of your space and its surrounding areas.

The Ch'i of the Land

As you gather information about your land, you will be looking for specifics as well as an overall assessment of all the exterior factors. Some of these things might have a significant impact on your health, while others, depend-ing on how they affect your interior Feng Shui and you yourself, may have no impact at all.

Keep in mind that as soon as you decide to begin the Feng Shui process for yourself or for someone else, *everything becomes important*. Pay attention to everything that comes to mind. Aspects of your home and surroundings that you have never noticed before may suddenly be brought to your attention as you become ready to decipher their hidden messages. So be alert as you start this process, and keep an eye out for everything that crosses your path, whether you are assessing a new space or just taking a fresh new look at your old digs.

1. *People, neighbors, events.* For starters, examine the types of people who have chosen to live in your neighborhood. I know this suggestion might sound "loaded" and raise a few eyebrows, but try to honestly observe who is around you without being too judgmental. Sometimes we are so invested in doing the "politically correct" thing that we overcompensate and avoid seeking the truth at all costs. The reason for looking at this factor is that from a Feng Shui perspective, the universal laws of energy always rule. Energetically speaking, one of the main universal laws is "Like attracts like." This law applies significantly to the ch'i of the land because the land existed independently before anyone moved onto it.

   So, if you find that you are surrounded by individuals who are angry, rude, emotionally unbalanced, constantly in trouble with the law, abusing drugs, unemployed, or violent, you need to acknowledge that this type of ch'i exists around you. This doesn't imply that you are bad or wrong, or that your life and health will be permanently affected in some way. But as you start your Feng Shui health assessment, it should serve as an alert about what might be happening with the ch'i of the land and the surrounding neighborhood, for that energy, left unchecked, will eventually find its way into your home and subsequently into your life.

   I am also aware that socioeconomic status at least partially determines where we live, especially in today's world. See if you can challenge yourself and look past your initial response to my suggestion. When I referred to "types of people," you may have thought I stopped just short of mentioning race and/or referring to a tenement slum, and that I was implying indirectly what I didn't have the nerve to say outright. If so, you were wrong. Everything I listed above, I have had to address in varying degrees in many of the neighborhoods I have worked in. Every problem that exists in society exists on *every* level of society. In the human race, no one is spared. I have worked in many affluent neighborhoods, with individuals who were very financially comfortable. What I found was that I never had to adjust my approach or my Feng Shui assessment process because of their financial status. They had the same fears, diseases, struggles, and worries that everyone else has. Actually, what I found was that it was even more difficult to wade through the denial and shame surrounding the white-collar crime, marital affairs, and substance abuse that came with certain neighborhoods and social circles.

So, with that in mind, step back and ask yourself about the quality and character of your neighbors. Energy is insidious. It moves around and affects all that it comes in contact with, *especially* people. And in turn, the people and their lives and life circumstances affect their neighborhood and all who live in it. And we also travel in "energy groups"; every neighborhood or apartment building is another "family of energy," a group of people who assemble for a period of time for reasons that may or may not be obvious. I believe there is a personal as well as a social karma that different groups choose to work on collectively. Sometimes those groups choose to expose themselves to certain environmental factors that trigger events they need to experience in their lives for their own souls' growth and sometimes for society's growth as well. The energy of external ch'i can attract specific experiences that can later manifest in one's life. Often one finds common characteristics in neighborhoods, such as high rates of divorce, unemployment, or certain diseases. Check for any history of specific or recurring events such as car accidents, robberies, muggings, and the like. If you are able to detect this before you move in to a place, great! Interview nosy neighbors; they love to tell all. Even the fact that you want to know the truth and that you are focusing on what you desire will move some energy, and a shift of consciousness can begin to occur. You still may find yourself moving into the neighborhood anyway, but you may not be at all affected by the exterior energy patterns; or, even better, the newfound awareness can encourage you to adjust the Feng Shui inside your home so as to offset any exterior concerns.

SOLUTIONS: Chapter 9 will provide you with two different "Transcendental Feng Shui Cures": one is called "Sealing the Doors" and the other is "Interior/Exterior House Clearing with Blessed Rice." Both can be used to offset any problem that seems bigger than what you think you can handle unassisted.

2. *Vegetation/animals/life force.* The next group of "earth ch'i indicators" to review will bring your attention to the type of life force that gathers or is able to grow on the land around you. This is an important indicator of "earth ch'i" regarding a potential health problem, because if plants can't grow there, it is an indication that the life force in that area is low or somehow being compromised. When any life force is compromised, it greatly contributes to lowering the ch'i force, which in turn contributes to disease, depression, hopelessness, and malaise. The questions that you have to start asking yourself are What is the vegetation like? Can food grow in this soil? Are there trees around? Plants? What kinds of animals frequent the area? (Stray cats? Homeless dogs? Crows or blue jays?) What is the condition of their life force? Are they well fed? Starving? What is the overall feeling that this neighborhood elicits?

Obviously, city living provides different criteria for what constitutes life force than rural or suburban living. For example, you wouldn't necessarily look for a lot of trees in an inner-city neighborhood, but you would want to see if there is a park nearby, and how green it is. There are many other indicators of earth ch'i that might be more appropriate for the area you are assessing.

SOLUTION: If you are living with a low earth-ch'i environment, bring more life-force elements into your house. Add plants and flowers, increase indoor lighting, or get a pet that will bring good energy to your life, home, and spirit.

3. *Spiritual occurrences/omens/metaphysical happenings.* While you're on your way to the house or apartment that you might rent or buy, it's important to stay very alert. The universe will often use this time to communicate something important to you about the ch'i of the land, and whether this particular apartment or house is the right one for you: for example, having to stop to let a funeral procession pass, finding a dead animal on the land, or an awning unexpectedly blowing off as you begin to enter the front door are all subtle signs from the universe. Sometimes it can show itself in the form of odd occurrences, like a light in the new space blowing out when you turn it on. Sometimes it is as simple as a

gut feeling, a sense that something isn't right or is at least a bit off.

You don't have to be frightened. The universe is simply giving you additional information. Only you can determine what it means to you, based on your interpretation of the event. For example, you might interpret the light's blowing out as a sign that something isn't right about the dwelling. For me, the same incident might mean that there is a lot of excess or stagnant energy that is in need of clearing. My personal energy system runs very "electrical," so it isn't uncommon for me to blow out many lightbulbs in a relatively short period. If I arrive at a site and a lightbulb blows out, I don't interpret it as an alarming signal. Stay alert and try to observe everything that comes your way, but try not to overreact or automatically assume the worst. Remember, you are learning these techniques so you can better assess invisible factors.

SOLUTION: If, after all factors are considered, you still feel that you would like to move into the space, first consult a Feng Shui expert. Besides providing an objective opinion, quite often an experienced consultant can explore the many ways that you can offset the problems. In addition, try the "Sealing the Doors" cure in chapter 9.

4. *Buildings/businesses/places of worship or burial.* Looking at the types of businesses and institutions that exist in and around your neighborhood is another way to assess the "ch'i of the land." This observation will bring you information from another energy perspective. The types of structures and businesses that have gravitated to a neighborhood are indicators of the energetic "pull" of the earth ch'i there. A neighborhood that has many churches, hospitals, doctors' offices, civic centers, colleges, or funeral parlors would indicate to you a possible energetic "pull" in one direction over another. A neighborhood with many after-school centers and senior citizens' programs would indicate that there is an abundance of community-minded ch'i. If the neighborhood has many funeral parlors or cemeteries, that would be an indicator of a lot of dead Yin energy. What about businesses—are they thriving or marginal? These are factors that would indicate the strength of the money ch'i of the area. If the neighborhood is the site of the city's main garbage

dump, or there are small waterways with stagnant waters, those are "red flags" signaling that the neighborhood has very toxic and unhealthy ch'i.

SOLUTION: Assess the impact that these different variables might have on you and your objectives and goals. If you are prone to depression, choosing to live in a neighborhood that is gloomy and gray may not be your best choice. We now know that from a Feng Shui perspective, your exterior environment can shape your energy, health, and life circumstances. Make the inside of your apartment as beautiful and uplifting as possible to offset the impact of the exterior ch'i. Perform the "Sealing the Doors" cure or the "Interior/Exterior House Clearing with Blessed Rice." In addition, use the "Shedding the Golden Cicada" cure on yourself. These are explained in chapter 9.

5. *Exterior electromagnetic energy fields (EMFs)/high-tension wires/transformers.* We are just beginning to understand the impact of electromagnetic energy on individuals who are exposed to it on a regular basis. The word *electromagnetic* actually represents two different energy currents: one electric, the other magnetic. EMFs may be caused by faulty wiring, high electric out-gaussing, or certain types of ungrounded currents. Studies show that frequent exposure to these potentially dangerous energy fields contributes to a decrease in immune functioning and a rise in the level of certain cancers.[2] EMFs can be caused in your home's interior by certain types of appliances, clock radios, microwaves, hair dryers, fluorescent lighting, etc. (You'll find more information later in this chapter, and in chapter 5, page 161.) But they also exist outside of your home, negatively affecting the ch'i of the land and your physical health. Sources include large transformers, substations, buried electrical cables, and high-tension wires. Several years ago in Long Island, New York, a very high rate of breast cancer was detected. The authorities at first considered this a coincidence, ignoring the environment as a contributing factor because it would mean accountability and major change, which would cost money. After much protest, the government admitted that there *might* be a connection between the elevated cancer rates and the high-tension wires and transformer cables found in large numbers in the surrounding areas.

SOLUTION: Check your surroundings for types of businesses and electrical structures that might be emitting high levels of dangerous EMFs. If you are concerned, call your local electric company. Many have free services that will dispatch a crew with sophisticated detection equipment to do an EMF reading on the structure you are concerned about. Please keep in mind that you may not get much cooperation. Many states do not provide this service, and those that do may have a tremendous conflict of interest. If they validate your concerns with factual testing data, it would mean they would have to make costly changes. Remember what is important to you, and if you suspect an EMF problem, don't be dissuaded. Hire a company that specializes in objective EMF testing.

The good news is that in some cases it will take only minor adjustments to lessen the impact of EMFs; quite often the best solution is distance. The potentially dangerous impact of EMFs on your health can be greatly reduced, if not eliminated, by creating a distance of several yards to several miles between you and the source. Then place nine potted plants, along with a 50-mm Feng Shui crystal on a nine-inch red string, in your living room, bedroom, or whatever rooms are of concern and closest to the EMF source.

Other Exterior Factors That Can Influence Your Health

1. *Trace your activity path.* Spend some time tracing your activity path. This is the route you take to and from your home, work, or any other daily or regular activity. Notice what you see along the way, for that will influence your health as well as your mind-set and ch'i. Are you passing by places that lift your ch'i or depress it? Is your path colorful, filled with life force, hopefulness, and inspiration?

A student of mine shared a story with my class about her son, who was having a lot of behavioral problems. Every morning, while driving him to school, she had to pass a cemetery. Even though it became routine and didn't appear to be an issue in his behavioral problems, this was a good example of an activity-path influence. She changed routes and applied a Transcendental Cure that I suggested, and over time his behavior improved significantly.

SOLUTION: Reroute your travel path; take a different road or walk down a different street. If you are stuck (not just inconvenienced) and can't change your activity path, apply the Transcendental Cure for Purification called the Orange Peel Cure, explained in chapter 2, and use the cure also in your car.

2. *Assess your view.* Take a look out of all of your windows and main doorways and make note of what you are facing. Do you face a brick wall, or a big tree? Do you see the local church across the street? (If so, is it a center for spiritual communion? Does it host many funerals?) Is there a large green park or a burned-out building? What you are exposed to over time will shape your ch'i and, in turn, your health.

SOLUTION: Create a visual bumper between you and what you don't want to see. Add hanging or tall standing plants to the window. Install stained glass or hang a 40-mm Feng Shui crystal on a 36-inch red string in the window to transform the negative ch'i. In addition, add a Bagua mirror outside your window, with the mirror side facing out, deflecting the unwanted exterior factor.

3. *Look for trees and foliage that block ch'i.* Very often, when we are looking for exterior factors, we look for things that would be considered bad by society's standards. Don't be lulled into this assessment trap! Even though trees, bushes, and beautiful foliage are a wonderful life-force adjustment, if they are unkempt or overgrown, or block walkways and entrances, they are not elements of good Feng Shui anymore. If a tree is directly outside your front door, its placement is not auspicious, since it is blocking the ch'i from entering your home. If it is blocking the front door, it can also create respiratory problems. The lack of care or inauspicious placement of otherwise positive elements will influence good versus negative ch'i flow.

SOLUTION: Cut, trim, and care for all outside bushes, branches, and trees. If you have a tree (or telephone pole) blocking the energy from smoothly entering your space, then place a small, round three- or five-inch mirror, or a red piece of paper that says "Raise Head See Happiness," on the tree or pole a few inches above eye level, and follow the procedure of the Three Secrets Reinforcement, found in chapter 9.

4. *Undesirable waters.* Water follows the same principles as trees. Although being surrounded by water can be very auspicious and great for health and money, remember that the body is made up of approximately two-thirds water, and it has a tendency to resonate to other water elements, especially if it is in close proximity. If the water is dirty, stagnant, and smelly, or too polluted for fish to live in, it is not a good exterior factor to have close by you, especially from a Feng Shui health perspective. This holds true for unkempt pools, ponds, fish tanks, and wells. Stagnant water can depress the immune system and make one highly susceptible to disease.

SOLUTION: If you have control over the offending element, then do whatever you can to clean it up. If you are not able to alter the problematic water at all, perform the "Sealing the Doors" and the "Interior/ Exterior House Clearing Cure with Blessed Rice," in chapter 9. In addition, if you can see the water, place a 50-mm Feng Shui crystal in the window (on an 18- or 27-inch red string) blocking the negative ch'i, or place a large plant in the window, blocking the view. In addition, place another 50-mm crystal on a nine-inch red string hanging from the center Health gua in your bedroom.

5. *Direct walkways and traffic flow/rushing ch'i.* There are very few if any straight lines in nature. God has created a beautiful world that surrounds us with wispy sunsets, wildly shaped flowers, and fruits and vegetables saturated with colors and sensuous curves. Ch'i is emitted from these elements of nature in a free-flowing, meandering, and unrestricted way. When we build and design man-made structures that produce ch'i that is angled, confined, accelerated, or linear, we distort energy from its natural flow. So, when walkways and roads are very linear and lead directly to the front door of your home, it creates a very stressful and aggressive flow of ch'i. Assess whether your house or front door is in

direct alignment with a nearby road, then check the walkway to your home and see if it was designed in a direct line with your front door. This combination may cause high blood pressure, strokes, and anxiety- and stress-related issues.

SOLUTION: Place a Feng Shui Bagua-shaped mirror (see chapter 3, page 97) or a five-inch octagonal mirror on your front door to deflect the aggressive ch'i. Add a brass wind chime over the front of the door to diffuse the intense energy. Plant trees, bushes, or flower beds to act as a buffer between you and the traffic flow. Add some large rocks or boulders to the front of the driveway or property facing the traffic flow. If you have "direct ch'i" from a direct walkway, add planters to recurve the walkway, or add round flagstones that change the walkway from a straight line to a curved path.

6. *Oppressive buildings/signs and other structures.* As you are reviewing the exterior ch'i, keep an eye out for factors that are too large, overwhelming, or disproportionate to your apartment building or house. First, look for "oppressive ch'i" buildings. These are structures that are much larger, very near your building, and tower over your home. Then look for buildings that are positioned at a 90-degree angle opposite your front door or a window to a major room in your house if the point of that angle is creating "cutting ch'i," a finger-pointing, knifelike energy that threatens you, your home, and your ch'i. Next, see if there are any structures such as overhead train tracks, large neon lights, and other energetically intimidating factors. Finally, look for other things that create negative psychological ch'i.

In Brooklyn, not far from where my office was located, there is a huge sign advertising a local law firm, approximately 20 by 5 feet, posted on a building and covering the exterior wall space of at least three different apartments. It says "Divorce and Bankruptcy for Under $300!" Every driver who passes that sign reads it over and over, reinforcing those negative thoughts. I can't help wondering what is happening in the lives of all those tenants, and what the impact is of having the thought of divorce and bankruptcy constantly reinforced by every passing motorist.

SOLUTION: Place a five-inch octagon or Feng Shui Bagua mirror on the side of the house or in the window facing out toward the oppressive structure or element, deflecting the image and its oppressive energy away. Apply the Sealing the Doors Cure in chapter 9.

Be Clear, Define Your Intentions

As you see, there are many things to start assessing even before you start looking at the interior of your space. We have been taught to look for the tangible and visible factors when we are looking for a home or a neighborhood to live in, but the intangible and invisible are equally, if not more, important.

So, if you are looking to move in to a certain neighborhood, go ahead and inquire about the local school system, the closest grocery store, and where the nearest highway is, but don't forget to assess the energetics of the people by whom you and your children will be surrounded. They might be pillars of the community, earning six figures a year, but where are their hearts, their souls, and their sense of integrity? Are their values similar to yours? What would be more important to you: an honest and friendly working-class neighbor, or one who has a doctor's degree and a secret mistress? Don't forget to look at all the ways the exterior environment can affect your ch'i. Gather all the information you can. You might be asking yourself whether we can really find out this information in detail before we move into a neighborhood. The answer is that quite often we cannot. But from a Feng Shui perspective, just by raising the questions in your mind, you give the universe permission to "interfere" more aggressively on your behalf in making one real estate deal fall through, while making another one happen. As you learn to work and commune with the spiritual aspects of Feng Shui, you will inadvertently open yourself to help, guidance, and direction in orchestrating an environment that is harmonious with all forces.

BEGINNING THE ASSESSMENT OF THE HEALTH-RELATED INTERIOR FACTORS

Even without knowing yet how to assess the interior factors regarding Feng Shui and your health, the following list of Feng Shui Health Principles will immediately get you started on your way to being your own Feng Shui health consultant. The list gives you a great head start in looking for problems as they manifest in your interior environment that may contribute to your specific health concerns.

Even if you are very healthy, I strongly encourage you to use these tips and take a proactive approach to maintaining and supporting your good health.

If you find that your home has some of the problems listed below, but you do not have the corresponding symptoms, or even if you don't have any illness at all, *adjust the problem areas anyway.* Why? Because it's important to make the adjustments as a preventive measure to keep yourself well. We are still looking only at the tip of the iceberg in exploring the connection between Feng Shui and health. Some of these principles might at first seem a bit odd, unrelated to health as you have come to know it, but if you remain open, you just might stumble into a whole new world in the invisible energy kingdom.

Nine Crucial Feng Shui Health Principles

1. ***No backs to the door.*** In Black Hat Feng Shui, we believe that in order to obtain optimal health it is very important not only to face the main doorway of the room that you are in, but to be able to see it as well. The ch'i of a space enters through the main entrance of your home and through all the individual doorways that lead into the specific rooms. Ch'i brings the life force that carries the energy and opportunities into all the aspects of your life. When you physically position yourself in a way that has you facing the door, you are also positioning yourself to actively "face your life." Not until you are ready to face your life are you able to take full responsibility for it. When we are not facing our entranceways, things can go on "behind our backs," including being "talked about," "stabbed in the back," and the like.

    The three most important pieces of furniture that affect your life are your bed, desk, and stove. These three interior objects influence your finances (stove), work and creativity (desk), and, most important, your personal relationships and your overall health (bed). *Position these three main pieces of furniture to face the door. It is extremely important, however, to make sure you do not position them in a way that would place you, while you are seated at the desk or on the bed, in direct line with the doorway.* Ch'i force is very powerful, and it would be too taxing for the body to be exposed to such a direct energy flow (see chapter 5, page 142, bed position 7). This layout weakens the nervous system, causes anxiety, and raises stress levels and blood pressure. In addition, if the bed crosses the door, the main area of the body that the ch'i hits directly will be compromised, or possibly develop an illness. Proper bed positioning is probably one of the most important principles pertaining to good Feng Shui Health.

(Although most people think this Feng Shui principle originated many years ago in China, as an Italian, I personally believe that it actually originated somewhere long ago in the backwoods of Italy, because every respectable Italian knows that you never sit with your back toward the door!)

2. **Repair all leaks.** Leaks of any kind can create a whole host of health problems, because our bodies are made up mostly of water. When the problems in our home are water-related, we have a natural inclination, physically, to resonate to that problem. All elements have a symbiotic connection to elements of the same nature. Water is no exception.

When the house has minor water drips or leaks, it experiences a process very similar to our human process of sweating. If you took a brisk walk every day in moderately warm weather (say, 80 degrees), you might work up a slight sweat; but if this walk didn't last just 30 or 40 minutes, but instead went on 24 hours a day, seven days a week, you'd find yourself sweating moderately but continually, each minute releasing more and more crucial body fluids with their sustaining life force, vitamins, and minerals, with no slowdown in sight and with no opportunity to refuel with more liquids. In essence, that's what happens to our environments when we allow drips and leaks to go unattended and eventually accumulate. Our bodies respond to the drain of energy, which over time can lead to fatigue and "runny" illnesses such as sinus problems, diarrhea, and urinary tract infections.

In addition, water in Feng Shui resonates to the same vibration as *money and our emotions.* So, to compound an already deleterious situation, leaks can also cause depression and emotional outbursts. They can also create financial instability, especially if they remain unchecked. These problems, in turn, can cause a lot of stress-related illnesses.

3. *Fix all doors.* In Feng Shui, entranceway doors are known as "the mouths of the ch'i," for they bring the life force into a space. The quality of that ch'i creates an environment that can either support the occupants' health or eventually deplete it. Each entranceway is a sacred place of transition that brings life support in the form of ch'i and oxygen. Doors that do not open all the way, close improperly, get jammed, or have hinges that are broken or squeak create energy patterns that adversely affect health. Doors and their hinges serve the same purpose in the home as the joints do in the body, in that they permit flexible movement. Joint problems related to the elbows, wrists, neck, hips, knees, and ankles are common fallout from doors remaining in disrepair. Problematic doors can exacerbate all joint diseases such as arthritis, rheumatism, multiple sclerosis, TMJ disorders, and neck and shoulder pain. Doors also oversee our head area in Feng Shui. For any related head problems, such as tumors, strokes, or migraines, check all doors and entryways for obstructions and clutter.

In addition, doors oversee the "mouths of the adults." Problematic doors disempower adults and create "power struggles" with adolescent children by shifting the authority from the parent to the overly empowered child. Doors also represent the adult's "voice." When a significant room such as a master bedroom has an entranceway but no physical door, it's like having a mouth without a tongue and an adult without a say! Doors that don't align, or face each other and are of different sizes, can also create problems between adults, such as constant arguing or an inability to assert oneself. On a physical level, doors also oversee the health of the teeth, gums, and mouth.

Though it is not uncommon to have at least one problematic door in one's home, what I find even more frequently are broken locks and latches, which affect our emotional security, and wobbly doorknobs, which affect our ability to "get a handle on things."

In order for the joints in our body to work well, they must be strong but flexible. When you are feeling stuck, off track, or find yourself acting rigid and "inflexible," check all the hinges, door frames, closets, drawers, and kitchen cabinets in your home. Act like the Tin Man did in *The Wizard of Oz:* Get a can of oil and lubricate all the metal hardware. If oil got his old, rusty body unstuck, just think what it can do for you!

4. ***Clear away clutter.*** If you follow only one piece of advice in this book, let it be this: *Clean out your home, office, garage, basement, and attic, for you cannot make a stronger adjustment from which your whole life and overall health will benefit.* The hallways, foyers, stairways, and entranceways are the arteries and veins that run through your home: they carry the life force to all the different areas throughout your space. When these crucial avenues are blocked with clutter, it's analogous to having high amounts of cholesterol in your blood, and it's just as dangerous to your health. It clogs up the life-force "arteries" in your home in the same exact way, resulting in illnesses such as high blood pressure, heart disease, angina, stroke, tumors, diseases of the blood, metabolic disorders, and organs that become sluggish and eventually diseased. My stepdad collected more nonfunctional electrical appliances and broken transistor radios in my parents' home than they had room for; eventually they had to use one of their guest bedrooms to create a "spare room" for all his "spare parts." The spare room, filled with clutter, oversaw the area of the body that corresponded to the heart and lungs. Over time, my mother developed water retention in her lungs and high blood pressure, my stepfather had to have quadruple bypass surgery, and several years later he passed away from cardiac arrest.

Clutter has many characteristics, depending on where it accumulates in your home. The energetic dynamics of clutter are often related to issues that you hide away and don't want to deal with, or for which there is some underlying shame. Clutter creates creativity obstacles in our lives. It helps to slow us down, sabotage our dreams, and throw a monkey wrench in the workings of the "divine order." We humans love to use clutter to avoid dealing with our life and our feelings. In chapter 4 I have addressed in greater detail areas common to clutter buildup, such as entranceways, attics, basements, closets, and drawers.

The specifics of the emotional underpinnings of clutter can be determined even further as you begin to assess the different Feng Shui areas of your home and determine the corresponding life areas (guas) that contribute to its creation. For example, if the clutter is in the family area of your home, then personal issues that are related to your family may be part of the emotional infrastructure that helped create the cluttered area to begin with. Not only can clutter keep a family matter from being resolved, but it can create many new problems as well. On the physical level, it can cause health-related problems of the feet, ankles, and legs, because the family area oversees those specific areas of the body. (To find out which Feng Shui areas oversee the various areas of the body, see chapter 3.)

I realize that we all need to hold on to certain stuff, and I don't mean to imply that you shouldn't have storage in your basement, attic, or closets. Just make sure it is organized, that it contains only things that you truly need, and that the space is kept relatively neat and clean. *Strive to keep the energetic integrity of all your possessions and the sacred spaces that house them.*

5. ***Check your electrical systems.*** All the electricity that runs through your home resonates to your own body's electrical system, your nervous system. Electricity flowing through the wires and into the outlets of your home follows the same pattern that ch'i does as it runs through the body. When the electrical system in your home is in disrepair, it adversely affects your level of energy and your ability to stay direct, focused, clear, and calm. It creates energy patterns in the home that quickly tail off or become blocked, which, in turn, cause burnout and malaise for all the individuals living in that space. It creates tension and amplifies the "short fuse" of anyone who has a short temper or is predisposed to stress, impatience, and arguing. From an energetic perspective, when the electricity is not working properly in one's home, it contributes to a lot of fighting over inconsequential things.

Any illnesses having to do with the nervous system, including depression, anxiety-related disorders, nervous or emotional breakdowns, hormonal imbalances, thyroid problems, adrenal burnout, and difficult menopause, will be exacerbated by a weak or faulty electrical system. *Make sure you check for frayed wires, broken outlets, broken sockets and switches, unfinished electrical work, and fuses and lightbulbs that often blow out. Then fix them.* Lamp shades and coverings that are torn or have lightbulb burn marks can mimic an irritated stomach lining and ulcers. All these things will mimic and re-create parallel problems on the emotional as well as the physical level in your life.

The other very important electrical-related things to check for are broken appliances—the old toaster oven that doesn't work, the juicer that broke down five years ago. If you have electrical gadgets or appliances that are broken, either repair them, give them away, or bless them and throw them out. Their presence, hidden away or visible, is a major energy drain on you and your family's life and health.

6. ***Illuminate dark areas.*** As you are coming to understand, the home directly mirrors the physical body and affects how it works. A home that has areas that are dark or not well lit will lack life-force energy.

The whole objective of Feng Shui is to bring more ch'i flow, in a balanced way, to an environment in order to enhance health and overall well-being. Think about the incredible power of light. It can move us in a split second from being in the dark to being able to see. It metaphorically illuminates our path, and in the real world it helps us to see and to navigate. Only when we can see obstacles can we figure out a way to manage them. What we can't see or choose not to see, we can't address.

Dark spots in the home can eventually create dark spots in the body, which can lead to disease. Think about what happens when a doctor reads an X-ray film. What he or she looks for are dark spots or masses, places that light cannot pass through. As you will learn in chapter 7, our spiritual anatomy consists basically of units of white light that existed before we were born. This spiritual light that exists within us needs its energetic counterpart of natural and incandescent light to fuel its "energy tank." The more of that light we can effortlessly bring into our life, the healthier we will be. The light in our homes and the light available to us in nature, given by the sun, help us support our need for energetic light.

Look for burned-out lightbulbs, and get into the habit of replacing them within 24 hours after they blow out. When you do replace them, always use the same wattage or higher. Never go lower in wattage, especially after you begin your Feng Shui process. The light around you actually becomes part of the adjustment items when you begin applying Feng Shui principles to your home. Add candles to empty candle holders, even if you don't light them all the time. Then, when and where appropriate, get into the habit of keeping them lit to enhance the life force in your space.

Keep in mind that you don't have to have every area in your home lit. Just look for areas that require more light, such as dark closets or corners of hallways (which oversee intestinal areas, including the colon), and basements or attics that are being ignored. For some reason we tend to tolerate and accommodate areas in our home that lack light, and over time we begin to ignore and avoid them altogether. When we ignore such areas, we are also ignoring all the corresponding life and health issues associated with them.

7. *Reduce all high levels of EMFs in the home.* Interior electromagnetic pollution is caused by the out-gaussing of AC and DC electric and magnetic fields from appliances and other sources. These leak into the environment, causing energetic toxicity, weakening immune systems, and inducing or exacerbating illness. Such energy fields can be dangerous, as opposed to the less toxic fields emitted by appliances that are properly wired, insulated, and grounded. Interior EMF sources such as microwave ovens, fuse boxes, cordless and cell phones, toasters, refrigerators, electric heaters and shavers, blow dryers, dishwashers, halogen and fluorescent lighting, computers, and TV sets are some of the most problematic ones.

Although it has become nearly impossible to avoid all these common appliances, it's important to try to avoid using them often and to stay at a relatively safe distance from them when they are in operation—eight feet or more. The motors of electric shavers and blow dryers are just inches from your head! Incandescent lighting is still the best, if it is wired properly and grounded. TVs and computer monitors give off high levels of EMFs. Utilize some of the newer products for reducing computer EMFs, such as monitor-screen shields and Smog Busters and other EMF reduction gadgets. These items help tremendously in reducing EMFs, but don't be fooled into thinking that they solve the core problem. The best solution is still prudent avoidance or keeping your distance from the offending sources; TVs should be a distance of nine feet from your body, and try to keep your computer monitors at least two feet from your keyboard.

The most dangerous EMF sources are those located in your bedroom. These are common appliances such as TV sets, clock radios, electric blankets, computers, and answering machines (see chapter 5, page 161, on how to reduce EMFs from these sources). The problems associated with EMFs are becoming a worldwide health concern. Studies are showing that many common household items can be a contributing factor to various types of cancers, blood disorders, and a host of autoimmune diseases.

Getting a wind-up clock or walking to the other side of the room to shut your radio off may be somewhat inconvenient, but cancer is a lot more inconvenient to your body and your life. It's your choice. Choose wisely and with awareness.

8. *Clear all sewers, plumbing, waterworks, and air-conditioning and heating vents.* Systems that run through the whole house, or at least through several rooms, always oversee systemic functions such as the immune, circulatory, and nervous systems of the body.

Such waterworks are an especially important part of your Feng Shui health assessment since they resonate specifically to the circulatory and immune systems in the human body. When the waters are flowing smoothly and the systems are clean, clear, and doing their jobs, they support the healthy ebb-and-flow of your blood.

Backed-up sewers and toilets are not only bad hygienically, but can also cause physical illness related to the colon, rectum, bowels, and other intestinal areas, and can trigger other immune- and blood-related diseases. In our homes, these are the passageways that take our bodily waste and release it for us. A sewage system that doesn't work properly can cause "backups" in our physical bodies, ranging from constipation to growths in the colon and rectum such as hemorrhoids, polyps, and cancer. Blocked plumbing can affect us very similarly to the way clutter does in our homes, causing our lives to slow down and get stuck. Emotionally, this type of sewage problem can mirror ways we are resistant to letting go of old issues, painful memories, traumas, and wounds.

When pipes are broken or rusted, it's important to check for ulcers and lacerations in the stomach and intestinal areas. These types of problems also spill over into the "water-leakage" problems: emotional upset, crying, and money loss. Faulty plumbing can quickly break down physical and energetic resistance to heart disease, high blood pressure, and many unpredictable and rare kinds of illness.

Women who are having a difficult time conceiving, or are suffering from gynecological disorders such as ovarian cancer, cysts, and ectopic pregnancies, should check their homes carefully for faulty waterworks.

Finally, ducts and vents, if not kept clean and unblocked, can affect one's respiratory system, blood pressure, and stress levels, and can create a variety of allergies, ranging from mold sensitivity to pollen irritation.

9. ***House maintenance is crucial.*** Our homes are regarded as very sacred places in Feng Shui. It is very important that we maintain them just as we maintain the hygiene and well-being of our bodies. All repairs, refurbishing, redecorating, and housework should be looked upon as labors of love, because each act of improvement is an opportunity for you to change and enhance the quality of your overall life and health.

This doesn't mean that in order for you to have great Feng Shui, you have to do all the labor and housecleaning yourself, but it does mean that if you have the luxury to pay for these services, you should offer respect and gratitude to the individuals who are providing them. Also make sure that you are happy with the service providers, and that they are competent, qualified, and careful with your home and valuables. Hire domestic help and contractors with the same level of standards and care you would use to find a nanny for your infant, a baby-sitter for your five-year-old, or a doctor to perform your surgery. Remember that every place in your home oversees another part of your body and subsequently your health. Be picky; it's your home and your body!

I'M OVERWHELMED . . . WHERE DO I BEGIN?

At first, as you begin your Feng Shui analysis, it can seem more overwhelming than helpful! Please don't be discouraged; this is a common feeling, and an important one in your Feng Shui process.

As you begin to absorb all this new information, keep in mind that the information itself is working very rapidly through the many different systems of your physical and energetic bodies. Your intellect is only one of the many systems that is being stretched and reset as it tries to comprehend a new way of understanding your home and your health. The process can be quite exhausting at first, as the conscious, unconscious, and subconscious parts of the mind get reworked.

The disease or illness that you are facing is inadvertently trying to fight for its life; it does not want to be cured, because a cure would mean annihilation. And although every illness has a life force, it does not have intelligence as we understand it. It doesn't know that your environment is helping to keep it alive, or that it is harming you. As far as your illness is concerned, it perceives itself as an energy form that is being annihilated, because you are reshuffling the energy patterns around it. With all the energy of the illness fighting you, it would make perfect sense for you to feel overwhelmed. It would be almost impossible not to! The important thing here is to remember that the resistance of the illness as well as feelings of discouragement and of being overwhelmed are part of the change process, not a signal that you should give up.

Closing Chapter Exercise

As you start to work more closely with your Feng Shui process, you will see why house maintenance is so important. Though you may not as yet understand the specifics of Feng Shui Design, I encourage you to take care of as many "behind-the-scenes" repairs as you can. Although some of the health principles mentioned above seem like good common sense, from a Feng Shui perspective they are crucial in setting the tone and the energy template for sound health.

The best way to approach this book is chapter by chapter, addressing all the information and suggestions as they are presented to you. Below is a sample of a basic maintenance chart to help structure and organize you, and get you on your way.

Items Needing Repair	Whom to Contact	Completion	Feng Shui Area
Repair leaky faucet	Superintendent	Two weeks	Relationship
Fix broken burner	Appliance store	One week	Fame
Repair windowpane	Handyman	Two weeks	Wealth
Tighten all doorknobs	Superintendent	Two weeks	Various
Repaint bedroom	Painter	One month	Children

UNDERSTANDING ENERGY PATTERNS AND THE ESPs OF ILLNESS

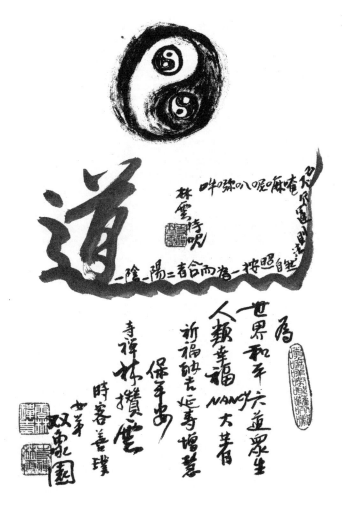

"Tao."

CALLIGRAPHY BY H. H. PROFESSOR THOMAS LIN YUN RINPOCHE

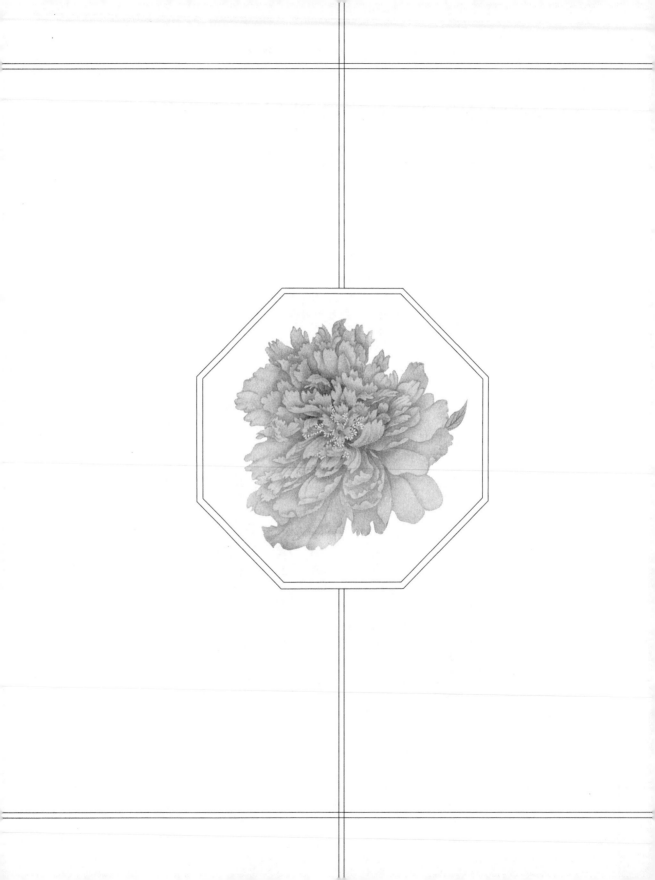

MANY OF US go through our lives thinking that our existence is unimportant or insignificant in the bigger picture of life. We try to do the right thing: be kind to others, live life fairly, and play by the rules. We pray, we meditate, we recycle, we eat low-fat yogurt and brown rice, and in spite of all our good intentions, *life happens anyway!*

Although many unpredictable things take place in our lives, nothing throws a monkey wrench into plans quicker than the reality of developing an illness. Sickness, no matter what it is or who you are, catapults you into your deepest, darkest unresolved fears regarding life and death.

In the past, and even now, many people have depended on their religious beliefs to give them a structure, a way to understand their illness. Although that works for some people, others who can't make sense of what is happening to them may blame themselves and eventually others for their sickness. Many people interpret illness as a punishment for wrongdoing. Still others struggle, believing in a God who unexpectedly and randomly doles out punishment even to good people who try hard.

YOUR ILLNESS IS ACTUALLY THE EXACT THING THAT YOUR SOUL ORDERED

I believe that to a certain degree we have all been misled. A whole spiritual generation of goodhearted, well-intended people have been lulled into thinking that illness or disease reflects a failure of some kind. Unfortunately, most of us do not understand all the variable factors that govern why a person gets sick, or how and why someone heals. Instead we have been scared and shamed into thinking that if only we had done something different, the illness wouldn't have occurred!

When we are under siege, stressed, or in tremendous fear, even the most enlightened among us will revert to primary ways of coping. By the age of six, most of us have already developed a deep-rooted sense of the psychological barter, or the dynamic known as "cause-and-effect." For example, "If you don't eat your vegetables, you don't get dessert," or "If you don't pick up your toys, you can't watch television." As we get older, the stakes get higher: "If you don't pay your electric bill, you don't get to watch *Who Wants to Be a Millionaire,*" or "If you don't show up at work, you don't get paid!" By the time we are adults, we have all thoroughly learned the psychological process of cause-and-effect, and our sense of logic has been well conditioned by it during our very early formative years.

When we are challenged by something as scary as an illness, we instinctively revert to those primary belief systems as a familiar means of coping with something that feels totally out of control. It gives us a temporary sense of power over the exact thing that is making us feel so powerless. If we are able to place the blame on something, even if only on ourselves, we regain a temporary sense of control.

The problem with using this means of coping with illness is that many people never get past the temporary feeling of being back in control. But in the absence of another set of beliefs or principles regarding illness, the cause-and-effect approach remains, becoming calcified into a faulty truth. This frame of reference often locks the individual in to a blaming or "victim" pattern, which in turn fuels the illness and hinders the recovery process.

The ironic twist in the above thinking is that many are now beginning to understand that it is *the illness itself* that draws to the individual the exact set of circumstances, and brings to light the personal needs of the sick individual that have gone unnoticed or unaddressed. When the person who is sick begins to address his or her unattended needs and wants, the process begins to slowly transmute the underlying problems or blocks that caused the illness to surface in the first place. ***The illness is actually the exact thing that the soul ordered for its next stage of growth.*** Understanding this spiritual principle helps to move the person away from a response that focuses on control and self-blame, to a more inclusive, expanded response that focuses on responsibility and the individual's soul's growth.

When people face overwhelming health challenges, quite often they are simultaneously facing old, conditioned ways of understanding their lives and health. A multilevel conflict can ensue, because initially when we are facing health problems and are afraid, we don't know that we are often trapped in old belief systems that don't serve us anymore.

In order for us to apply new teachings and solutions to our health problems, we first need to grasp some of the ways that our understanding of illness has changed and how to utilize the new paradigm for understanding health and health-related issues.

OUR BODIES ARE MADE OF ENERGY

As we grow into other levels of understanding and awareness, the energy of our bodies shifts, too. The physical makeup of who we are on a cellular and DNA level changes also because energetically, in order for any species to survive on a planet, they have to resonate vibrationally with the vibrational composition of that planet. As we grow as spiritual beings, the planet around us energetically expands also; and as the planet's overall consciousness expands, it indirectly encourages us to grow into a greater awareness. We are the most technologically advanced machine on the planet, complete with hard drive (body) and tons of software programs (information and knowledge). When we accept and acknowledge that we are multidimensional beings with a physical and spiritual body, we move closer to understanding the complexity that goes into developing an illness and sometimes healing, too.

WHAT GIVES US LIFE?

From a scientific perspective, the different organs in our bodies, such as the heart, lungs, respiratory system, and blood, work together and collectively activate themselves in a way that gives us life. But if you examine a cadaver, you will see that it too contains a heart, lungs, blood, and a respiratory system, even if the physical body is dead. Therefore, technically having those systems in one's body isn't enough to create life; instead, another kind of force needs to be present in order to bring a life force to what would otherwise be a dead body. In Black Hat Sect Feng Shui, we believe that the force that turns an otherwise inert body to life is ch'i.

Ch'i is the energetic force that runs through our bodies and keeps us alive. It's the life-force spark that turns an egg and a sperm into an embryo; that provides the energy that pumps the heart, and the fuel that makes the brain think. Ch'i flows through the body along invisible pathways called meridians. The Chinese have known of and worked with strengthening this energy force since the beginning of time through many different "vibrational medicines" such as acupuncture, flower essences, aromatherapy oils, shiatsu massage, Tai Chi, and Chinese herbal medicine.

WHAT MAKES US SICK?

People are born with different amounts and balances of ch'i, and although its core essence is unchangeable, its quality, constitution, and status may be altered or, under certain circumstances, fluctuate at times. This energy flows to all different parts of the body, including the organs, blood, tissues, bones, and every strand of hair. When this flow is moving smoothly and in a good rhythm, health is at its best. When there is an interruption in its flow, or when it is not reaching all of the body's different areas, a state of dis-ease can occur. Any energy disruption in the emotional, spiritual, and physical bodies, the meridian systems, or the environment can put the body in a state of imbalance and cause sickness.

Although several sources contribute to nurturing the ch'i flow that runs through the body, one of the main sources is the surrounding environment. Through breathing, the meridian system in the body relays the ch'i from the environment to the blood, the organs, and so on, which in turn helps create good health. If any of these sources are compromised, so is the ch'i. The same energy force that exists outside your body also exists inside it; the exterior life force and its impact on people is what we refer to as Feng Shui. Feng Shui Design is essentially the study of both the natural and man-made energy patterns that exist in the environments that surround you, and how those patterns interface with your life and influence your health.

THE TWO TYPES OF ENERGY SYSTEMS
THAT PROFOUNDLY AFFECT OUR LIVES

There are basically two kinds of systems that help support our life force. The first of these are the systems of visible energy patterns. These are the systems that appeal to our sense of logic and are easily identified. Many of these systems exist in our body: the respiratory system, the neuromuscular system, and the digestive system, to name a few. These are the systems that are visible, tangible, and are able to a certain degree to be scientifically measured. These systems are crucial and vital to the support of our life force, and volumes have been written about them from medical, scientific, and evolutionary perspectives.

Research about what causes diseases and what we can do to prevent them has given us insight into how to keep these energy systems functioning well. In the past several decades we have made numerous medical breakthroughs, ranging from organ transplants to laser surgery. These were all great discoveries that further enhanced human life. The problem we have run into with all these various medical technologies is that in our well-intended effort to heal what ails humankind, we have inadvertently locked ourselves in to a certain way of thinking, and when we limit ourselves to only one way of treating illness, we limit our own process of learning about other kinds of treatment, and we prevent true healing. Like a research scientist who has lost the ability to be objective, we have stopped looking for other factors that might be contributing to the outcome of our situation. It is at this point that Western medicine and Western thinking start to become ineffective. With all our advanced technology and monies going into research, we are still not making the kind of breakthroughs that we should be making. As we come to this realization, it is very important for us to finally acknowledge that there may be other contributing factors to why people get sick.

The second set of systems that profoundly affect our lives are the invisible energy patterns. Although there are many, the two that are the most influential are expressed in two ways: externally by Feng Shui, and internally through the Chakras, which are the seven energy centers located in the body. By learning how these invisible energy systems affect us, we can learn how to strengthen and utilize them as preventive approaches to keep us well.

The Feng Shui of your environment is the invisible energy system that affects everything in your life, from your career to your overall health. As we become more knowledgeable about the impact of the systems of invisible energy, we begin to understand that certain vibrational patterns, inadvertently created through specific design layouts, can energetically mimic the vibrational patterns of certain diseases, both chronic and acute. When a person who has a particular illness or a predisposition to a specific illness is living in a house that resonates to the same vibrational frequency as that illness, it can create a vibrational dovetail match. The environment acts likes a mirror holding the same energy pattern and frequency as the illness, thus keeping that illness alive, making it very hard for that individual to recover. Feng Shui can help us identify those vibrational patterns as they exist in our environments, and restructure their makeup, disarming their hold on your illness.

The Chakras are the invisible-energy system that exists internally in your body. These energy centers directly influence the types of people, places, things, and even illnesses that you attract into your life. By learning to work with your Chakras, you can learn to assess their level of functioning and diagnose how and why you are storing certain illnesses in your body. By applying certain techniques, such as creative visualization and "color breathing," you can address your illness from the inside as you shift it externally through the Feng Shui Design system.

Because both the Chakra and Feng Shui energy systems are invisible to the untrained eye, their validity is often questioned. Your mind must understand these systems' existence and power for you to be open to receiving their benefits. As we grow and expand into these higher levels of understanding, our mind and senses can also expand, making us more open to experiencing other ways of perceiving life. These other levels of perception have always existed, but not until we grow consciously will we be able to experience them personally. The first step is to accept that there are many things around us that we are not able to see with our physical eyes, hear with our ears, or smell with our noses, but that do exist and are as important as all the other "invisible technologies" we use in our daily life. Our TV's remote control is a simple example of an invisible technology. We have become so dependent on it that almost every home with a TV in it uses one. When you press different buttons you can turn the TV on and off, adjust the volume, or change stations. When we press those buttons, what we are really doing is changing the frequency of the signal that the remote is sending out. Each invisible signal is programmed. Shift the frequency, and you change the outgoing signal; change the outgoing signal, and you change its response. Does this make sense? Well, learning to work with Feng Shui and the Chakras teaches you how to decipher the energy signals of your life, and how to rework them so you can change the signals and thus change the outcome.

AN ENERGETIC UNDERSTANDING OF ILLNESS

A more expansive perspective on invisible energy fields, including the metaphysical and scientific changes that are taking place around you, will empower you with the ability to connect with Feng Shui and the Chakras, these new and powerful vibrational medicines that are now available to you. Embracing the understanding that there is science in the metaphysical, and metaphysical in science, you won't run the risk of pushing away tools, theories, and knowledge that have been specially designed and made available to help you heal. Without an understanding of how Feng Shui Design and the Chakra Energy System tie in to your illness and your healing process, utilizing them to improve your health will seem to you risky at best, superficial at worst.

As you read through the rest of this chapter, I encourage you to do so with an open mind, for some of this exciting information will radically alter how you currently see your life and some of the causes of your illness. I invite you to put aside linear, analytical thinking for just a little while and join me in what may prove to be one of the most informative and eye-opening experiences you may have regarding your illness and disease today.

All Matter, Both Physical and Subtle, Has a Specific Vibration and Frequency

Everything—thoughts, feelings, success, money, birds, cats, butterflies, illness, disease—has its own vibrational pattern or unique set of frequencies to which it resonates. The speed and the density of each specific vibration will determine how that vibration will manifest. We, too, are made up of many variations of vibrational patterns. Actually, human beings are a combination of complex energy systems that are sustained in a "dynamic state of equilibrium." Many of Einstein's theories were based on these principles.[3] As you come to understand this very significant concept, you will be able to start applying all the theories and solutions that are offered in this book.

Two Different Types of Vibrational Patterns

Each vibrational pattern consists of many different variables that come together to create a frequency. Most frequencies can be categorized into two distinct types, which I refer to as *general* and *specific*. Certain energy patterns are constant and affect all groups of people (general frequencies), while other patterns affect only a specific person, place, or thing. For example, each human being has a specific energy frequency to which his or her body vibrates. Some of the factors that make up that frequency are hair color, weight, biochemistry, height, personality, thought processes, core issues, spiritual path, past lives, race, religious beliefs, gender, and sexual orientation, to name a few. Together these characteristics make up not only who you are, but the total composition of your natural specific frequency. No one else has this frequency, just as no one else has your DNA, fingerprints, or handwriting.

When you or someone you know is ill, it is because the innate biological homeostasis that exists in the body has been somewhat altered, causing illness to occur. When the body is strong and surrounded by supportive energies (including people), good health has a good chance of reigning. But, as I have mentioned, the body's frequency is very much influenced by the ch'i of the surrounding area. If the Feng Shui of that environment is unbalanced, it can shape and trigger weaknesses within the body and disease or illness can occur.

Vibrational Patterns Create the Feng Shui of an Environment and an Illness

Vibrational patterns are created in the environment by different variables coming together: the color and shape of a space, the positioning of furniture, the locations and numbers of windows, and how close the stairs are to the doors, to name a few. These variables, when placed together in a room, unite in "vibrational patterns" that are either health-supportive or health-diminishing.

Every illness or disease has its own vibrational pattern. When an individual has a family history of, or predisposition to, a certain illness, that person carries the potential illness in the form of a vibrational pattern in his or her physical body, and in its energetic field. The Feng Shui of an environment can also re-create energy patterns that vibrate to specific illnesses. An individual might unknowingly move into an apartment or a house that has a similar vibrational pattern to a disease for which he or she has a propensity. When those two factors dovetail, they can trigger a dormant illness and disease can set in.

Unbalanced energy patterns don't affect everyone who comes in contact with them, because energies of different frequencies can coexist in a space and never affect one another. The illness vibration in house has a general frequency, which means it resonates to a weakened energy pattern that can cause certain types of illnesses; but in order for it to actually participate in the triggering of an illness, it has to resonate directly with the specific frequency of an individual who has personal contact with that pattern and is predisposed to that illness. That is why several people can live in the same house with the same general frequency illness potential, and only one of them might come down with the illness.

Illnesses can also occur under the influence of Feng Shui patterns when an individual without a predisposition to a specific illness is put under great stress. The unbalanced energy patterns of the environment turn opportunistic and, during a weakened time for that individual, can help create illness.

Unbalanced energy patterns in the environment can also slow down your recovery process if you are trying to get well, trigger frequent relapses, and weaken the impact of your treatment plan. That is why it is very important to analyze and support the Feng Shui of your home, for it can provide you with yet another puzzle piece toward understanding the nature of your illness.

A New Paradigm for Understanding Illness

We all exist on many levels, which, when combined, create who we are. Decades ago, we were simply thought of as physical beings with a body, separate from our minds. Then, as time passed, we started connecting the mind with the body. We began to get a glimpse of a new reality that suggested that the mind and the body were one, inseparable and interconnected.

In the past decade or so, we have begun to give credence to the concept that the mind can directly influence the health of the body and the body can influence the health of the mind. The old ways in which we interpreted illness and tried to heal are not working anymore because they were made to treat only the physical body or the physical manifestation of the disease, and not the whole person. Now we are starting to realize that we are multifaceted beings who need all aspects of ourself, including our spirit and emotions, to be acknowledged and addressed if true healing is to occur.

The ESPs of Illness™

Often when an individual gets sick, especially if the illness is sudden or perplexing, it is not uncommon for that person to spend a lot of time trying to "figure out" what happened and what might have caused it. It's human nature to want to know, because knowing puts us back in control, even if only for a short period of time. The more ways we can honestly take a good look at our illness, the more we raise the probability that the illness can be transmuted.

All Illness Is a Threefold Dis-ease

If you want to know about your illness and the different ways it might be trying to speak to you, then it's important to thoroughly explore what I call the ESPs of Illness, for they are the three main components of every disease. The ESPs of Illness are the *Emotional* aspect, the *Spiritual* aspect, and the *Physical* aspect of every sickness. Every illness has these three underpinnings that together create a vibrational matrix that allows the illness to manifest and thrive. By dissecting your health concern into its ESPs, you are breaking it down into manageable pieces, which is a powerful first step in disempowering it. Just as illness becomes more resilient and may be prolonged when it has similar groups of vibrations supporting its inner structure, the different ESP aspects, when addressed collectively, can speed up the recovery process.

1. **Emotional aspects.** These are defined as unresolved feelings and/or personal issues that might still be eating away at you, or that you haven't

entirely made peace with on a deep level. The operative word here is *personal*. These issues are germane to *you*. It's all the stuff you stored inside of you, hid away, or didn't consciously remember, which has lain dormant until now: old hurts, abandonments, betrayals; fear-based feelings such as jealousy, anger, and powerlessness; unprocessed grief, losses, disappointments, and traumas; along with painful memories of emotional, physical, and sexual abuse. Our current life issues may reflect memories that go as far back as into the womb and beyond.

2. *Spiritual aspects.* These are the parts of the illness that hold the energetic space for you to soul-search and find the spiritual reasons behind this particular dis-ease as it relates to you in your current life. It's the part of the illness that helps you find your way back to the last place you were in before you "separated from your healthy self." Reclaiming these aspects helps you hit the spiritual reset button and gives you a new lease on life. It also helps you to reconnect spiritually and get back on your life's path. This part of your illness can help you to fulfill your commitment to service as part of your life's work while here on the planet. Some souls have actually made a contract to develop a particular disease and make their contribution to humankind through providing that service for others to grow. The key concepts here are bigger-picture issues, spiritual lessons, service, past lives, and karma.

3. *Physical aspects.* All disease has a physical component by which it manifests in a certain way, through a certain organ or area in the body. Although this is the stage that gets the individual's attention first, it is usually the last place where disease and illness surface. Most individuals are already in a state of disease emotionally and spiritually before any illness erupts in the physical body. Often we have ignored the signals for some time, allowing our emotions, thoughts, and spirituality to fall by the wayside. When a physical illness surfaces, it's usually the universe's last resort to get our attention about something. Although this is not exclusively true (as you will see in the next few pages, there are many different ways and reasons why we get sick), quite often it is. Another

common reason why an individual contracts a certain illness is that his or her soul has made a conscious choice to contract that illness, for it is in that particular illness that the exact lessons the soul needs to experience will emerge. This decision oversees all hereditary factors of physical issues, predisposition to certain illnesses, the individual's physical body, and potential exposure to miasms.[4] It also connects to the physical environments that surround us, and in turn influences and is influenced by the Feng Shui of a space. In order for this part of the illness to transform, you need to attend to the physical body and provide for medical treatment to care for the physical manifestation of the disease.

All Aspects of Yourself Need Attention

Each of the above aspects of any illness, acute or chronic, constitutes one-third of the energy pattern that holds that particular illness in place. Each of these three energy patterns contributes to holding the illness in place and keeping it from being transformed. As you start to address each area separately, and then in combination, you will begin to break the invisible energetic gridlock that keeps the illness and its dynamics alive. Each area needs your attention and care if you want to accelerate your healing and recovery process.

People who are ill tend to focus on one or two of these areas. It's usually based on one's comfort zone and his or her familiar way of approaching sickness, crisis, and life. For instance, individuals who are used to going to doctors will act upon that part of the equation—i.e., the physical aspect—and possibly not address the emotional or spiritual underpinnings of their illness. People who tend to meditate, on the other hand, might examine the spiritual underpinning of their illness. And still others, who have had experience with psychotherapy, are more comfortable with processing some of the emotional issues that contribute to holding the disease's matrix in place. It all depends on what makes rational sense to you, and the types of experiences and support systems that you bring to the illness.

The truth is that if you really want to heal, you have to address all three areas. All too often I see people addressing just one area—the spiritually evolved person ignoring the need for medical treatment for his or her body, and the individual who will run out to get assistance from their doctors ignoring the need to look at the underlying emotional and spiritual issues.

When I first became ill with my virus in the late 1980s, I was a practicing psychotherapist, and it colored my approach to my treatment. For the first year or so of my illness, instead of going to a medical doctor, I processed all the emotional issues around why I was feeling so exhausted. I connected it to the stress in my life, a relentless conflict centering on my mother, and a host of other things that were very real and would have had to be addressed eventually, but which sidetracked me from getting the medical care I needed for my physical body. Without recognizing the severity of the illness that was upon me, that first year ended up exacerbating my condition and putting me on the road to hell for many extra years.

That experience taught me a lot about leaving no stone unturned. I now always try to explore different options and approach all problems multidimensionally. The ten years that I was sick, and the lessons that my illness taught me, became the core of my work and the premise of this book.

The point I am trying to make is that when you are sick you can pray, meditate, and process all you want, but if you don't remember to care for the physical body, you run the risk of a slower recovery process, relapses, and having that illness show up in another form, at another time, and in another place in your body. The same thing is true if you choose to deal with the illness from only a physical perspective; you will run the same risks during the illness or at a later, unanticipated time.

THE EMOTIONAL COMPONENT: DEALING WITH THE B.A.D. EMOTIONS IS *GOOD*!

These emotions are bad not in themselves, but only in the sense that either we have been told not to have them or we feel shame about having them because they are "spiritually incorrect," especially if you consider yourself an enlightened being. But no healing can ever truly happen without inner cooperation. Your body, your home, and all your feelings must live in cooperation with one another for physical health to thrive. Otherwise the resulting chaos can create illness and disease. By honoring your emotions and creating for yourself a safe space to have them, you ultimately assist the transformation of your illness and subsequently your life.

The BAD emotions are *Betrayal, Anger,* and *Despair.* To further complicate things, family, friends, and society discourage these feelings also. If we want to get well and heal, we are told that we have to stay positive and have only positive thoughts. I do not agree with that theory, because it assists you in suppressing those feelings, helping you disconnect from them and making you feel flawed and inept that you are still having them. Not a single person I have worked with, including myself, while dealing with the ESPs of their illness, didn't eventually have to process some of these feelings that were lodged and buried deep down inside. Certainly I believe in positive thinking and affirmative action, but if you do not allow yourself to experience all your feelings as they come up, those feelings will eventually have to surface somewhere, and quite often it's as an underpinning of an illness.

In my opinion, the problem is not in *having* these feelings, but in *avoiding* having them. However, working on understanding and processing our feelings until we feel complete is one thing, but getting lost in those feelings and never moving through them is something else. In the new approach to illness, everything is valuable and part of the lessons that you need to experience and process. There are no junk experiences! Even the not-so-comfortable feelings and issues are part of your healing process, not an obstacle to it.

As you explore your feelings of betrayal, anger, and despair and some of their emotional underpinnings, make sure that you keep a close lookout for shame. This is probably the most insidious of all feelings because it comes up and does its thing long before you know it's there, and it is often a by-product of the BAD feelings. It's an upward emotional flush that runs through your body at lightning speed, telling your mind and your heart to react in a different way so you do not have to feel the shame that is surfacing for you. Keep in mind that shame will attach itself to any emotion or feeling and shut it down, along with the individual to whom it is connected. When I was a practicing psychotherapist, I always said that out of all the feelings my clients brought into the office, shame was the hardest one to uncover and work with, because it was so visceral and camouflaged itself as so many other things. Ninety percent of all shame is learned; the other ten percent is given to us by God, just enough to keep us from going to the grocery store to purchase a container of milk naked. The ten percent that we get from God is what I refer to as "healthy shame," and is needed to maintain certain boundaries and keep our integrity intact. The other ninety percent is learned, and then internalized.

Betrayal is a very important feeling to acknowledge and process when you are ill. Often this is a harder feeling to face than to have, because in processing it, you have to look at the ways that you have been weakened by a situation or person and made vulnerable. *If you are ill, it's very important to your healing process that you begin to look at the ways that you feel and have felt betrayed.* Sickness was something that was supposed to happen to other people, other families, and other lives! Its reality can turn your world upside down as you start realizing that you have been betrayed by your own wisdom, intuition, Feng Shui process, body, prayers, and God. Illness has a way of sneaking up on and pulling the rug out from under you as you begin that long journey through shock and betrayal, trying to figure out what went wrong and why this happened to you.

Anger is the other significant feeling that we never quite get a handle on. We are either shoving it far down in our bodies and working hard to avoid it, or trying to express it inappropriately. It is the least "spiritually correct" of all the emotions, and it always comes with some past baggage as well. It's the emotion that has really gotten a bad name because in a so-called civilized society we think we should be able to control it and talk things through.

When anger is used as a catalyst to get to another place, to help you advocate for yourself or set a needed boundary, it becomes a very necessary emotion for healing to occur. The problem with anger comes when it is not expressed, dealt with, or discussed. When it is avoided or denied altogether, it can then surface in many destructive ways. Accumulated unprocessed anger can be implosive and can eventually turn into illness because the anger has a vibrational energy field around it with a life force, and like anything else, it needs to be expressed. When we deny that expression, we force the anger to surface elsewhere, and that place is usually in our bodies.

Over time, accumulated and repressed anger can inappropriately be expressed in the form of rage. It's important to have all your feelings, and this means the willingness to face the uncomfortable ones, too. As you begin your healing process, a good way to gauge whether you are really in it is when you start feeling your anger. Make sure, as it starts to surface, that you find a healthy way of having all those feelings, and do not repress them again. Most of us will find at the bottom of our illness some anger, if not a lot of it, waiting to be heard and dealt with. Don't stuff it back down, for in its ugliness is an important message for you about your life, health, illness, and innermost pain. Honor it, because it finally feels safe enough with you to come forward and make itself known so the healing can begin.

Despair is another important emotion for your healing, because once you get to it, you know that you are well on your way to transmuting the energy around the illness. It is very important to maintain a positive outlook and keep faith that things will change for the better. But if, deep down inside, you are frightened and feel bone-chilling despair, it's vital that you get to those feelings as quickly and as honestly as you can. Often I have worked with individuals who were ill and felt that remaining positive and keeping a stiff upper lip was the way they were going to barrel through it, but deep inside they felt incredible despair. Without giving that despair a voice, they remained in that part of their illness that much longer. If you truly don't feel the despair, well, that's a good thing; but you have to keep an eye out for "pseudo-feelings" that disguise themselves and convince you that that's not what you are truly feeling.

Avoidance Equals Powerlessness

All these feelings will render you powerless if you don't confront them head-on. Deep hurts, small lies, and heart-wrenching infidelities have to rise to the surface, for when they do, they represent a significant stage in your spiritual growth and healing process. Many of these feelings are at the core of our diseases, and illnesses, and we must deal with them if we are to move forward and to higher ground. Allowing them to come up actually shows that you are well into your healing, and that you are working in a co-creative process with the energetic forces that are assisting you in your healing. Your emotions are going to be the key to your healing process, so welcome them with open arms and congratulate yourself for letting yourself have them, because the amount of emotional distance you keep from your feelings will equal the same distance that you have from your healing.

Clearing Away Stagnant Energy and Old Emotional Carnage

The energy contained in your feelings is very powerful, so powerful that they become a contributing component to the ESPs and matrix of your illness. When you start releasing their intensity, you release their power over you and your body. As you purge them, you also discharge them from your body, to be absorbed back into the environment in which you live and work. These hard-to-purge emotions now exist in your environment, only to be reabsorbed back into your body and your emotional-energy field. During times of illness, crisis, or healing, it's important to keep your body and the environment as clear as possible, so that spirit and life force can come through.

The Transcendental Cure given below is from the Black Hat Sect and Grandmaster H.H. Lin Yun's teachings. This healing and body-clearing "scent cure" attempts to adjust your internal ch'i and the external ch'i of your home through the sense of smell and through your skin—which, by the way, is the body's largest organ.

The Orange Peel Cure: For Clearing Home and Body

Home: To clear all stale and negative energy from a home or office, or to clear the energy field of a newly purchased or rented home, you can employ Professor Lin Yun's cure for clearing the energy of a space. First, purchase a fresh orange. While sitting in a peaceful, quiet spot in your home, with or without a knife start to peel *nine small, round, disklike sections* of the rind off your orange and think about the energy that you would like to clear out from your home and all the things from which you would like to be released. Then place the orange peels in a small bowl of water and, starting at the front door of your home, walk through each room of the house and sprinkle water with your hand in an "Ousting Mudra" position (see chapter 9) where you extend your pointer and pinky fingers, using your thumb to pull back your middle and ring fingers at the same time, creating a flicking motion. Apply the Three Secrets Reinforcement Blessing nine times (see chapter 9) to ensure a successful clearing process. Make sure you visualize positive and uplifting ch'i meandering through your house clearing all negative emotions or stagnant energies. (Also, see the Purification by Fire Clearing Method listed in chapter 9.)

Body: Prepare a warm, soothing bath, play some healing music, and don't forget to light some white candles. Turn your bathroom into a "sacred space" as you prepare to use the Orange Peel Cure as a sacred ritual for cleansing your energy field and physical body of stagnant or leftover emotions. Prepare the nine round orange peels as mentioned earlier and squeeze them gently, one at a time, over the water in the tub, then bless the bath with the Three Secrets Reinforcement Blessing (see chapter 9), visualizing that the bath and the oils from the orange rinds will absorb all the energy fields and elements that no longer serve you, and that they will purify your being through the sacred healing waters. Afterward, take a quick shower to wash off the energies that remained in the bath. Discard the orange peels. To strengthen the cure, do this for nine consecutive nights.

THE SPIRITUAL COMPONENT: REASONS WHY ILLNESSES MANIFEST

Illnesses appear for many reasons. Most of the time, although we can speculate and guess, only the soul's consciousness truly knows why. But it's still important to review some of the reasons that illness does occur, in order for you to flush out any preconceived notions, judgments, and issues of self-blame. Above all, it is most important that you realize that *illness does not always mean unresolved blocks, and death is not a sign of failure.* If that were true, we could all start looking forward to becoming failures someday, because we are all going to die!

As you start to look at the different components of your illness, your concepts and conditioning about health, healing, death, and dying will need to be revisited and revamped. Most of us have been conditioned to believe that when an individual who is sick either gets better or finds the right medication or cure for his or her malady, that means the person has been healed; and that when someone is sick with a prolonged illness, or dies from that illness, it means the person did not get better and was not healed. Those are leftover beliefs from our old ways of thinking, which never really addressed the possibility of other reasons for sickness, life, or dying. In that mind-set, healing means that the physical body has gotten better and recovered. Many of us now understand that there is more to us than just our physical bodies. So sometimes the healing we receive from the sickness or the disease takes place in another one of our energy bodies, such as the emotional or spiritual level.

Often the soul gets the exact healing it needed from the disease that it has taken on, but our old thinking sometimes interprets it as a non-healing (physically), a sad loss, or an untimely death. That is why we need to reframe our goals and our win-lose definition of healing. Instead, we need to strive toward transmuting the illness into a higher form, respecting the lessons that it has brought us for our souls' growth, even if at first it's hard to pay homage to it. It is important that we remain open and rethink some of our original conditioning so we can truly embrace the challenge of ill health from a broader, more spiritually diverse perspective.

Remember, *illness creates a powerful schoolroom for transformation to occur.* When the lessons are learned and the soul experiences what it is in need of experiencing, there is no other need for that illness to be active. At that point in the transformation process, the individual will be physically, emotionally, or spiritually healed, and the illness will then dissipate or return to spirit. During these times the person can have a spontaneous healing, find the right cure, or leave the body, passing over from the Yang life (living) to the Yin life (afterlife). In the bigger picture of things, every illness will be eradicated and every "cure" that is needed will be discovered when that particular illness is no longer needed as a teacher on our planet.

Seven Reasons Why Illness Can Manifest

1. The individual might have missed prior messages, emotional and spiritual, regarding some aspect of their life, path, or work. Perhaps they were in denial or avoiding the truth about certain situations. Such reactions or nonreactions to life and life situations will cause a backup and eventually a block. The illness was the soul's inner wisdom and last attempt to get one's conscious attention.

2. The illness may be programmed into an individual's vibrational field before he or she is born. The individual might have decided to use the illness as a "reset button" if certain things go wrong. The individual, prior to incarnating (during a state of total consciousness and awareness), reviews the illness and the potential that it will bring if those experiences are suddenly needed by the soul to grow and expand further. This poten-

tial manifestation may draw upon stored genetic factors, predispositions, environmental factors, or a prior health history to trigger the onset of a preprogrammed illness.

3. The illness occurs in that individual's life at the exact time and under the exact conditions for which it was programmed. The individual needs to experience this particular illness because it will bring the perfect set of circumstances to further the growth of the soul. The illness was supposed to occur, according to the individual's higher plan, to address personal and past-life karma issues.

4. Manifesting the illness is actually one of the soul's main responsibilities and reasons for incarnating at a specific time. The soul, fully aware of the complications that come with having a given type of illness, still chooses to commit that lifetime to doing service for humankind, as part of the soul's work on this planet. It is through the use of its physical body that it acts as a conduit for teaching. In addition, the soul will be working to rid the planet of this illness, breaking down mass "group illness thought forms" that are holding in place the matrix of the particular disease. This type of illness addresses issues related to personal, as well as social, karma.

5. A certain type of illness occurs when a person has gone so far off the track of his or her incarnation, and is so out of alignment that the only way he or she can grow or get back on track is through manifesting some type of physical illness. The illness may be an intervention by the universe when an individual is in a landslide or full breakdown. This type of illness may have also been preprogrammed by the individual to act as a "spiritual awakening."

6. An illness may occur as a result of an energetic *miasm*.[5] A miasm is an energetic mass that lives outside of a person's life system and under most circumstances never makes contact with that life system. It can live outside that being for lifetimes and never become activated until one day a series of weakening events occur, making the person vulnerable and allowing the miasm to find its way in. This connection activates the

miasm, and with it the particular illness or disease it is carrying. This miasm can stay in a person's energy system for a very long time, until it is transmuted or somehow purged. Because of all of the major energy changes on the planet, energies that are otherwise stable have been placed in constant flux, weakening their bigger-picture energy fields. This shift has allowed certain bacteria and viruses to mutate and proliferate, resulting in "new" illnesses such as chronic fatigue syndrome, autoimmune disorders, and HIV.

7. An illness may occur as a "rite of passage" when the soul has completed its work here, and no new lessons are to be learned or contributions made. The soul uses the illness as a vehicle to take it back home and return it to spirit. If you see all illness and death as a negative thing or as a failure of some kind, you are only heeding the limitations of the conscious personality and not supporting the inner wisdom of the soul's purpose and mission.

THE PHYSICAL COMPONENT: GOD IS IN THE DETAILS . . . AND IN THE MEDICINE

It is very important that we tend to the physical body and provide for it all the possible treatments and care that it requires so that a complete healing or transmutation of an illness can occur. However spiritually or emotionally astute you are, you still have to remember that you have incarnated into a physical body that needs to be cared for, and doctored when needed.

I am often asked what my position is on homeopathic, naturopathic, and allopathic medicines. I feel very strongly that God exists in all types of medicine. It is a very personal decision that we each have to make in sickness and in health regarding what type of treatment is best. No type of medicine is always right or always wrong. Throwing the baby out with the bathwater stops us from taking the best of all worlds and creating the complementary medicines of the future.

No one medicine or treatment plan is right for healing everyone. That's why we have been given all these empowering choices—not so that we can debunk something we don't personally believe in or care to use, but so we can freely expand our access to a variety of complementary medicines that can make us better. True technology gives us options to help us expand, not choices dictated by misconception and outdated fears. Abuse and misuse are possible with all medicines, and occur among doctors who practice both traditional and nontraditional modalities. You must find a treatment plan or medication combination that works for you, no matter what magazines say or your friends might think. Make it your goal to get well, and never take your eyes off that ball! There are many wonderful doctors who are open, caring, and very adept at combining medicines, interfacing them skillfully with all the other vibrational medicines now available, such as homeopathy, flower essences, color therapy, sound balancing, and Feng Shui Design.

The more you understand about the ESPs of Illness and all the vibrational medicines that are available to you, the better you will feel, the more manageable your illness will become, and the more sense it will make.

When your soul no longer has an emotional, spiritual, or physical need for the particular illness it has encountered, your healing will begin. One day you may be eating a peppermint stick, and that will be the medicine that begins your healing process; or the healing can come from finding the correct homeopathic remedy or doctor's prescription. As you will soon begin to see, healings come in many guises.

Our Personal ESPs Mirror Collective Thought Forms of Illness; Collective Thought Forms of Illness Mirror Our Personal ESP Thought Forms

Every illness has a vibration, frequency, and thought form that is unique to it. Thought forms are highly charged pieces of energy that collectively can resonate to a particular illness. They connect to an individual only if the individual has a matching "specific frequency" that dovetails with the illness. If the individual does not have a specific connection to the "illness thought form," that illness can never occur in that individual's life because the lessons it would bring would have no value or meaning to that soul. From an energetic and spiritual perspective, this provides a very simple explanation of why many people can be exposed to the same virus and only a few will become sick. Or several siblings may be exposed to the same genetic factors, but only one of them will develop a given hereditary disease. On the other hand, to heal completely from an illness, one has to seriously alter the matrix of one's own specific illness frequency that was tapping in to the frequency of the bigger vibrational pattern that resonated to the specific disease. Collectively, the ESPs of Illness take on a bigger picture meaning, acting as a gatherer of human thought forms and an energetic mirror to what's happening on a more personal level with the society that is being challenged by the disease.

The ESPs of Illness gather all the thinking, judgments, hates, abuses, jealousies, anger, fears, and skewed energy patterns, and combine them into various groups that then turn into "energetic masses." These masses then collectively create the general frequency to which an illness or disease vibrates. In turn, these energetic masses or diseases act as a mirror reflecting back to us, through the various illnesses that exist on the planet, all our unconscious, subconscious, and conscious thoughts, feelings, and fears. The illness holds the space for all those aspects of the human condition that are in need of healing individually as well as globally. Every illness that exists on the planet first exists in separate ESP pieces inside many different individuals.

From an energetic point of view, if a disease exists in the world, it has already existed for a long time in each of us. As units of energy and beings of light, we have collectively created every illness that has ever existed. Our thoughts are powerful, and energy always follows thought. We have not spent much time looking at and addressing the collective thought form that holds each illness's matrix in place. Our frustration and limited progress in the areas of research and cures have been hampered because we have attempted to heal the illness in its physical component only, thus leaving out other important emotional and spiritual components of the healing equation. This slows down and interferes with the actual healing process itself. By understanding this perspective, you will lend more dignity to the illness and grace to the person who is ill, for it lifts us out of our prior understanding of illness, which kept us in a victim role, to a position of trust, honor, and self-empowerment. This is the promise of the new paradigm for redefining illness. What lies on the other side of our hard work and endurance is a better world, with less disease of mind, body, and spirit to pass on to the next generation of people.

Break the Matrix, Disarm the Illness

The best way to disarm any illness is to "break the matrix" in which it lives, because all the ESPs of that particular illness need to be present and working together for that illness to exist and thrive. When you begin to loosen and break down this grid by addressing its separate components, you disempower the illness at its core, where it is at its strongest. By addressing the ESPs of your illness, you are actually addressing the essence and consciousness of the disease itself, engaging all of the pieces of your illness to assist you in your healing process.

My Client, My Teacher

A few years ago I was blessed with the opportunity to work with a wonderful family and their son, whose health was being challenged by AIDS. Although his family initially asked me to do a Feng Shui consultation of his home for him, not long into the first hour I began to talk to him in detail about his illness, how he was dealing with it, and the potential reality of his passing. After several hours we had covered everything from why he thought he had contracted the illness to his feelings and fears about death, dying, and being a homosexual man in today's world. During what proved to be the most vulnerable time in his life, he let me into his deepest and darkest thoughts about what he was facing. Although he was my client, he also became my teacher, for which I feel honored and grateful. His bravery in looking within himself during a very difficult time proved to be one of my greatest lessons in working with individuals during their healing process. When he discussed with me his personal struggles with his shame about being ill and some of his leftover feelings regarding his relationship with his father, he was addressing the issues that created some of the emotional underpinnings of his disease. When we discussed his "life after life" beliefs, his fear, and his concept of God, along with the bigger-picture reasons why he'd contracted the AIDS virus, we were addressing the spiritual component of his illness. When we discussed his choice of medical treatments, medicines, and the betrayal he was experiencing with his body during the few months prior to my visit, we were discussing the physical component of his illness and the different ways he had to care for himself.

In a concentrated effort, as we addressed many of the different aspects of his illness, we were defusing the specific frequency around it, which was providing an energetic electrical charge that held the matrix of his illness in place. My Feng Shui work with him that followed was then to find the ways the ESPs of his illness were being energetically re-created in his apartment.

After much review, I suggested that he hang several 30-mm crystals to add rainbows and light force, a few wind chimes in strategic places to move the stagnant ch'i, plants for additional life-force energy, and an altar in his "Helpful People" corner. Why the "Helpful People" corner? Because in my exploration of the Feng Shui of his home, I discovered that the place where he spent most of his time listening to music, watching TV, sorting through his medication, and eating his dinner was in the area that oversaw the Helpful People section in Feng Shui Design. (This will be explained further in chapter 3.) The Helpful People section is the area that oversees the relationship with one's father. He was spending a lot of his time in his home in the Feng Shui section that carried the energetic vibration of the exact thing that was weighing most heavily on his heart and mind, his dad.

One of the more significant cures I suggested to him was to write an unedited letter to his father baring all feelings, good and bad—all the things he needed and wanted to say, but, for whatever reason, didn't get to or was holding in. In addition to a special transcendental blessing that I did, I suggested that he place his letter on the altar in his Helpful People corner.

Several weeks after my Feng Shui consultation, his health began to decline very rapidly, and shortly after that he passed away. In many ways, from the viewpoint of traditional medicine, his physical health was much better before I did the consultation. But through his inner exploration, soul-searching, and willingness to address some of the deeper issues that lay heavily on his mind, I believe he was able to let go both emotionally and spiritually, and move on with the next part of his existence in the afterlife. We broke the matrix, and although we didn't get the physical healing that he and his family and I truly wanted, I do believe that his higher self learned what it was here to learn and contribute, and when the work was over and the lessons were completed, his soul decided to return home. The Feng Shui consultation supported him in his process and helped him to move toward closure of his life. I thank him, bless him, and think of him often. His passing served to remind me that there are many courageous soldiers among us, and that Feng Shui can be used to assist people at all stages of their lives and in many important rites of passage.

How Our Personal Healing Influences
the Healing of Our World

In 1997 I founded a nonprofit program called Feng Shui Across America (its current name is Feng Shui Around the World; for more information, e-mail FSAW108@aol.com). This program utilized Feng Shui consultants from around the world to provide free Feng Shui consultations for individuals who were facing life-threatening diseases. During that time I had the opportunity to talk with several consultants who were very interested in joining the Feng Shui Across America program, but were experiencing some difficulties along the way in trying to get their efforts off the ground. Often they would tell me they had a hard time finding others to get involved, or that certain AIDS sites had turned down their offer of free Feng Shui services; still others felt a bit overwhelmed about taking on extra work.

I thank those individuals who were candid with me and expressed their frustrations and conflicts, because it was through their experiences that I started to understand the vibrational nature of AIDS and develop some of my theories on illness, vibrational patterns and, specifically, the ESPs of Illness and general versus specific frequencies.

As some of them talked to me about their frustrations and the obstacles that they were facing, it became clear that they were having a difficult time and facing lots of resistance. It made perfect sense to me, because AIDS is a disease of Resistance! It has baffled doctors and scientists alike for 20 years with a virus that has been resistant to almost every kind of medicine with which they have attempted to combat it. Given the nature of its emotional structure, it would be preposterous to think that as consultants and volunteers we wouldn't be faced with and confronting the same type of energy field that was holding the matrix together. So I began to look at the energy and emotion of resistance as a core issue inseparable from its ESP matrix.

If we were doing our jobs right, then on some level we *must* eventually encounter resistance, within ourselves and within the various project sites, for that was the exact energy we had to start working with in the small of the matrix, if we wanted to transmute and alter the disease at its core. I believe that emotionally and psychologically HIV/AIDS is a disease of *resistance* born of a matrix of individual hate and judgments.

If we truly want to find a cure and transmute the virus, we have to find ways of transmuting its ESPs, as well as the thought forms that have helped create it. By taking a multilevel approach to dismantling an epidemic, or any disease for that matter, we will accelerate a true healing process that includes all aspects of the illness, and not only the physical components.

The healing that I foresee, and the thing that I believe can turn this disease of AIDS around, is to uncover where resistance, homophobia, and judgments are lurking in our own hearts and in the energy of some of these institutions. We need to do this for every illness that we face; instead of backing down from it or getting discouraged, we must apply gentle persistence and move through it to the other side—for the other side of resistance is release, and through release transformation and healing become possible. This is the alchemy of disease; this is how we will all contribute to healing this epidemic—by walking through individual pieces of resistance. Every illness has a vibrational pattern. By learning how to understand and decipher such patterns we are given the power to change the core of illness itself, by changing our thinking, attitudes, and ourselves first.

Closing Chapter Exercise

The following exercise is crucial for exploring the next stage of your Feng Shui health process.

Before I or any of my associates begins a Feng Shui consultation, we always ask from each of our clients that they submit a personal biography and a floor plan of their home. The reason why both things are so important is that they force you to stop, think, and personally get involved with the process that you are undertaking. The biography gives you the opportunity to pause and think about what's happening in your life at the time of the consultation. We request a current day biography reflecting all the things that are of concern right now, including relationship issues, career options, financial challenges, and any health concerns. This gives the consultant an overview of what is going well in the client's life and where he or she is blocked or struggling.

In preparation for the next few chapters of this book, I'm going to ask you to do a one- to two-page biography that specifically focuses on any health-related issues. Think about any emotional times, crises, chronic conditions, acute illnesses, injuries, or nagging health problems. Make sure you ask yourself if there was a point, prior to or during your illness, when you felt compromised or you lost your integrity. Think about this, for it was at that point that your illness began, or your healing started to unravel. Write down whatever it means to you, and whatever concerns you have about it. Everything that comes to mind should be included, even if it's just a brief mention. The actual task of sitting down with pen, paper, and a willingness to tell your story is a wonderful signal to the universe that you are ready to begin your process of disclosure and subsequent healing.

Everybody Has a Story . . .

Find a nice quiet place where you will not be interrupted and have some privacy, and bring lots of tissues. Be still, light a candle, and reflect on your life for a few minutes. Start writing a story about your life: key points, traumas, frightening times, significant events, turning points, and your health history and issues. Try very hard not to edit it or to worry about grammar or proper sentence structure. For just a little while, let go of your intellect and the rational thinker inside you. No one else has to read this writing unless you let them. Give the "committee" in your head the day off and just freely associate, write, and cry if you need to. Let all your thoughts be heard and written down, even if they seem totally unrelated to one another.

At the end of your health biography, think about one particular illness that has plagued you for a while, or about which you have some concerns. Create three separate columns, and label them "Emotional," "Spiritual," and "Physical." Then list under each heading issues that you feel fall under that category and constitute the specific frequency of your illness. Then list the things you might need to do to start dealing with the underpinnings of your health concern. Remember, every illness or health-related problem needs to be attended to emotionally, spiritually, and physically in order for you to truly begin to transmute the illness and break its matrix.

CHAPTER THREE

TOOLS FOR BEGINNING YOUR HEALTH ASSESSMENT PROCESS

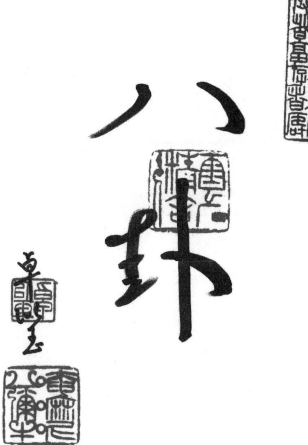

"Bagua."

CALLIGRAPHY BY DR. CATHERINE YI-YU CHO WOO

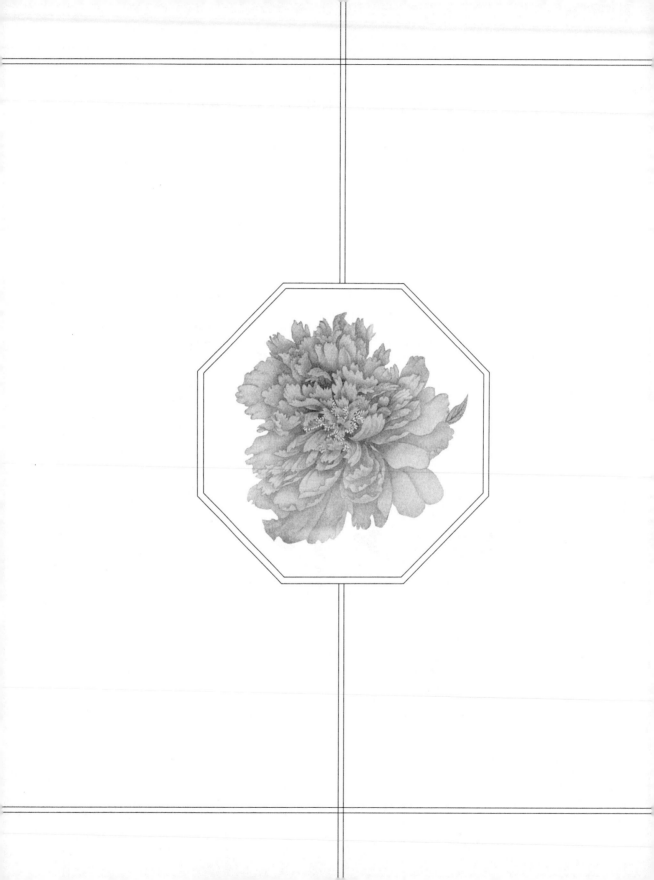

AS YOU START to work more with the process of Feng Shui, you will begin to develop a deeper level of understanding of what Feng Shui is, and how it actually works from a personal perspective. As we work toward integrating this information into our lives, it requires us to rethink our notions and understanding of what we deem visible and invisible. Through exploring the world of invisible energy fields, we are challenged to push aside our rational thinking and spiritually trust the information that is currently being made available to us through Feng Shui.

When I first learned about the principles of Feng Shui, I was very sick and desperate, but even in that very painful state of duress, I felt I needed to understand what I was learning at all levels of my being, including my intellect. The challenge of processing the logic of Feng Shui actually strengthened my spiritual knowledge and personal understanding of energy and how it works. Logical thought enabled me to integrate the teachings on a deeper, more comprehensive level and, in turn, have greater confidence in sharing it with others.

As you read through this book and sort through other available information on Feng Shui, it's important to ask yourself questions that will help you arrive at your own level of understanding and personal truth. Why? Because crisis, especially when it involves one's health, tends to make even the strongest of people quite vulnerable. In addition, if your illness is life-threatening, it is an already frightening situation and can lead even the most stable person into sheer panic and desperation.

When we are sick—and I know this from my own ten-year illness—we're willing to try anything. When a treatment plan fails, fear and desperation are opportunistic feelings that are never far behind. When desperation is combined with fear and panic, together they become a very dangerous emotional cocktail. This bag of mixed emotions increases the likelihood that even the most logical among us can fall prey to believing in "magic bullets" and "quick fixes."

The good news—and perhaps the bad news—is that *Feng Shui is neither.* It's a design system that teaches us how to interpret the invisible patterns of energy in our surroundings, understand their impact on our health, and show us what to do to rearrange these patterns to support our well-being.

Learning how to detect the flow of ch'i throughout your dwelling allows you to locate the areas where energy is blocked, stagnant, oppressive, or flowing too strongly. Any energy imbalance can trigger or lead to illness. The assessment of ch'i in your home will give you the information you need to make the proper adjustments and bring the ch'i back to its natural balance. It may be as simple an adjustment as moving your desk into a better energy position, adding extra light to a room, or simply changing the color of your bedroom. By learning how to work with energy to design the interior of your home, you can ultimately shape and alter your health and the many different situations in your life. If you are using it properly, Feng Shui should serve as an adjunct to your other medical treatments of choice.

The following information will start you on your process and provide you with the tools that you will need to begin your Feng Shui health journey.

The Feng Shui assessment of your home begins with a step-by-step walk-through, reviewing everything from the location of your front door to the colors used in each room of your house. All of these things affect the way ch'i flows through your home and workplace, thus affecting your personal ch'i and specific vibration. This is very important because your personal ch'i dictates the overall quality of your health and life.

HOW DOES FENG SHUI CONNECT
WITH THE ESPs OF ILLNESS?

As I have previously stated, everyday life patterns that emanate from the internal energy field of a human being are mirrored and held in place by the external energy field in the environments that surround you. That external energy field is known as your Feng Shui. Feng Shui holds in place, reflects, and then re-creates in the environment all the unprocessed and unbalanced energy patterns that make up the ESPs of Illness for the individual who resides or spends a lot of time in that environment. Feng Shui re-creates the vibrational pattern of an illness and sustains its energy pattern until a part of the energy equation has been altered in a way that will weaken and disarm the illness. When the disease or illness pattern is reinforced externally, it locks the illness in to a higher, stronger, and more resilient vibration that becomes very hard to treat and transmute. The exterior environment, and its Feng Shui, then become factors in why individuals become ill and stay ill, and have a slower recovery process and relapses.

In addition, the ch'i in your body is then influenced by the quality of the ch'i in your home, workplace, and surrounding environments. Once influenced, the ch'i in your body acts very similarly to the way the energy of a transmitter works, attracting the same type of energy signals that it sends out. It receives the same type of energy that it generates. For instance, if your ch'i is sending out energy signals that resonate to a sense of harmony and balance, then it will draw to it objects, events, and opportunities that will reflect that feeling. That's why it is so important to work with and balance the ch'i in your environment: it influences the relationships, finances, career opportunities, and health challenges that you will draw toward you.

THE BAGUA, YOUR FLOOR PLAN, AND
NINE BASIC CURES

The three most important tools needed to begin the next part of your Feng Shui health assessment are (1) your understanding and appropriate use of the Bagua (your Feng Shui map), (2) a simple floor plan of your space, and (3)

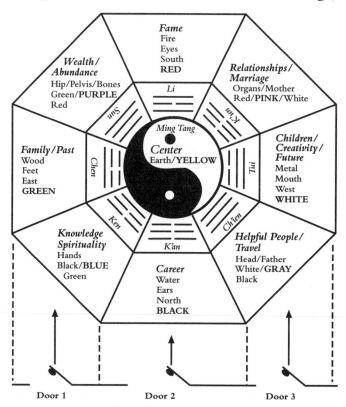

Bagua Feng Shui Map
Fig. 2. Three Door Positioning

Fame
Fire
Eyes
South
RED

Li

Wealth/ Abundance
Hip/Pelvis/Bones
Green/**PURPLE**
Red

Sun

Relationships/ Marriage
Organs/Mother
Red/**PINK**/White

K'un

Ming Tang
Center
Earth/**YELLOW**

Family/Past
Wood
Feet
East
GREEN

Chen

Children/ Creativity/ Future
Metal
Mouth
West
WHITE

Tui

Knowledge Spirituality
Hands
Black/**BLUE**
Green

Ken

K'an

Ch'ien

Helpful People/ Travel
Head/Father
White/**GRAY**
Black

Career
Water
Ears
North
BLACK

Door 1   Door 2   Door 3

a grasp of the Black Hat Sect Nine Basic Cures. Together these three components will give you the basics to structure your process. The more quickly you understand and use these tools, the more quickly you can allow yourself to open up to the healing.

As the ch'i moves closer to the individual, it breaks down into nine compartments, eight of which specifically correspond to different areas of your life, and one that oversees all other issues and, specifically, health. The map that we use to illustrate this information is called the *Bagua* (pronounced *Bah-gwah*). The Bagua, which means "eight-sided trigram map," evolved from the *I Ching,* the ancient Chinese oracle that has been used for thousands of years for divination. These principles are believed to govern all uni-

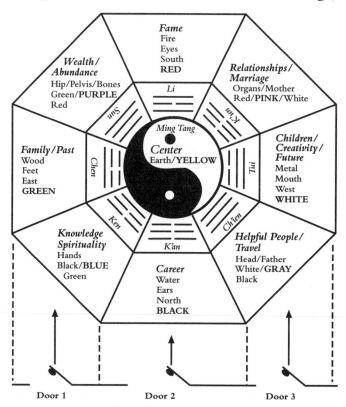

versal laws. Various healing modalities, such as traditional Chinese medicine (TCM), acupuncture, and shiatsu massage, are directly derived from these basic laws of nature. Feng Shui also has its roots in this belief system, for its objective is to try to assist people in understanding different aspects of their lives through their living environments. Feng Shui uses your physical environment as a schoolroom to teach you about yourself and provide you with the tools you need to resolve the conflicts and challenges that you face daily.

The Bagua is the whole eight-sided diagram illustrated on page 78. When we want to refer to just one section of the Bagua map, we call this a *gua* (pronounced *gwah*). There are nine main guas or areas in Feng Shui that break down and correspond to various components of your life. In addition, each gua oversees other specific aspects and attributes. These aspects include colors, elements, areas of the body, individual family members, and health-related issues.

The Nine Areas of the Bagua

(from the perspective of the Black Hat Sect Tantric Buddhism school of thought)

1. **Fame.** The Fame area of the Bagua is located in the middle of the top section of the map. Its Chinese name is *Li,* and it represents who you want to be known as or what you would like to accomplish in this lifetime. It refers to the kind of fame that comes with being a well-known actor, doctor, or businessperson, but it also relates to the important roles in our society that usually don't receive that kind of acknowledgment, such as being a loving mother, a nurturing father, or an inspirational schoolteacher. This area oversees all issues relating to the eyes, and to the middle daughter in the family. It also oversees one's ability to be successful and have a good (or not so good) reputation in the world. It is ruled by the element of Fire, and is strengthened by the color Red.

2. **Marriage/relationships.** The Marriage area on the Bagua chart is the upper right-hand corner. Its Chinese name is *K'un,* and it most strongly represents the marriage ch'i in your life, and your ability to draw on a successful, loving partnership. It is also the area that conducts the energy flow for other types of relationships, including dating, living together, and nontraditional unions such as gay and lesbian relationships. Individuals

79

who choose not to be in a relationship can still utilize this gua as an area that represents their relationship with themselves or issues regardding their mother or female siblings. This section also oversees all issues related to the organs of the body, and to the mother in the family. It doesn't have a ruling (five) element, but it does resonate to the color Pink.

3. *Children/creativity.* This section of the Bagua, located in the middle on the right side, represents the future and all the life-affirming things that we give birth to. Its Chinese name is *Tui* and it represents all your descendants, in particular your children and the children you plan on having, and any issues related to them. Difficulties regarding fertility or pregnancies can be addressed here, also. In addition, this area oversees all issues of creativity, including new thoughts and ideas, art, writing, and inspirations. This gua allows all individuals to utilize it because the energy it generates serves the same purpose for everyone: to manifest the creation principle. The area of Children also represents the youngest daughter and is ruled by the element of Metal. Its corresponding color is White, and it oversees all issues related to the mouth and teeth.

4. *Helpful people/travel.* This section is located on the lower right-hand side. Its Chinese name is *Ch'ien,* and it oversees two main categories in your life. The first is the energy that draws on the helpful people in your life. Helpful people are all those we come in contact with who help us and direct us along the way. They can include friends and family members who support and love us on a daily basis, or a counselor who helps us through a difficult time. Many times these helpful people show up quietly, without a familiar face or name. One of them may even appear to us as the person who conveniently pulls out of the parking space just when we're in need of one! This section also represents the energy needed to attract opportunities and to help others. Clients, students, and other supportive people are pulled into your life from this gua. The other category this section oversees is that of Travel. All aspects and opportunities related to traveling (business or personal) are generated from here. The head area of the body, the father, and the color Gray are represented in this gua. It doesn't have a ruling (five) element.

5. ***Career.*** This section of the Bagua, located directly in the center at the bottom of the chart, provides the foundation energy that stabilizes the rest of the guas. Its Chinese name is *K'an,* and it oversees all matters concerning one's career, hobbies, life-path work, community service, volunteerism, and your personal skills. This is the gua holding the energy that helps us connect with our "personal genius," unique to each individual for his or her work and journey during this incarnation. This section differs from the Fame area, because it represents what you do, as opposed to who you want to be known as. This section generates the ch'i force pertaining to the type of work you do or aspire to do. For instance, work-related issues like being hired for a job you applied for, or getting a long-awaited proposal at work, is generated from this gua. Our careers give us a very important way to provide service and return something to the world. The ways we contribute to society are very personal and wide-ranging, and can include such things as raising a family or volunteering at a local hospital. This gua represents the middle son in the family and the ears on the body. It is ruled by the element of Water and corresponds to the color Black.

6. ***Knowledge/spirituality.*** This area is located at the bottom left corner. Its Chinese name is *Ken,* and it oversees all types of self-knowledge and ways we are able to enrich our understanding of who we are. This is the gua that generates the energy that brings us our opportunities and lessons for spiritual growth. It oversees all areas of spirituality, and when used for such practices as yoga, meditation, self-reflection, and prayer, it can become a very powerful healing area in your home. This area helps us to open up and develop our intuition, which is our source for personal knowing and truth. This section also supports all aspects of educational pursuits ranging from academic to more informal and nontraditional types of study. The youngest son is represented here, as well as both hands on the body. This gua is not ruled by a primary (five) element, but does correspond to the color Blue.

7. ***Family.*** This section is located in the middle on the left-hand side. Its Chinese name is *Chen,* and it oversees all issues related to your ances-

tors and the history connected to the many generations of your family lineage. This area primarily represents biological, reconstituted, and nontraditional family units. This section also includes support groups, religious congregations, and your inner circle of friends that you consider to be like family. In addition, it represents and provides the cohesive energy for your family of co-workers and other work-related units or organizations. Because it represents the past, all family secrets and childhood issues are stored here. This gua oversees aspects that relate to the eldest son in the family and the feet in connection with the body. It is ruled by the element of Wood, and corresponds to the color Green.

8. *Wealth.* This area is located in the upper left-hand corner. Its Chinese name is *Sun,* and it generates the ch'i that draws on the energy that oversees finances and all the things that we perceive as connoting wealth. Wealth in our society is often associated with greed, excess, and luck. The presence of this gua reminds us that money, complicated as it might seem, is just another type of energy. Having the amount of money that you need or want should not be seen only as a luxury but as a birthright we are all entitled to. This is the nest-egg area of the Bagua, thus a great section in which to store all your valuables, such as piggy banks, stocks, coins, stamps, and savings account books. This section oversees the energy and all issues related to power. Shoring up this area will help strengthen your ability to draw on the power source that connects us with the abundant universal supply. This will help us develop our internal sense of "healthy power" and release the "unhealthy power," a learned response that implies we must take from others in order to give to ourselves. The pelvic area of the body, the bones, and the eldest daughter are represented here. This gua does not have a ruling (five) element, but it corresponds to the color Purple.

9. *Center/health.* The center is located in the middle of the Bagua. It connects all the other eight sections and is represented by the Yin/Yang symbol. Its Chinese name is *Ming Tang.* Although it oversees all the other issues and life situations that are not represented in the eight other guas, its main focus is on health. All health-related issues can be addressed and

reinforced in this section. Although health issues are a very big concern for most people, you'll notice that health is not specifically addressed in any of the other eight areas of the Bagua chart. The reason for this is that many factors influence the outcome of good or poor health. From a Feng Shui perspective, health is not seen as something that can be easily adjusted in just one gua. Instead, health is represented in the middle of the chart, connecting to all the "supporting and influencing spokes," represented by the other eight areas. Hence we interpret good health as a result of all the different areas in your life (guas) being in balance. You can also use this area to reinforce an issue or a life situation that has already been represented in one of the other guas. This center space also oversees all other family members and areas of the body that are not addressed in the other eight guas. Its ruling element is Earth, and it corresponds mainly to the color Yellow.

The above nine areas and their corresponding aspects can be located by superimposing the Bagua map over the floor plan or the layout of your home, apartment, or office space. In order to determine how to position the Bagua correctly on your space, you first have to establish where the doors and entranceways are located in relation to the rest of your home.

Drawing a Floor Plan

Throughout this book we are going to be exploring many different ways of working with the Feng Shui process to strengthen your health and enhance the invisible patterns of energy that exist in your environment. Before we can move into chapter 4 and more approaches to assessing health, you'll first need to begin your own process by drawing your floor plan. I can almost feel you holding your breath as the fear kicks in, and hear you saying to yourself, "But I can't draw!" Hang in there with me for a minute, because this doesn't have to be a scary experience. For as long as I have been practicing and writing on Feng Shui, this is the part of the process that always stops people dead in their tracks. It doesn't have to be, so please try not to run from it.

If it makes you feel any better, I make all my clients, whether on-site or by phone consultations, draw a floor plan of their space and send it to me before I do *any* Feng Shui consulting for them. Besides needing it for practical reasons, there is also a very important metaphysical reason why this step is crucial. From a practical standpoint, you need to have a floor plan to look at in order to correctly assess the different aspects of the Feng Shui of your home. Otherwise it is difficult to learn what might be creating a risk to your health. The other, more important, reason, in my opinion, is that when you finally stop the excuses and sit down to draw up your plan, you give the universe permission to work with your healing process through Feng Shui Design. It's your etheric "green light" that says that you are ready, emotionally, spiritually, and physically, to look at your space and all the hidden issues you might uncover . . . and uncover them you will!

To begin this process, start by drawing your floor plan. If you have more than one floor, draw a plan for each floor and, if applicable, a plan of your lot and/or yard. Make sure you label very clearly where all the entranceways are, and specifically indicate the swing of the door (e.g., "door opens right to left"). What you might find helpful is to use circles and squares to indicate the main pieces of furniture in each room, slits to show window locations, and boxes to illustrate closets.

Walk through your house, look at each room, and follow the wall lines as you visually trace the shape of each room. Do not assume that a room is square, even though it appears to be. Follow the parameters and try to draw what you see as opposed to what you thought was there.

Remember that this floor plan does not have to be perfect or to architectural scale, just something you can work with. Your well-being and recovery are worth the time and angst.

If you still feel you need a little help, the opening chapter of my first book, *Feng Shui: Harmony by Design* (Perigee, 1996), walks you through every step of drawing a floor plan. It illustrates in a very user-friendly way how to draw the shape of your rooms, and even which symbols to use to indicate where the clutter spots are. Have some fun with it. If you wish, invite a friend over to help. Do whatever you need to do to get started.

Now comes the fun part. Take out your floor plan. If you haven't yet drawn one, now's the time to face your resistance and get going with it. Having a floor plan not only puts you in your process, it also makes this section much more visual and personal. If you are really feeling stuck or immobilized, try drawing just one room, preferably your bedroom. If you are in a studio apartment, then draw the main room or area where you sleep.

Feeling stuck and fearful is often a signal indicating how much you are actually on the right track. The amount of resistance you feel is usually equal to the amount of healing and change you will experience once you pass through it and get to the other side.

Getting It Right

This is a very important part of your Feng Shui assessment process. If you misinterpret the correct way to lay the Bagua down on your home or property, you will incorrectly "read" the corresponding areas in your home and, in turn, the corresponding areas of your health.

The following example provides a testimonial to the importance of proper Bagua placement. Many years ago I got a call from a client who was in dire straits. After several years of doing her own Feng Shui, she was perplexed by the amount of misfortune and illness that continued to fall upon her and her husband. She was sick with stomach-related illnesses, her husband had been unemployed for over a year, and overall her life was in chaos. To make things worse, once her husband finally found work, she lost her job a week later! To her it seemed as though it would never end.

My client was so responsible and efficient that when she sent me her floor plans to review, she also included a computer printout of the Bagua map, which she electronically superimposed over each floor and room of her home. This was the Bagua layout she had been using for the past year or so to make adjustments in her home with the intention of improving both her health and that of her husband. When I reviewed it, I understood immediately what the problem was. She had accidentally placed the Bagua incorrectly over the entire second floor, where all the bedrooms were, and had inadvertently skewed all of the energy patterns! Based on this layout, she was making Feng Shui adjustments and placing her intentions in all the wrong guas. Although there were other problems, the scrambled energy patterns contributed to a lot of the downslide and continual madness. By reapplying the Bagua correctly and making some modifications in her adjustment items, together we were able to get her life back on track.

The Three Levels of a Home Assessment

As the Circle of Life chart in chapter 1 illustrates, all environments have an impact on our lives, but the three environments that will have the most profound and immediate influence are (1) the rooms in your home, (2) the floors in your home, and (3) the lot or yard that surrounds your property.

When you superimpose the Bagua map over each area, you will discover where the nine different areas of the Bagua are, and whether any of them are odd-shaped or missing completely. This is important information and figures significantly into the "health quotient" of your home. Now you can begin to develop a profile of your home and the quality of energy that actually runs through your home and property.

Three Door Positioning

If you look at the bottom of the Bagua illustrated on page 78, you will see broken lines and arrows. You will also see three sections labeled "Door 1," "Door 2," and "Door 3." These doors correspond to the three lower guas on the map, Knowledge, Career, and Helpful People. When you superimpose your Bagua over any level of your floor plan, it's crucial that you align the front door, second-floor landing (or any other floor), doorway to any room, driveway opening, or the entranceway into the lot with one of these guas. Determining proper Bagua placement will depend upon whether the door, opening, or gate is located to the left, right, or center of the property. The illustration and the placement tips below will guide you through this next step.

Level 1 of Your Home Assessment
Placing the Bagua Over Individual Rooms

Take the room plan of your bedroom (or any other room) and find the wall that runs parallel with the *main* doorway into the room. **For purposes of instruction only,** label the four walls in your room with the four compass directions. First, stand in the entranceway into your room; assign the south direction to the wall that runs parallel to the doorway. Now assign the east wall to the wall in your room that is farthest to the right, the west wall to the wall that is farthest to your left, and finally assign the north wall to the wall that is farthest opposite your entranceway wall. Then take the Bagua map and superimpose it over this room plan with the Fame areas paralleling the north wall, the Career area lined up with the south wall (entranceway wall), the Children area paralleling the east wall, and the Family area paralleling the west wall. The Wealth area will always be in the upper left-hand corner of the room, if you are standing in your entranceway facing into the room. The Relationship area will always be in the upper right-hand corner of the room if you are standing in the entranceway facing into the room.

Tips Regarding Interior Doors

Sometimes you'll find that there are two or more entranceways into a room; use the following rules to help you determine which doorway is the main entrance and should be used to orient the Bagua:

1. Open archways and openings with no physical doors are still considered doorways, since they are an entranceway into a space.

2. If you have two doorways that lead into a room, select the doorway that is used most frequently. If they are both used equally, use the one that is physically wider. If they are both used equally and are the same size, then use the one that a guest entering your house would use.

3. If you have exhausted the above rules and still aren't sure which one to declare the main door, use the door that has the most traffic outside or passing it. The busier side is referred to as the "Mother Side," as opposed to the lesser-traveled area, called the "Son Side."

4. To determine whether a door/entranceway that is on a diagonal in a corner is either the Helpful People or the Spirituality gua, use the Mother/Son activity rule (rule number 3, above) to assist you in defining how to lay the Bagua down on that room or floor plan. The side with the most activity will become the wall/line of entranceway that will run parallel to the three lower guas: Spirituality, Career, and Helpful People.

5. If you are still at a loss, then pick the door that intuitively feels correct. Actually, this step is very important, because the more you understand the principles behind Feng Shui and why you're doing what you're doing, the more you can make intelligent decisions in situations that do not fit the common protocol.

Fig. 3. Placing the Bagua Over Individual Rooms

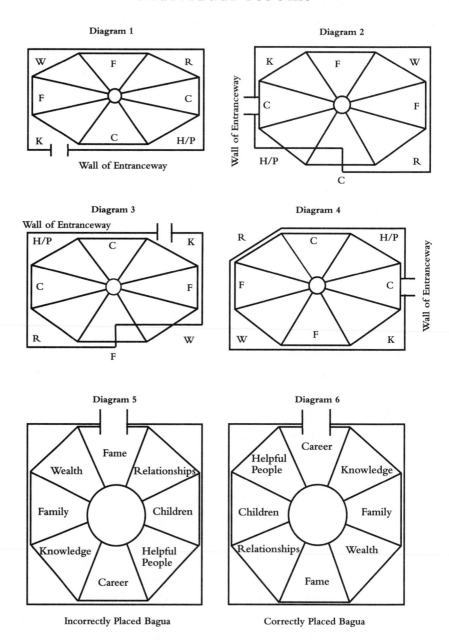

Diagram 1

Wall of Entranceway

Diagram 2

Wall of Entranceway

Diagram 3

Wall of Entranceway

Diagram 4

Wall of Entranceway

Diagram 5

Incorrectly Placed Bagua

Diagram 6

Correctly Placed Bagua

Level 2 of Your Home Assessment
Placing the Bagua Over Each Floor
of Your Home

Find the main entranceway into the first level of your home. Place the Bagua over the *entire floor,* with the three lower guas falling along the line that runs parallel with the entranceway door, assigning the Fame section to the top farthest wall on that floor, the Children section to the farthest right wall on that floor, and the Family section to the farthest left wall on that floor. Now connect these lines. This layout should give you a larger picture of where the different Bagua areas are on your overall house. This will also show you where areas are missing and/or odd-shaped and problematic. *If your home has more than one floor, place the Bagua on each floor at each entranceway or landing.* The Bagua layout of the second floor can be completely different from the Bagua layout of the first floor, and vice versa. Each floor's Bagua layout is determined by where the *entranceway* is to that specific floor. Depending on how the stairs are positioned, you can have a Relationship area of the Bagua on one floor while on the floor above it, in the same location, could be the Wealth area. That's why we call it "the ever-changing Bagua." It moves around depending on where the entranceway, or "mouth of the ch'i," is.

Front Door Placement Tips

Even if you use the side door, back door, or garage door regularly to enter your home, you should still use the *architectural front door* of the house to properly lay the Bagua down for the correct reading of the overall floor plan. For additional information, you can position the Bagua over the specific room that you pass through first and most frequently depending on the entranceway door that you are using most often to enter your house, such as the side, back, or garage door. Please note that traditional Black Hat Sect teachings by H. H. Professor Thomas Lin Yun Rinpoche assigns each floor of one's house with the same Bagua layout as the first-floor configuration. For example, the location of the Wealth area on the first floor will also be consistent with the guas on all the above floors.

Fig. 4. Placing the Bagua Over Each Floor
of a Home with Several Levels

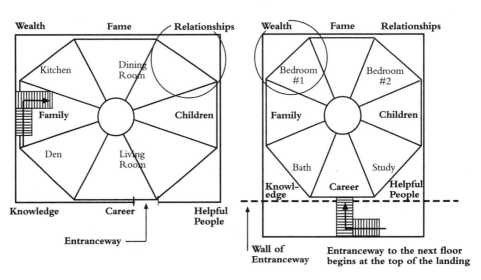

FIRST FLOOR

SECOND FLOOR

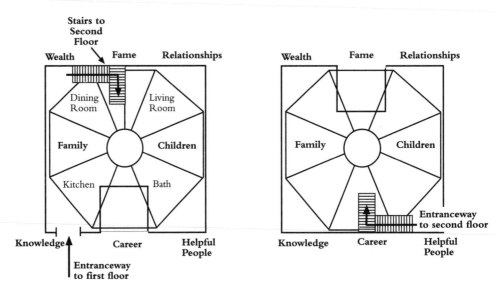

FIRST FLOOR

SECOND FLOOR

Level 3 of Your Home Assessment
Placing the Bagua Over a Lot or Yard

This third step also follows the same "four walls" rules. Instead of physical walls, use the property lines as defined on the site plans. The important thing, again, is to position the Bagua correctly over the site or lot plan. This can be a challenge because, more often than not, there are several ways to enter a property, with no clearly dominant entranceway. When this is the case, the following rules often help:

1. Determine the main entranceway onto the property and use it to align the Bagua. This can be the main road in, or the driveway or main walkway. Use the "four walls" concept mentioned above.

2. If there is more than one entranceway or roadway onto the property, pick the one that has the most traffic flow and energy (follow mother/son side rules in Tips Regarding Interior Doors, page 87). That will become your "entranceway wall," and you should use it to determine the proper placement for the Bagua on your lot or yard.

3. If both entranceways have the same flow of traffic, identify the closest main highway and use the road from that highway to your property to determine how you position the Bagua. Align its "entranceway wall" with the Knowledge, Career, and Helpful People guas.

Fig. 5. Placing the Bagua Over a Lot or Yard

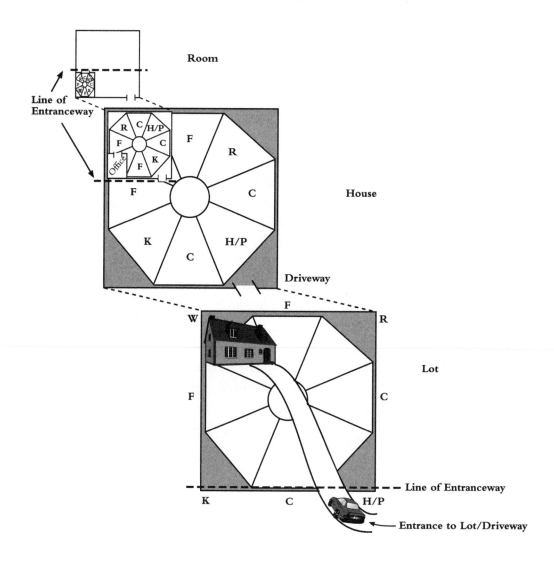

Although there are many different floor plans and house layouts, Figs. 6a–6h will indicate some of the more common concerns or spatial problems and how to correctly lay the Bagua over each one.

Figs. 6a–6h. Various Bagua Layouts

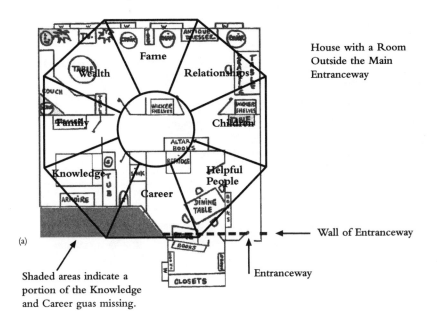

House with a Room
Outside the Main
Entranceway

Wall of Entranceway

(a)

Entranceway

Shaded areas indicate a
portion of the Knowledge
and Career guas missing.

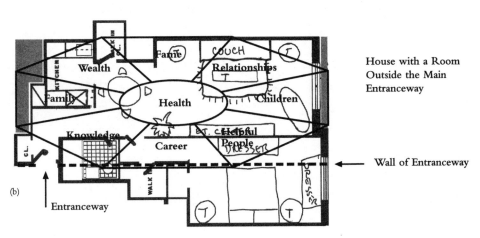

House with a Room
Outside the Main
Entranceway

Wall of Entranceway

(b)

Entranceway

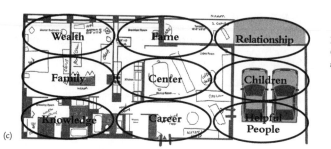

Laying the Bagua
Over a House with
an Attached Garage

(c)

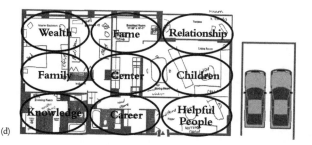

Laying the Bagua Over
a House with a
Detached Garage

(d)

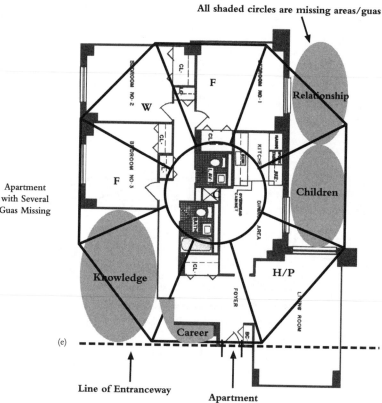

All shaded circles are missing areas/guas

Apartment
with Several
Guas Missing

(e)

Line of Entranceway

Apartment
Entrance

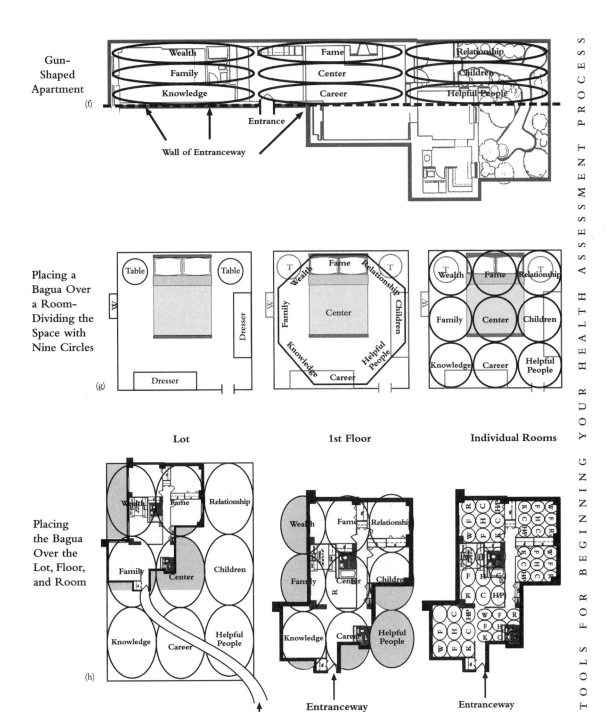

Gun-Shaped Apartment (f)

Wealth / Family / Knowledge / Fame / Center / Career / Relationship / Children / Helpful People

Entrance

Wall of Entranceway

Placing a Bagua Over a Room—Dividing the Space with Nine Circles (g)

Table / Dresser / Dresser

Wealth / Fame / Relationship / Family / Center / Children / Knowledge / Career / Helpful People

Wealth / Fame / Relationship / Family / Center / Children / Knowledge / Career / Helpful People

Lot

1st Floor

Individual Rooms

Placing the Bagua Over the Lot, Floor, and Room (h)

Wealth / Fame / Relationship / Family / Center / Children / Knowledge / Career / Helpful People

Entranceway Driveway

Entranceway

Entranceway

Exploring the Nine Basic Cures

As you continue to read through this book and work with the Feng Shui process, you will repeatedly encounter the term "adjustment items." An adjustment item is a specific object that is hung or placed in a particular area of your home, office, or car (or on your body as well), to help adjust an area (gua) that has been deemed imbalanced or "energetically problematic." Depending on the situation at hand, one's own intuition, and various other factors, a cure will be recommended to correct it and restore balance. These cures are powerful, and when placed with intention and purpose, they rework the energy patterns of a space to restore harmony.

Feng Shui is often referred to as "acupuncture for the home." The acupuncturist follows invisible lines of energy, called meridians, that run through the body. These are passageways that carry the life force, or ch'i, to different parts of our bodies. When these meridians are blocked or overactive, the flow of ch'i in the body is altered and illness and disease can occur, especially in areas that are cut off or are experiencing diminished life force. To rebalance those meridians, the acupuncturist places small needles in specific spots on the body along them, to adjust the flow of ch'i. In Feng Shui, when we use an adjustment item, it works in a similar way. After we locate the energy patterns that are blocked in a home, we then use adjustment items the way the acupuncturist uses needles on the body. We place these adjustments in specific areas of your home or on your property to restore a natural flow and reset the energy pattern.

Although there are hundreds of adjustment items or cures, during a consultation I often suggest the ones listed below, which are most commonly used by Black Hat Sect Feng Shui practitioners and laypeople alike. These are applied according to a method known as *Sye-dz,* or "minor additions," based on the Chinese principle that states "it takes only four ounces to deflect a thousand pounds."

Feng Shui Adjustment Items
Lights/Bright Objects
(These items lift up and expand the ch'i)

Lighting (the brighter, the better)

Feng Shui crystal ball (man-made), round and faceted—20 mm–60 mm (All crystals should be hung on a red string measured in multiples of nine ([e.g., 9, 18, 27, or 36 inches.])

Candles/lanterns

Objects that sparkle

Others

Mirrors (multi-use)

Bagua or octagon shape (deflects negative ch'i)

Convex (expands narrow areas)

Concave (turns oppressive images upside down, e.g., towering buildings)

Round or square beveled (expands or deflects depending on your intention)

Decorative/framed (reflects and draws in positive images, expands space, etc.)

Sound (keeps energy moving and flowing)

Wind chimes (brass or copper are best)

Music (audio equipment or musical instruments)

Chanting (music and mantras)

Life Force (stimulates ch'i)

Plants	Fish tanks	Birds
Bonsai/trees	Flowers	Pets
Color	Bamboo Stalks	Others

Heavy Objects
(diffuse fast energy or hold down issues)

Rocks

Statues/Sculptures

Heavy vases

Large potted plants and trees

Color
(These schemes are used to enhance and/or soften ch'i)

The Nine Trigram Colors of the Bagua (red, pink, white, gray, black, blue, green, purple, yellow)

The Five-Element Color Theory (red, yellow, white, black, green)

The Six True Colors (white, red, yellow, green, blue, black)

The Colors of the Rainbow/the Chakras (red, orange, yellow, green, light blue, indigo, violet)

Vibrant Colors (red, yellow, orange, black; these enhance ch'i)

Pastel Colors (light greens, blues, and pinks; these soften and hold on to the existing ch'i)

Movement/Mobile Objects
(These disperse negative ch'i and circulate ch'i)

Mobiles

Wind chimes

Tassels (red and gold)

Flags or wind socks

Windmills

Fountains

Weathervanes

Power and Energy Objects
(These convey strength and power)

Firecrackers (ward off negative ch'i)

Arrowheads (power objects)

Talismans (spiritual protection)

Photos/statues/images of deities (create sacred space and safety)

Water (circulates ch'i, activates wealth)

Indoor or outdoor fountains

Fish tanks

Brooks, streams, and trickling water

Ponds with goldfish

Vases/bowls of water

Yu (a small, round bowl with earth stones and blessings inside)

Others
(Most important, these expand on the basic cures)

Bamboo flutes (lift oppressive ch'i)

Beaded bamboo curtains (act as a ch'i diffuser and divider)

Ten Coins of the Ching dynasty (enhance wealth)

Crystals/gemstones (raise energy and vibration levels)

Fragrances (incense, oils, flowers, and orange peels; these clear negative energy)

Touch items (art objects, soft fabrics, nurturing objects)

Others (your personal touches and various Black Hat Feng Shui Transcendental Cures)

Interior and Exterior Factors List

As you begin to see all of the variables that go into a Feng Shui health assessment process, you will quickly gain a new level of respect for all that is considered. Below is a partial list of what Black Hat Feng Shui refers to as Interior and Exterior Factors. These are the various elements that must also be considered as we create an overall profile of your home and the impact, for better or for worse, that these elements are having on your life and your health. Throughout the rest of the book I shall discuss these factors and how to determine their influences on your life.

Facing Your Life and Doing Your Work

Everything that exists around us was a thought in someone's mind first! This is where we store all our unresolved issues, pains, memories, and the ESPs of our life and illnesses that help create diseased vibrational patterns. Our objec-

Feng Shui

Interior and Exterior Factors

INTERIOR FACTORS	EXTERIOR FACTORS
Position of bed	Roads/streets/slopes
Position of desk	Lighting: Natural and man-made
Position of stove	Trains/subways
Entranceways	Traffic direction and flow
Staircases	Trees
Pillars/posts/columns/structural corners	Bodies of water: river, ocean, swimming pool
Exposed beams	Bridges
Colors	Roof shapes/pointed roof ridges
Lighting	Temples/churches/cemeteries/funeral parlors
Voids/empty spaces	Telephone poles/flagpoles
Ceilings	Nearby buildings/skyscrapers
Doors/windows/skylights	Noises/sounds
Fireplaces	Colors
EMFs: computers/clock radios/answering machines/transformers/microwaves	Neighbors and neighborhood
Aesthetics	Surrounding businesses/signage
Shape of room	Gardens
Location of room	Garage location
Furniture placement	Patio/terrace/deck
Clutter/obstructions	EMFs: Transformers/high-tension wires
Computer location	Ch'i of land
Interior 5 Elements and their shapes	Shape of house
Others	Shape of lot
	Cutting ch'i
	Rushing ch'i
	Exterior 5 Elements on the land
	Others

tive is to bring into harmony our inner and outer environments, so that balanced energy patterns can be achieved.

It's almost impossible to have good Feng Shui in your home or office without your inner environment being somewhat at peace. Sometimes that just means taking more responsibility for your life and its overall quality, including all levels of your health. Keep in mind that solving your life's problems and making an effort to transmute your failing health is a very important part of your life's work and spiritual growth, not something that happens outside of it. This is part of the overall reason why we incarnated into our current existence. Even though looking at our issues may be painful and scary, we must commit to doing it on some level if we want to approach our health and healing in a whole new way.

Living authentically and in the present, with integrity, means that you have to be willing to do your own personal work, especially if you truly want to get well. Doing your personal work makes an energetic statement that says you are willing to step up to the plate and be part of your own solution rather than part of the problem.

Closing Chapter Exercise

Finishing Unfinished Business: Nine Steps to Better Health Through Using the Feng Shui Wheel of Life

The following Wheel of Life Chart will give you a list of thoughts and questions to help jar your memory and review different aspects of your life and the Bagua that still have business left unfinished or issues left unresolved. Please feel free to add your own thoughts and concepts to each gua.

Find a place that is quiet and light some candles, burn some incense, and have with you a pen and some paper. Take a look at the Feng Shui Wheel of Life on page 102, and begin at number 1, the Family gua. Read all the issues that are connected to that gua, and make a list of all the things that have been left unresolved or unfinished. Write about losses you still carry, family members who have hurt you or with whom you still have differences, issues related to past family members, etc. Write as much as you can tolerate, then write some more until you feel complete. Please do not try to edit this, or worry about proper grammar or sentence structure. This is an exercise in moving ch'i and dislodging energy blocks.

Fig. 7. The Feng Shui Wheel of Life

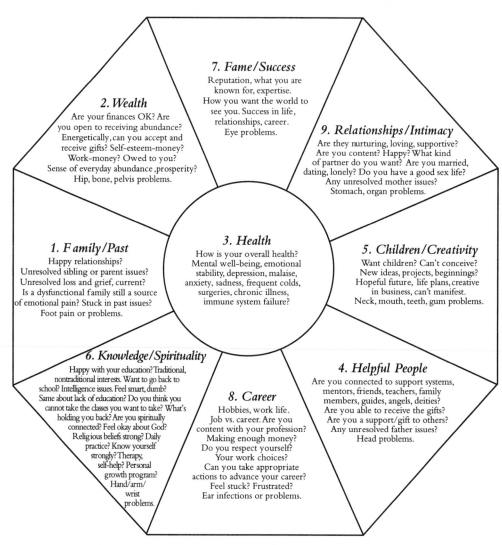

7. Fame/Success
Reputation, what you are known for, expertise. How you want the world to see you. Success in life, relationships, career. Eye problems.

2. Wealth
Are your finances OK? Are you open to receiving abundance? Energetically, can you accept and receive gifts? Self-esteem-money? Work-money? Owed to you? Sense of everyday abundance, prosperity? Hip, bone, pelvis problems.

9. Relationships/Intimacy
Are they nurturing, loving, supportive? Are you content? Happy? What kind of partner do you want? Are you married, dating, lonely? Do you have a good sex life? Any unresolved mother issues? Stomach, organ problems.

3. Health
How is your overall health? Mental well-being, emotional stability, depression, malaise, anxiety, sadness, frequent colds, surgeries, chronic illness, immune system failure?

1. Family/Past
Happy relationships? Unresolved sibling or parent issues? Unresolved loss and grief, current? Is a dysfunctional family still a source of emotional pain? Stuck in past issues? Foot pain or problems.

5. Children/Creativity
Want children? Can't conceive? New ideas, projects, beginnings? Hopeful future, life plans, creative in business, can't manifest. Neck, mouth, teeth, gum problems.

6. Knowledge/Spirituality
Happy with your education? Traditional, nontraditional interests. Want to go back to school? Intelligence issues. Feel smart, dumb? Same about lack of education? Do you think you cannot take the classes you want to take? What's holding you back? Are you spiritually connected? Feel okay about God? Religious beliefs strong? Daily practice? Know yourself strongly? Therapy, self-help? Personal growth program? Hand/arm/wrist problems.

8. Career
Hobbies, work life. Job vs. career. Are you content with your profession? Making enough money? Do you respect yourself? Your work choices? Can you take appropriate actions to advance your career? Feel stuck? Frustrated? Ear infections or problems.

4. Helpful People
Are you connected to support systems, mentors, friends, teachers, family members, guides, angels, deities? Are you able to receive the gifts? Are you a support/gift to others? Any unresolved father issues? Head problems.

You will need nine red envelopes for this cure. The envelopes can be any shape or any size. You can make them out of any kind of red paper. (The ritual of the red envelopes will be further addressed in chapter 9, page 313.) When you have completed the Family section, reread aloud what you wrote, and apply the Three Secrets Reinforcement Blessing using the Ousting Mudra and the *Om Ma Ni Pad Me Hum* mantra, while visualizing that all the stagnant energy and blocks are released, as instructed in chapter 9. Do this nine times, then place the papers in a red envelope and clearly mark the back with a brand-new black marker, writing the name of the energy gua that it belongs to (Family), and place it in front of you on a table or the floor, in the middle section on your left-hand side. Envelope by envelope, you will be creating a "red-envelope altar" on the floor or table in front of you in the shape of a Feng Shui Bagua mandala.

Now go to the second area on your chart, number 2, Wealth, and do the same. Write out all the thoughts you need to release. Read it out loud, place it in the red envelope, and bless it with the Three Secrets Reinforcement Blessing, and then add that red envelope to the Wealth position (diagonally to your forward left) of the Bagua mandala you are creating. Then go on to the next section, number 3, in the center, which represents Health, and follow the same procedure. Do this for all the other six sections that follow, blessing each envelope separately and adding it to your red-envelope altar.

It is very important that you follow the numbers in order of the sequence that they have been listed. This sequencing order in Feng Shui is known as "Tracing the Nine Stars" (see chapter 9, page 318). It is a sacred order that raises your intentions and purifies your thoughts and wishes regarding those issues. Each vertical, horizontal, and diagonal row of three adds up to the number nine or a multiple of nine. Nine (and its multiples) is the highest of the Yang numbers connoting power and completion. These are the auspicious numbers that we work with as often as we can incorporate them in our Feng Shui process.

When you have gone through all nine sections and your red-envelope Bagua is complete, then visually walk through the Nine Star Path as it sits in red envelopes before you, do the Three Secrets Reinforcement Blessing on the whole mandala, and then, starting with the envelope in the number 1 position of Family, start to dismantle the layout by removing this envelope first. The next one you will take would be number 2, and so on until you have collected all nine in the same Nine Star Cure order.

Take the envelopes to your bedroom, and starting with number 1, place that envelope in the Family gua on your bed between your box spring and mattress, then take the next envelope, Wealth, and place that in the Wealth section between your box spring and mattress. Continue this process until you

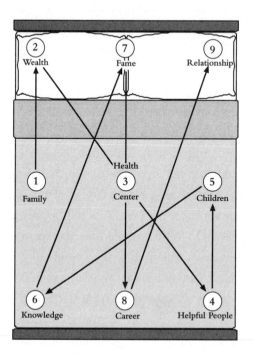

Fig. 8. Tracing the Nine Stars on the Bed

have re-created the Red-Envelope Bagua Mandala underneath your mattress. After they have been reassembled, perform the Three Secrets Reinforcement Blessing on them again and sleep on these envelopes for the next 27 nights in a row. (Make sure you are going to be home for this 27-night cure.)

On the morning after the twenty-seventh night (try to do this between the hours of 11:00 A.M. and 1:00 P.M. for the strongest results), take the envelopes out, again starting with the Family envelope and following the Nine Path sequence all the way to the Relationship envelope, and then wrap the bunch of envelopes together with 99 windings of red string or ribbon. Take the envelopes to a river, ocean, or lake (moving waters), do the Three Secrets Reinforcement Blessing nine times, and toss the package into the body of water, releasing it and with it, everything that was acting as underpinnings to your emotional, spiritual, and physical well-being. If you cannot get to a body of moving water, then bury it at least nine inches down in the earth or place it outside under a potted plant.

CHAPTER FOUR

TEN FENG SHUI METHODS FOR DIAGNOSING ILLNESS AND ADJUSTING CH'I

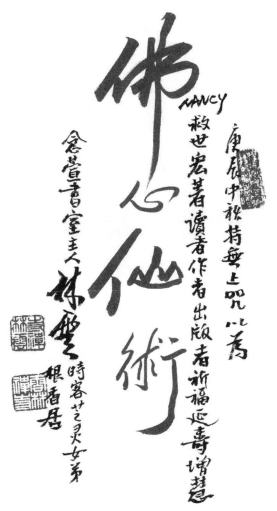

"Buddha's Heart; Divine Skills."

CALLIGRAPHY BY H. H. PROFESSOR THOMAS LIN YUN RINPOCHE

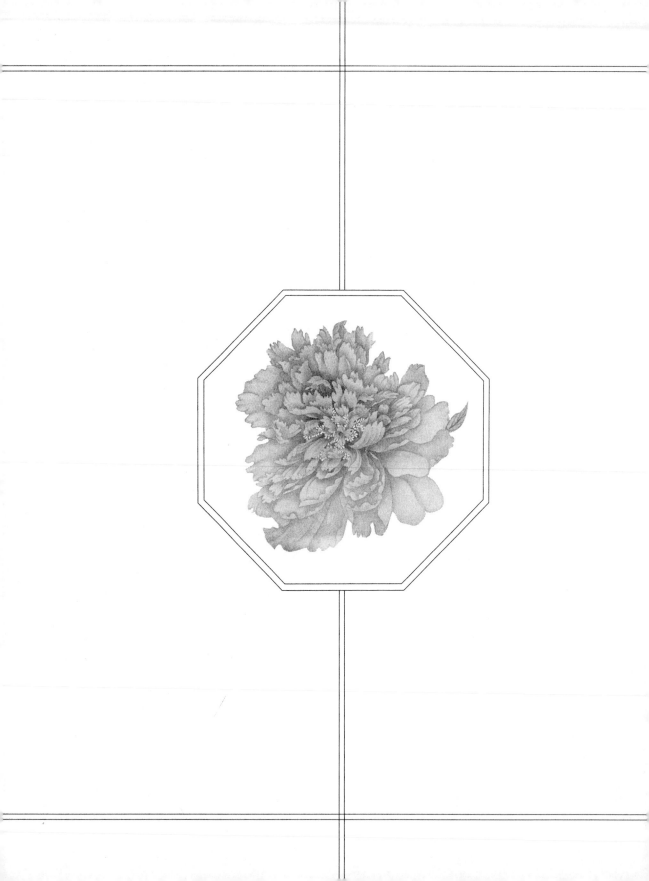

THE MORE WE UNDERSTAND the nature of the invisible energy patterns that surround us, the more quickly we can resolve our own skepticism about Feng Shui as a real and tangible entity. Although we strive to be open, trusting, and spiritual believers, often it goes against the grain of our rational thought. Unfortunately, we hold on to that ability to rationalize, and instead of serving us, it eventually leads to our demise. The mind was given to us as a tool for navigating the world, but instead we gave it too much power and allowed it to make all the decisions for us. In turn, it then became our dictator. In many ways this is actually a misuse of its function. When we over-empower the mind, we create a big bully that, when active, intimidates the other navigation instruments we were gifted with, such as our heart, intuition, and feelings.

LETTING THE OBSTACLES RISE
TO THE SURFACE

When we or someone close to us becomes sick, it is a very scary and vulnerable time for all involved. As we race for the cure, we often leave behind unattended issues that eventually surface elsewhere in our lives. Those issues, when left unresolved, often surface in the subconscious ways we design our homes or in the apartments and houses that we are drawn to rent or purchase. The more we reveal these hidden pieces of our lives, the greater the probability that we will heal and transform our overall health.

Most of us would agree that something traumatic, such as chronic financial stress from job loss, can contribute to illness. But more often I find that illness results from the accumulation of a lot of little things that at first seem benign and unrelated. You might find yourself thinking back to a small incident that happened when you were five, and wondering how it could be contributing to an illness developed forty years later. As I write this, one particular story comes to mind. Many years ago a former therapist of mine shared a personal story with me when I was in the throes of trying to uncover my own issues regarding my illness. She told me that when she was at the end stage of recovering from lupus, an autoimmune disease, and while she had been working on some of the emotional underpinnings of her disease, she had uncovered a long-buried memory. She remembered that when she was a young child her family had moved, and in her new neighborhood she'd felt left out and couldn't find anyone to play with. In a loving attempt to speed up the process, her mom offered a couple of the children in the neighborhood a nickel each to play with her daughter. My therapist found out about this shortly afterward from her newfound friends and became very ashamed about herself, and doubtful of her ability to be liked just for who she was. This incident, although long past, calcified in her energy field and had a great impact on her ch'i. Years later it resurfaced as an important piece buried deep in her psyche and as a key factor in her adult-onset illness.

Who knows why we hold on to what appears to be benign events, and release other things that appear to be even more traumatic? By making a commitment to uncovering as many of the pieces of the illness picture as we can access, we give our healing process the best prognosis possible.

Below is a list of ten different ways to begin your Feng Shui health assessment. As you do this and begin to explore and treat your illness in psychospiritual and vibrational ways, you too will start to unravel some deep-seated memories and energies that are very much ensconced in your illness. Make sure you allow those thoughts, memories, and feelings to come up, even if at first they don't seem interrelated. The Feng Shui approaches in this chapter will try to break the matrix in your home in which your illness thrives. Be brave and dare to heal!

These ten methods will walk you through a step-by-step approach to assessing the Feng Shui health quotient and diagnosis of your home. It will also guide you in how to make adjustments that will enhance your ch'i and disarm your illness.

TEN FENG SHUI METHODS FOR DIAGNOSING ILLNESS AND ADJUSTING CH'I

Method 1: Explore the Predecessor Law

Energy patterns, once created, cannot be destroyed, only transmuted. Left to its own devices, energy will not change on its own and needs a catalyst or stimulus to be altered. In a home, energy patterns are created through various interior and exterior factors, along with the individual's personal karma and house history.

When someone moves or vacates an apartment or house, they leave behind both the house's ch'i and traces of their own energy, too. The vibration of the house holds the energy patterns of all the successes, failures, joys, sorrows, and issues of the prior owner. If their successes and/or failures were influenced by the Feng Shui of their space, that energy would remain intact even after they moved, because energetically it was embedded in all aspects of the house.

Whenever you rent or purchase a space, if at all possible, try to obtain all the information you possibly can about the previous owners or tenants. Inquire politely about their reason for moving, their level of success, and their relations with their children. Ask about any unexpected deaths or bankruptcies, and try to determine the status of their health. This information will give you deeper insight into the invisible energetics and possible preexisting conditions in the space. This invaluable information will help you make a more conscious decision about taking the space or not.

Keep in mind, though, that if you find a space that has a negative history, it doesn't mean you shouldn't move there. Instead, go in armed with knowledge and apply what you know, continuing to assess the Feng Shui and health quotient of the space. If you feel stumped or unsure, hire a Feng Shui expert to help you make the final decision on whether or not the space can be cleared and transformed. Often, with the right advice, adjustments, and

Transcendental Cures, the bad Feng Shui of a space can be transmuted into auspicious Feng Shui. The information that you acquire from the real estate broker, owners, and nosy neighbors will help you determine whether some of the corresponding problems overlap with your own medical and personal history.

Unless you're lucky enough to design your home from scratch, most homes today come with some major Feng Shui problems; this is the norm. The objective in Feng Shui is to find those aberrations and improve on them, but if the information you gather indicates many different problems leading to the same concern, you may want to rethink your decision to move into that particular space. For example, say that you find out that the prior owner died prematurely of heart disease, and on further inspection you discover that the Fame area of the house is falling apart (in Five Element Theory, Fire oversees the heart); and the center of the house has a spiral staircase (the center of the Bagua oversees health). If you also connect the fact that both you and your partner come from families that have a history of heart disease, you may want to reconsider your options.

You can alleviate the problems by utilizing the principles in this book or hiring a professional Feng Shui consultant to help turn things around. It doesn't mean you can't take the space, but without the Feng Shui changes, you may be walking directly into the shoes, via vibration, of the former occupants. On the other hand, it is a very positive thing when shopping around to hear that the former residents were all healthy, moved to purchase a bigger house, received a promotion, became pregnant, or healed a long-time illness.

If you are already living in a space or have just purchased a new one and were unable to get much information about the prior owners, as a safety measure, you should sage (see chapter 9, page 317) and space-clear the whole house or object(s) you want deprogrammed (see "Space-Clearing Rituals" in chapter 9). Transcendental clearing cures such as Sealing the Doors and the Rice and Jusha House Blessing are explained in chapter 9.

The predecessor law also applies to objects, including gifts, furniture, and cars. Know who owned it before you did, for you will be the beneficiary of their energy. When purchasing used objects or antiques, remember to sage or Jusha them (see "Space Clearing Rituals" in chapter 9) or find other ways to disperse the old or stagnant energies.

Method 2. Utilize the Bagua: The Feng Shui X Ray

One way to approach health-related problems is through the use of the Feng Shui Bagua map (see chapter 3). Each of the nine areas of the Bagua has a corresponding body area that it energetically oversees:

Fame oversees the eyes
Relationship oversees the organs
Children oversees the mouth
Helpful People oversees the head
Career oversees the ears
Knowledge oversees the hands
Family oversees the feet
Wealth oversees the hips, pelvis, and bones
Center oversees overall health and all other body areas

Use the map to direct you to the particular area of the Bagua that coincides with the area of health that is of concern to you. For instance, let's say that you are going to have surgery done on your foot. Go to the Bagua map and locate the gua that oversees the ch'i of the foot (the Family gua).

Then take out your floor plan and locate the area that oversees Family on the overall floor plan of your house and locate the Family section in each individual room. If applicable, check the Family area on the outside lot. First, check those areas for missing corners, clutter, or situations of concern. Check for leaks, accumulated newspapers, obstacles, dead space, things that you might trip over or might "trip you up," and so on. See if anything seems out of place or problematic. If it does, then clean it up and make the necessary changes. In addition, do one of the Nine Basic Cures, perform the Three Secrets Reinforcement Blessing (see chapter 9), and visualize the operation being a success.

The above method is one you can use for all your health-related problems and concerns; just modify it to fit your particular situation. Remember, all parts or areas of the body that are not clearly listed in the eight surrounding guas are assigned to the Center area of the Bagua. This means you would follow the same procedure as above, but locating instead the center of your home and then the Center areas of each individual room. The Three Secrets Reinforcement Blessing is the spiritual backbone that reinforces and enhances this process.

Method 3. Assess All the Centers

After adjusting the specific corresponding guas discussed in method 2, take your floor plan out and locate the Center gua of each room, each floor, and, if accessible, the land on which the structure stands. The center of the Bagua is a very important area regarding health, because it acts as the hub and energetically fuels all the spokes to the other guas.

Three Different Uses

Although each of the eight guas oversees a specific health and body issue, the Center gua represents overall health and can be used for these three purposes:

1. As the primary adjustment gua for *all* health issues.
2. As the secondary adjustment gua, to reinforce energetically the adjustment and intentions you have made to a specific gua regarding a specific health concern—for example, adjusting the Knowledge area to help reduce the arthritis in your hands, since the Knowledge gua oversees the hands, and then adjusting the Center/Health gua in your bedroom to reinforce the intention.
3. To adjust for any illness or body area that is not related to any specific gua.

Two Ways to Adjust Center Gua Energy

1. ***Reduce, repair, and refurbish.*** The first thing you want to do is explore the area of every center and look for things that are old, no longer of value, broken, or faded. Make sure you check the ceiling and the floor area as well. Be on the lookout for cracked ceilings, peeling

paint, light fixtures that are old or not working, frayed wires, water or pipe leaks, and burned-out or missing lightbulbs. In addition, check for torn or tattered furniture, creaky floors, and worn-out rugs. Do whatever is needed to repair the area in question.

2. ***Augment and raise the gua's ch'i.*** After you have cleared out and repaired your Health guas (if applicable), make adjustments to the areas to strengthen the flow of your ch'i and your health. Adjustments can range from hanging a faceted crystal or a brass wind chime, to adding color to a room or raising the wattage of lightbulbs. If you are confused about how many Center guas you should adjust, begin by repairing all the guas that need major repairs, then augment as many Center areas as seem appropriate or are available. If you're still not sure, augment the bedroom first, because it is the most important room for health. Then adjust the Center areas of each floor of your home. Reinforce and bless all steps taken with the Three Secrets Reinforcement Blessing as explained in chapter 9.

Method 4. Taking the Clutter Challenge

One of the most influential factors governing your health today is the amount of clutter you have amassed in your home (especially the bedroom) and workplace. Even if at first the clutter doesn't seem to be causing a health problem, over time it tends to have a cumulative effect on the body. It becomes what I call an opportunist interior factor waiting for a particularly stressful time in your life to do its thing and zap a specific area of the body or organ that was rendered vulnerable. If you are already ill and are trying to recover, then clutter can not only sabotage your treatment but even bring your recovery to a complete standstill.

The issue of clutter is very important. Even if you follow all the other suggestions throughout this book, but avoid addressing the issue of clutter, you'll stand a very good chance of negating all the other Feng Shui adjustments, no matter how well intended they may be. Certain health adjustments might even exacerbate the already existing health problems. For instance, if you use mirrors as a Feng Shui adjustment item and cure, you may actually be *doubling* the amount of clutter energy that you already have in that room because one of the many things mirrors do is double what they reflect, or multiply the already existing energy. This is a very common error, so always check what is being reflected in the mirrors you hang, and make sure when you do use them that you reinforce the specific intention with the Three Secrets Reinforcement Blessing.

In all my years working with people who were "clutter challenged," I never had a client whose only issue was that they had "accidentally accumulated too much stuff." The more we explored all the different reasons why they accumulated what they did (when it first began, what the circumstances were, where in the house the clutter was located), the more layers were peeled away and the more we were able to reach a better understanding of what the real issues were. And for most clients, the thing they are most embarrassed about with regard to their homes is clutter, because it triggers an enormous amount of personal shame. For the most part this shame has less to do with the type of physical objects being hoarded than with the emotional baggage that is attached to them.

There are two easy ways to determine whether there are any underlying emotional or psychological issues attached to your clutter. First, try getting rid of it. If you make lots of excuses why you can't get to it, struggle with making the time, or can't peacefully make up your mind on what to keep, what to toss, and what to give away, it usually means that deeper emotional or psychological issues are at work. If even the thought of cleaning out your mess puts you on overload and has you courting panic attacks, that should be a major clue that something's off.

Second, if you are able to muster up enough courage to finally take the plunge to start sifting through the rubble and really clean things up, only to find that days or weeks later the clutter has returned, this is another telltale sign that other issues are present. If this has happened to you, you'll be happy to know that you are in very good company. Because when other issues are attached to the "stuff," those unresolved issues will continue to create an energy field that will pull in visible chaos (clutter) until the issue is addressed or resolved.

If you have lots of clutter, you will have to challenge yourself vigilantly to be honest about why you have it and what it means to you. Most of us would like to believe that we have the ability to be honest when called upon to do so. This might sound like a manageable request at first, but asking people to be honest about issues that are ingrained in their subconscious is not always easy. Often we practice our belief systems until we fail to see the inherent blocks that perpetuate the exact behavior we are so diligently trying to overcome. Please think twice when you are sifting through your clutter and you hear that little uninvited committee in your head saying things like "Don't throw it out, you'll need it someday." Know that this is a yellow warning light signaling that you are about to ignore your common sense and keep something you truly don't need.

We in the West have adopted a rather neurotic attitude that "more is better." We act as though we live 300 miles away from the nearest drugstore and a serious emergency may occur in the middle of the night. As we search for the only possible remedy to the situation, to our dismay, we discover that we ran out of shampoo!

Go ahead, I know you may be laughing, but I urge you to take the "clutter challenge." Go into your bathroom and look around (particularly in your medicine cabinet). You might be surprised at what you find. How many bottles of shampoo do you have? Old, expired medication? Lipstick colors that you will never wear again? We all have our personal clutter objects of choice, things we collect over time and then eventually forget about. If the bathroom is not your issue, then try checking your refrigerator, kitchen cabinets, closets, junk drawers, and my old favorite, under the bed. Your healing assignment is to make yourself see the insanity in the behaviors you've come to identify as normal. Your health and overall well-being will depend on your willingness to take charge of the clutter, a situation that can and will run amok, energetically and physically.

Clutter can also paralyze. If you are truly frozen and just cannot get started or cannot find someone to assist you, use the following Transcendental Cure to help you get over the hump and to locate some supportive help from someone who cares.

Hang a brass wind chime or a set of nine small brass bells over the area that is particularly challenging to you or has accumulated the most clutter. Make sure you bless it with the Three Secrets Reinforcement Blessing, and visualize that all the physical clutter and its emotional underpinnings are being lifted and freeing you from the blocks and undertow.

Different types of clutter create different types of health problems. The form clutter takes, its predecessor's history, and where it is located in the house will all determine its impact on your health.

Clutter: Types, Location, and Impact on Your Health

Attic. The attic corresponds to the top cavity on the vertical "Mystical Being" (see Figs. 11a–b). It oversees the head area and any type of head-related injuries, strokes, migraines, headaches (both emotional and physical), eye-related problems, impaired vision, difficulty in not being able to see issues and problems clearly, foggy thinking, scattered energy, everyday pressures, and a sense of uncompleted issues that are "hanging over your head."

Basement. The basement corresponds to the lower-cavity portion of the vertical Mystical Being (see Figs. 10a–b). It oversees the genital area, bladder infections, uterine cysts, vaginal infections, hemorrhoids, difficult pregnancies or problems in conceiving, prostate problems, menopausal problems, illnesses of the blood, any lower-body cancers and tumors, sciatica, edema, gout, and foot and leg problems. Keep in mind that energy, like smoke, rises. The foundation of your house, each floor above it, and the foundation of your health are affected by whatever is collected and stored in your basement.

Entryways/behind doors. The entranceways allow the life force and the breath of a space to enter and flow. They set the tone for the quality of the Feng Shui of your home. If they are blocked or constricted in any way, it becomes even more serious from a health perspective, and the fallout is profound. For pregnant women the risk factors are even higher, because the entranceways re-create the uterus and birth-canal areas, and blocked ones can cause everything from premature births to difficult deliveries. They can exacerbate respiratory problems, asthma, heart disease, lethargy, and fatigue; they can increase depression and anxiety, or create an overall sense of hopelessness. Doors need to open as fully and as completely as possible. We tend to put things behind the door, either for lack of space or mindfulness. Shirts, robes, and jackets are all common offenders that eventually pile up and keep the door from opening fully. One or two shirts, a jacket, or a robe is okay as long as it doesn't compromise your ability to easily access the room or foyer.

Clutter in various guas. No matter what challenges you are facing regarding your clutter issues, it's important that you take the time and locate which guas contain the most clutter. That should help you understand what underlying emotional issues are attached to the clutter, and it will allow you to check the health of the different body areas that the gua corresponds to. For example, if the closet in your guest room is so incredibly stuffed with clothes and junk that just opening the door runs the risk of setting in motion the biggest avalanche this side of the Himalayas, there's a problem. What you need to do is get your floor plan out and locate the gua that the closet falls into. For instance, if it falls in the Relationship area of the room, then you want to explore any floating issues regarding relationships, your mother, and all the organs in your body. These issues are either serving as the emotional underpinning contributing to the clutter or they are the specific issues being directly affected by it.

Drawers, closets, cabinets. "Hidden-clutter syndrome" is clutter with a twist. We stockpile, hoard, overstuff, and then hide all our madness away from others and eventually from ourselves. Even if clutter is hidden away and you are not regularly exposed to it, it still affects your health or some other significant aspect of your life. Hide it away if you must, but eventually it will have to be addressed. Make the time now, as a preventive measure, and take an honest look at what you are holding on to and why, then decide if you really need to keep it. If not, give it away or toss it. Check the floor plan and room plan, and locate the overall and room gua that the clutter or drawers are in. That should give you more information on what some of the underpinning issues are. Otherwise it's a losing game, with clutter always winning at the end—usually by a landslide!

Energetic clutter. The other type of clutter that is equally disruptive, if not more so, is energetic clutter. This is the kind of energy that permeates a room, stagnating the natural ch'i and health of a space. Because it is invisible to the untrained eye, it very often goes undetected. Although most people know something is wrong, without the proper language they just can't seem to put their finger on it. Stagnant or dense energy fields can be caused by negative emotions or by events such as trauma, death, or illness. A sad period, a breakup, depression, constant arguing, or sickness can create heavy energetics in a space, especially the bedroom, which, in turn, results in a very sick environment that depletes all who come in contact with it.

Bedroom/under-bed clutter. This is the worst kind of clutter, especially in relation to your health, because we spend one-third of our life in the bedroom. Having clutter in your bedroom contributes to your illness, but the reverse is also true: removing the clutter can significantly influence your getting better.

Collectibles versus clutter. Please keep in mind that it's really okay to treasure collectibles and have possessions. That isn't clutter! How we store our possessions, where we store them, and what they mean to us is how we can determine whether the energy they are emitting is supportive, oppressive, or acting as stagnant clutter. The most important thing to remember is that you always need to honor and take conscious care of the things you acquire, and their energy will happily support you.

Cluttered areas need to be space-cleared. Removing the physical clutter isn't always enough. Even after all your efforts at removing and reducing your clutter, quite often you still have to do an energetic clearing of the space itself, especially if you've been sick. All rooms in the house will need a clearing, but particularly the bedroom or whichever room you have spent a lot of time in. Areas that contained a lot of clutter in your home, including basements and attics, also need to be space-cleared before, after, and sometimes during the excavation process. There are several excellent methods and substances to use for conducting a space-clearing session. These include, but are not limited to, essential oils, sage, incense, Jusha, realgar, alcohol and epsom salts, and sound. See chapter 9 for further instruction.

Method 5. Superimpose the
Mystical Being

The Mystical Being is an imaginary human body used in Black Hat Feng Shui as another health-assessment method similar to method 2, the Feng Shui Bagua. It is superimposed, in both horizontal and vertical positions, over the lot, each floor, and each individual room of your house. The Mystical Being is then used to locate corresponding areas of your body as they appear in your home. It can also be used to locate other areas that may weaken your vital ch'i or contribute to your failing health. By laying this figure down properly, you will be able to find the areas in your home that oversee specific areas of your body. When used correctly, these methods together provide you with two different but equally important ways to learn how your health is being reflected in the Feng Shui layout of your home.

This method allows you to review the area that oversees your health concern, giving you another way to check for problematic health-related areas. When you locate the area of concern, physically go to it and check its Feng Shui to see if there are any problems—leaks, broken windows, doors that stick, clutter—and then make the needed adjustments accordingly. When assessing for health, you should apply both methods 2 and 5 to receive a complete and thorough diagnosis of your space.

As Figs. 9a and 9b indicate, the Mystical Being is placed on the layout according to the location of the entranceway into the space you are assessing, just like the other Feng Shui concepts that revolve around the importance of the door. The first approach to placing the Mystical Being is the horizontal-application method. First, locate the entranceway to the lot, to each floor, and then to each room. Then take your floor plan out and superimpose the Mystical Being over the areas you would like to assess. Draw a body (head, torso, two arms, and two legs) spread-eagle, facing down, with the head and neck aligned with the entranceway door or opening that leads to the area that you want to assess. Follow each body part to the area that it rests over, and check the Feng Shui of that area. If you locate an area in your home that needs repairs or some kind of overhaul, adjust that area with one of the Nine Basic Cures in chapter 3. Also look for other problematic interior factors—spiral staircases, large columns, low lighting, etc.—and make the necessary changes to improve its energy flow. If applicable, go to the specific areas that relate to your health problem or genetic predisposition, augment them (with wind chimes, crystals, and plants), and adjust that area also.

Figs. 9a and 9b. Mystical Being (Horizontal)

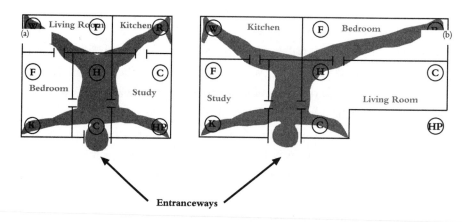

Entranceways

The next way to apply the Mystical Being is by placing it vertically (see Figs. 10a and 10b) over your home or apartment building. This approach allows you to assess the health of a space from yet another angle, in that it allows you to see the energy layout from a frontal and elevated view. This second method is used mainly for homes and apartment buildings with more than one floor. When applying this second approach, be sure to include the basement and the attic as part of the diagram. Place the front of the head facing into the house, with the back of the head flush up against the main entranceway, extending the arms into the basement and the feet into the top floor or attic. Note: You can also try placing the head facing forward in the attic and the feet and legs going down into the basement. Sometimes the illness or problem will show itself this way also, even though this positioning is not depicted in the illustrations that follow.

Figs. 10a and 10b. Mystical Being (Vertical)

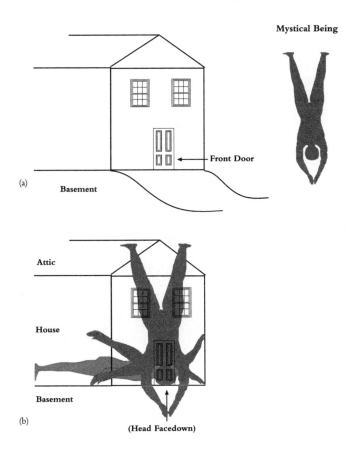

Mystical Being

(a) Basement — Front Door

Attic

House

Basement

(b) (Head Facedown)

Method 6. Assess the Three Visceral Cavities

This next method shares some of the same concepts as the Mystical Being in Method 5. It is based on the Black Hat Sect concept that the physical body can be broken down into three specific sections referred to as the Three Visceral Cavities. Each cavity oversees an important life-sustaining system of the body. The Upper Cavity oversees the circulatory system, and includes the heart, lungs, neck, and head; the Middle Cavity oversees the digestive system, which includes the spleen, stomach, liver, gallbladder, pancreas, and small intestine; and the Lower Cavity oversees the excretory system, which

Figs. 11a and 11b. Visceral Cavities—
Horizontal/Vertical

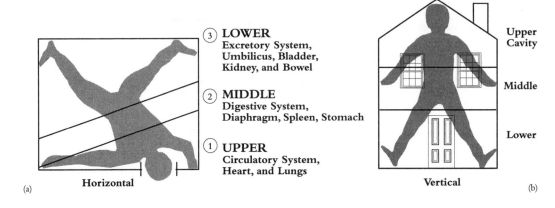

(3) **LOWER**
Excretory System,
Umbilicus, Bladder,
Kidney, and Bowel

(2) **MIDDLE**
Digestive System,
Diaphragm, Spleen, Stomach

(1) **UPPER**
Circulatory System,
Heart, and Lungs

Upper
Cavity

Middle

Lower

(a) Horizontal

Vertical (b)

includes the bladder, kidneys, large intestine, and rectum (see Figs. 11a and 11b).

When you assess the Three Visceral Cavities, what you are actually doing is applying the Mystical Being as learned in method 5, and assessing an overall body section rather than a specific body part or area. You are looking for how the overall section of your home fares in terms of its Feng Shui and the corresponding system that it oversees.

First, place the Mystical Being face downward horizontally in the area or space that you are assessing, and then divide the Being into three sections, or Visceral Cavities. Assess the three areas collectively, being sure to analyze as many interior factors as you can gather. This method gives you the overall picture of the strength of that area and how it is influencing your corresponding system's health. For example, if the Middle Cavity of a floor has a leak in the ceiling, a spiral staircase running through it, and plants that keep dying, collectively the poor Feng Shui of that space can be very weakening to your digestive system. To adjust and strengthen the ch'i, and to prevent a potential health problem, you should space-clear and augment that section of your home with the Nine Basic Cures. Potential cures might include repairing the ceiling, hanging a faceted 40-mm crystal on a nine-inch red string from the ceiling above the spiral staircase, and installing a bright overhead light at the top of the staircase to raise the ch'i and nourish the struggling plants.

If you already know that you have either a digestive problem or a genetic predisposition to one, you can go directly to these areas of your house and check them to see if they are energetically contributing to your particular health challenge. If they are, make the necessary changes, clear the energy fields, and enhance the healthy ch'i by augmenting those areas with the Nine Basic Cures.

For best results, use both the horizontal and vertical methods. When applying the Mystical Being vertically, be sure to include the basement as well as the attic, if applicable.

Method 7. Analyze the Shapes of Your Floor Plans and Drawings

If you have not already drawn your floor plan (I know you're out there!), or you have been using a version from your realtor or landlord, this is probably a good time to put the book down and create your own hand-sketched version. If you don't create your floor plan before reading this next section, you might miss out on the objectivity needed to get the benefit of this approach.

Before going on any Feng Shui consultation, I always ask my clients to send me two copies of their floor plan (as discussed in chapter 3). Most of them send me a hand-sketched version, and although the official floor plan is usually more accurate (and legible), I have found that the "rough version" provides me with much more information, because it is influenced by the client's subconscious mind.

Early on in my practice as a Feng Shui consultant, I found myself utilizing my former training as a psychotherapist and analyzing the hand-drawn floor plans of my clients. I was looking for any hidden issues or underlying messages that my client's artwork might reveal. What I found was that what my clients were not able to articulate fully or express consciously often surfaced through how they designed their homes. Because the Feng Shui of your home reflects everything that is manifested in your life, it can act as a wonderful window providing insight into all the nooks and crannies of your life. One of my very dear clients had to have her lung removed due to the unexpected and shocking find of a cancerous tumor. A closer look at her floor plan revealed the shape of one lung. Being able to interpret the invisible energy fields and patterns around you gives you a greater understanding of the nature of the problem or health concern and what you can do about it.

Method 8. Calculate the Life-Force Quotient

What do we really mean when we refer to the life force of a home? Many of us, if we even considered the concept of life force, would associate it with a tangible living being. So it's understandably a confusing thought at first, especially if you do not see your home as a living entity that has a metabolism and spirit of its very own. But your home *is* alive and does have its own personality based on the combination of the many interior and exterior factors I have already addressed. All these things combine to contribute not only to the way the house feels, but to how well it is able to support you, especially when you are ill.

When we are working with and addressing the life force of a home, we are actually assessing the interaction between the house's energy field and those of the individuals who reside there. These combined energy forces act as very significant factors in why and how we develop certain illnesses, and in turn they provide us with a wealth of information on how those same illnesses can be transformed.

The quality of the Feng Shui and the energy flow of your environment will determine the strength of your own external life force. The quality of the ch'i, or energy, in your body will determine the strength of your internal ch'i. When we get sick, what actually happens is that the inner life force in our bodies becomes diminished. The Feng Shui of your environment creates the force that interfaces with, and nourishes, your internal ch'i. From a Feng Shui perspective, one of the main contributing factors to good health is strong internal ch'i reinforced by an environment that has good Feng Shui.

When we get sick or develop an illness, what happens to us is that the natural flow of internal ch'i is diminished. It is during these times, when it is not able to produce a strong flow on its own, that the body instinctively attempts to extract some additional life force from the environment. That is why it is so important to assess the overall life-force quotient of the home you are living in, not only so you will have supportive energetic backup when you need it, but also to help prevent certain illnesses from manifesting to begin with.

Three Types of Life Force

1. *Living life force.* These are the elements that are actually alive and bring with them, wherever you place them, their own supply of life support. The life-force elements are plants, flowing water (such as indoor fountains), fish, birds, pets, rainbows, fresh air, sunlight, candlelight, and certain full-spectrum lighting. These elements provide strong and steady life-force energy wherever they are placed. They constantly enrich our environment and create an overall positive feeling in our homes while giving out the constant message that this house is alive. Life-force elements fill up our senses and remind us that another living entity is present in our space. Trees, plants, dogs, birds, cats, and water fountains force us to connect with them on a daily basis and create an opportunity to have contact with their ch'i and exchange some love.

In Feng Shui Design we fully understand the importance of first impressions and how to create a visual impact that will boost a person's life force. By placing plants, flowers, a small fountain, a fish tank, or by being greeted by a zealous pet at the entryway, we help create a magnificent life-force feeling from the entry point on. As an additional perk, these life-force adjustment items have built-in healing properties that positively affect other areas of your life such as finances and work opportunities. (For more about this, see my first book, *Feng Shui: Harmony by Design* [Perigee, 1996].)

Plants or flowers are a wonderful energy adjustment to any room in the house, especially the bedroom. Some Feng Shui references say that placing plants in the bedroom is not a good thing. The Black Hat Sect, however, fully supports the use of plants as a life-force adjustment in the bedroom or anywhere else. If they are flourishing and cared for properly, they represent growth and new life, and are a constant source of life force.

Sometimes, even with your best efforts, your plants will die. If your plants die because you forgot to water them, then you might decide that this is not the best type of adjustment item for you to use. But if you can find a way to gain mastery over your absentmindedness or brown thumb, I promise you that this will be a big personal step, for you have then mastered an inner block about your own ability to care for yourself and things that you are responsible for. If you want to make the extra effort, find the easiest plant to care for, get a watering schedule down pat, and install indoor plant lights. This would be a very good gesture toward your healing process.

Remember that even if you care for your plants very well, some might die anyway. This reflects the natural life-and-death cycle of all species, and it doesn't necessarily mean something horrible. Native Americans believe that when a plant dies, it is honoring you by sacrificing its life for you, absorbing the negative or unbalanced energy in the environment before your physical body absorbs it. It is quite a common occurrence for plants to die during times of stress, great transition, or illness. When plants die at nonstressful times, it may be a signal to you, letting you know that the ch'i of a particular space is unhealthy or unbalanced. Try not to let this alarm you, but instead see it as a wonderful gift, making you aware that you should adjust the life force in that particular gua or area. Observing this will give you an even clearer sense of some of the emotional underpinnings and physical areas of concern in your life. For example, if the plant dies in the Relationship corner of your room, it might mean that a relationship has ended or is about to, or that a new type of relationship energy may come into your life. Other significant factors could be that the organs of your body are tired and in need of healing or cleansing (the Relationship gua oversees the organs) or that you need to check out current or past mother-related issues (the Relationship area also represents the mother).

If you find that your plants keep dying, especially in a particular place, immediately replace them with a healthier or larger plant. Recheck the lighting and rethink your watering schedule. Do whatever you can to improve the ch'i of that area. Don't just toss a plant out and not re-augment the gua, especially if you are ill, because that could create an energetic drop in life-force ch'i. See these mishaps as opportunities, and always try to improve on the life-force quotient of your home, as much as you possibly can.

2. *Aesthetic life force.* This is the overall visual effect of the aesthetics of your living space on you and your health. When we talk about aesthet-

ics in Feng Shui Design, it is important to note that this is a design system based on energy flow and object placement. Traditional interior design builds most of its concepts on form and function. ***But good interior design in the usual sense does not necessarily mean good Feng Shui, and good Feng Shui does not always mean good interior design.*** But when you are able to blend the two, you can create an incredibly wonderful place to live, work, and heal.

So you need to ask yourself how you feel about your decor. Is it colorful, full of life force, vibrant? Or is all the furniture old, torn, and faded? What are the messages that your aesthetic surroundings are giving you? How do they mirror your illness and your state of mind? How does your environment contribute to your healing process? Is it delaying your recovery? What type of art do you have on the walls? Do you like being there, or do you dread coming home? Remember, you don't need a lot of money to make a beautiful home that will support your health. What you do need to do is to start looking at the important influence of your environment on your life and health, then begin to shift your priorities and learn to honor your environment. Keep it clean and orderly, and treat it with respect, regardless of how old your possessions are!

My great-grandmother from Naples always used to say, "Soap and water doesn't cost much," meaning that you don't have to be rich to be clean. Whatever you have, no matter how tattered, treat it with the same care you would give something brand-new. Your health will improve if your attitude improves, because everything is interconnected and one thing has a profound effect on another, especially your home and your health. That is the message of this book.

3. ***Energetic life force.*** The energetic life force, or lack of it, is a little bit more difficult to detect because it requires a certain amount of awareness and sensitivity. This is the type of energy that you sense or feel, perhaps without any tangible clue that something is wrong or, conversely, that something is right. This is the initial unprompted feeling of "Gee, this place feels great," or "Gee, this place feels eerie!" What you're actually experiencing is information that you're picking up intuitively. It's the energy field of an environment that has stagnated or flourished by ener-

getically recording the various events that have occurred there, as well as the impact, for better or for worse, that the Feng Shui has had there.

So, if an environment has been exposed to lots of fighting, sad events, loneliness, fears, death, and sickness, the energy that these events give off, if not cleared away, will remain and stagnate the flow of healthy ch'i. If the environment has been cared for and repeatedly exposed to positive people and joyful events, you will feel good too, because the ch'i is positive. Even if you don't particularly like the style of furniture or the layout of the house, if the space has good energetic life force, you'll know it. This feeling is the type of energy field that you want to have around you at all times, but especially during a time of illness, because a good environment will help you heal and contribute to you staying well.

Method 9. Follow the Daily Activity Path

The daily activity path that I spoke about in chapter 1 is the exterior activity path that any individual follows to and from work. This path is the route that we take into, out of, and around our homes. It is a very significant factor in the type of health or illness we experience. Because we walk through certain pathways in our homes over and over again, several times a day, seven days a week, 365 days a year, we condition our sight lines, ch'i, and Chakras by what we see each day.

When you are doing a health analysis, start at your front door, and, with a discerning eye, look at all you see and pass by through the route that you take each day. Because we pass through these routes so frequently, we develop metaphorical blinders and often no longer notice what we are seeing or not seeing. Our path becomes routine, and the awkwardly placed table that we have to squeeze by, the door that doesn't open fully, or the hallway narrowed by clutter no longer bothers us. We don't replace blown lightbulbs, litter boxes remain full until we can't tolerate it any longer, and we never have any time to fix the drip or unclog the drain. We are creatures of habit, and will go out of our way to accommodate dysfunction, rather than change the layout or situation that's no longer working.

So, take an honest inventory of what you are visually seeing and/or avoiding seeing, and think about its impact on your energy and your health.

Look for low or burned-out lighting; dirty walls; lack of color; low life force; tight, cramped entryways and hallways; frustrating locks that you have to struggle with; windows that are jammed shut; drawers that are broken; knobs that don't stay on; furniture that you have to practically jump over to get by; oversized accessories that are too big for the space; dirty and dusty areas; mats and carpeting that are old or that you constantly trip over. Really scrutinize your daily activity path and make the needed changes or adjustments to create an environment that your subconscious mind can commit to memory as a safe, loving, and health-enhancing place to live, grow, and heal. Let your environment vibrationally resonate to a place that reflects your intentions and your goal of healing and transformation.

Remember, your home is an externalized, mirrored reflection of you and your inner home, and if you want the space inside to heal, you have to represent that in the outside energy system as well.

Method 10. Analyze the Bedroom

The bedroom has a significant impact on our lives and our health because it's where we spend one-third of our lives. The impact that this has on our ch'i, health, and relationships is huge. It is such a vital room that I've devoted the next chapter to it exclusively. Below is a list of significant factors we will cover and elaborate on in chapter 5.

- The Bedroom, an Overview
- Keep All Work Out of the Bedroom
- Remove TVs
- Rethink What You Are Reading
- Relocate Towering, Dark Furniture
- Space Clearing and Clutter Reduction
- The Four Conditions of Proper Bed Positioning
- Adjust the *Center/Health guas*
- Life-Force Quotient
- Other Interior Factors
- Analyzing Bedroom Layouts
- Remove or Reduce All Electrical Items from Bedroom Area

About five years ago I was called to do a consultation for a very well known doctor of holistic medicine. She was installing a fountain in the backyard of her home, and wanted me to make sure it was positioned in the proper place. Her assistant told me she wasn't interested in having the rest of her home analyzed; she just needed some advice and direction for her fountain. At first I was going to decline and refer her to one of my associates, because I normally do not do piecemeal Feng Shui—my core belief is that for Feng Shui to be done properly, you have to assess the whole place— but I was strangely compelled to do the consultation.

Because my client was so busy with her practice, and all correspondence was conducted through her assistant, I did not get a chance to speak with her directly. The one thing I insisted on was that she had to personally draw and send me a hand-sketched floor plan of her space before our appointment. Right under the wire, the day before the consultation was to take place, the floor plans arrived via Express Mail. When I sat down to do my preliminary review of her floor plan, I opened up the envelope and looked at the floor plan. My gut reaction was "Oh my God, she has breast cancer!" Enclosed in the envelope was a hand-sketched drawing of the exterior area around her house. As I looked at it, I immediately saw a frontal image of a woman's torso with one arm and only one breast! (See Fig. 12.)

In retrospect, I know that this image could have been interpreted in a number of ways, but I sensed intuitively that the issue was cancer. My next challenge was to decide how to handle the information I was receiving, and how to present it to her with respect and compassion. It was at that point that it became clear to me why I was called to do the consultation and why I uncharacteristically decided to take it. The fountain was just a catalyst, a lure to get me there so I could work with this person. At the time I didn't know if the cancer had been diagnosed, or how far it had spread. I was somewhat apprehensive about even bringing it up for fear that she wasn't aware of it—and of course there was always a possibility that I was wrong.

When I arrived at her place, she immediately took me to the fountain in her back-yard. It was still in the process of being erected. As I guessed, it was already auspiciously placed in the Wealth gua of her yard, and it looked great. I made some suggestions on how to incorporate altars within the stone structure itself, but the truth was that my work was done regarding the fountain and she was doing fine without me.

Once inside, we sat down and I said to her, "I'm concerned about your health. How has it been?" I was both relieved and saddened when she replied, "I have breast cancer." She also shared with me that she had not told anyone else about the cancer and was waiting to decide what to do, how to treat it, and how to proceed. We spent the next two hours talking and doing some very introspective spiritual counseling. After much resistance, we set a goal: Each week she had to tell someone significant in her life that she had cancer, including a doctor, a close family member, and at least one good friend. That's what our initial Feng Shui work was about. That's why I was called in, to help her move forward and get the help for herself that she has so generously been doling out to others throughout her whole career. To get the process started, my suggestion to her was to plant flowers in a half circle in her front yard to symbolically replace the other breast that was missing on the outside landscape of her home. Energetically speaking, her healing process began by allowing all these issues to come to the surface to finally be addressed.

From a Feng Shui perspective, we needed to adjust the image of the missing breast and change the inherent imbalance in the inauspicious design in her home. From a psychological perspective, she needed to physically redo that image that was embedded in her psyche, implying that she was going to lose her breast and maybe her life. All the painful and frightening feelings that go along with those images had to be released too. Upon my last contact with her, the doctor was doing well and running her health center.

Fig. 12. Client with Breast Cancer

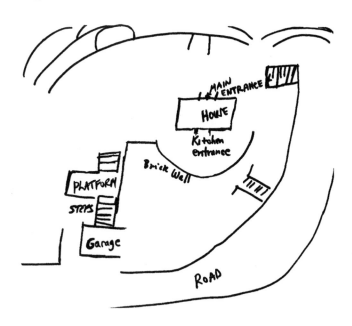

CHAPTER FIVE

THE BEDROOM

A Sacred Place . . .
A Healing Space

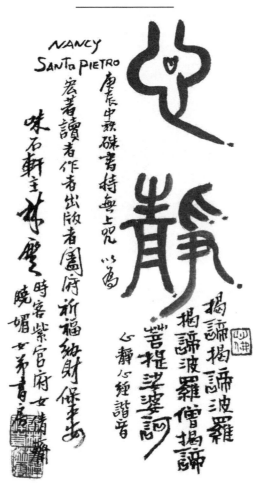

"Calming Heart."

CALLIGRAPHY BY H. H. PROFESSOR THOMAS LIN YUN RINPOCHE

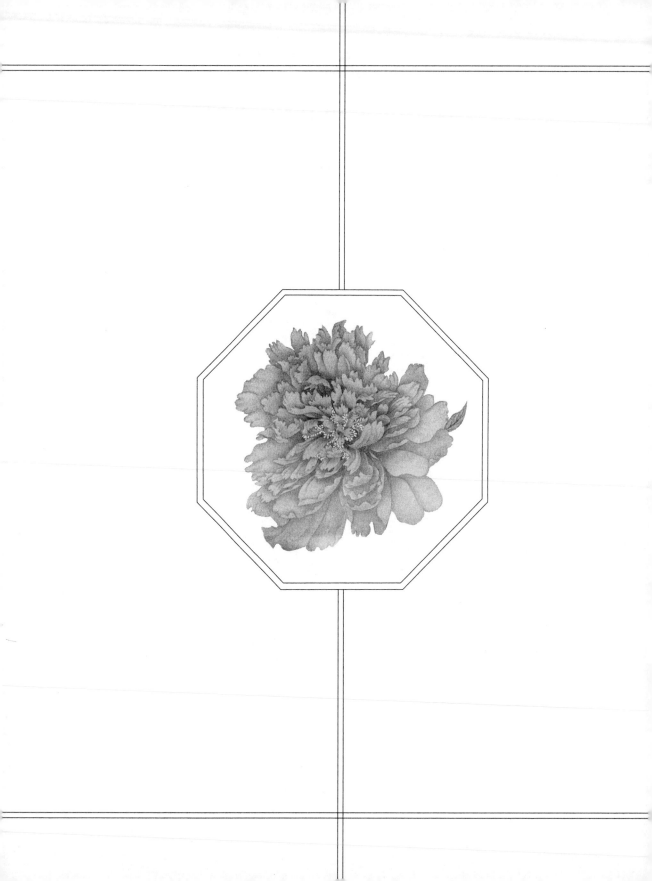

THE BEDROOM: AN OVERVIEW

WHEN WE ARE SICK, whether at a friend's house, at work, or at school, the first thing we want to do is go home, and the next thing we want to do is get into our own bed, because no matter what the circumstances are, there is nothing more familiar and comforting than your own pillow, blanket, and favorite pajamas. Anyone who has ever been in a hospital will wholeheartedly agree that their main goal, besides getting well, is getting back home!

It would be a shock to most of us to discover some the hidden dangers this wonderfully nurturing room can conceal. Having a bedroom with poor Feng Shui can very quickly become one of the main contributing factors to how illness develops. Our bedroom is vital to our health, but it can harbor many invisible energy imbalances. So, when we turn to our bedroom as a safe place to heal and recover, what we might actually be doing is sending ourselves back to the actual space that contributed to the developing of our illness in the first place. If you are looking to reinforce your good health or help support your healing process, then making necessary changes in your bedroom is paramount.

Of all of the rooms in your environment, the bedroom is probably the most important space in regards to your health. Because we spend one-third of our lives sleeping, this places us in the bedroom for more hours than in any other room in our house. Also, during sleep our bodies become less guarded as our ch'i seeks to rejuvenate and replenish itself for the following day. While in this passive, reparative state for several hours each night, we become more susceptible to the surrounding Feng Shui of the room we are in. The bedroom, and in turn the bed, create an energetic atmosphere that has a profound effect not only on your health, but on the quality of your intimate relationships.

As you begin to think about the design and the Feng Shui arrangement of your bedroom, it's important that you start training yourself to think in terms of vibrational energy patterns and not just in terms of traditional interior design, which is based mostly on aesthetics. The first thing you need to consider is the energetic concept of your bedroom: how it is laid out, what it should be used for, and what should be avoided. Below is a checklist of different aspects that should be considered when assessing the health quotient of your bedroom.

Keep All Work Out of the Bedroom

In my opinion, the bedroom should be used primarily for two things, love-making and sleep. With a few exceptions, all other activities should be performed elsewhere. This is an important concept to grasp, especially since we are living in such a fast-paced time in which multitasking has become a prevailing mode in our lives. We make business calls over lunch, exercise while watching TV, and bring our work home so we can catch up. As we over-stretch our boundaries, we slowly find ourselves reading office memos, doing backed-up paperwork, and bringing our laptop computers into the bedroom. This crossover of energies creates the antithesis of what the bedroom is meant to do—help you rest, recuperate, and heal.

Energetically the bedroom is considered a Yin room; i.e., a room where activity is slow and the energy should encourage us to be still and go inside. Work or office ch'i has a Yang ch'i, very opposite energy, one that encourages activity, thinking, and action. The stress that can come along with that particular kind of Yang energy should have no business in this healing, nurturing, sacred place. From a Feng Shui perspective, what you are actually doing when you bring work into the bedroom is re-creating a work-energy field that you have already been exposed to throughout the day but now find yourself sleeping in it all night. Your body, your personal stress level, and any illness or disease you are trying to heal will not have a fighting chance in an environment that suggests otherwise.

Remove TVs

The other mind-set we create in the bedroom that can negatively influence your mental and physical well-being is our love affair with the media. We get in bed, relax, turn the TV on, and often tune in to the late-night newscast. The last things we hear before we doze off are stories of tragedy and horror from around the world. You may not think that these events create lasting imprints on your psyche, but as you begin to understand the impact of energy, you will see how those stories create negative energy patterns and indirectly instill a sense of hopelessness about your own illness or struggles.

TVs also contain other energetic problems that can contribute to poor health and bad Feng Shui. They are a very high source of the electromagnetic energy fields discussed in chapter 1. A TV set and its wiring emit EMFs even long after the TV has been shut off.[6] Be prudent. If at all possible, move the TV into another room. And be sure you don't place the TV (or any other appliance, for that matter) on the opposite wall behind your bed or headboard. EMFs can travel through walls, curtains, and wooden cabinets. If you must have a TV in your bedroom, then put a couple of "smog buster beads" (these are EMF-reduction devices) on the top of the screen, keep the set at least twelve feet from your physical body, and, when it's not in use and especially at night, *unplug it.*

The above is also true of computers, clock radios, answering machines, and so on, near your bed and especially near your head. Move these devices at least six to eight feet from the circumference of your body. Make sure that you are not using an electric blanket, or sleeping on a water bed that has a motor attached. All these gadgets produce very high levels of EMFs and need to be eliminated or drastically reduced if your immune system is ever going to strengthen and stay strong.

Rethink What You Are Reading

You should also think about the books you are reading before you go to bed. Are they love stories with sad endings? Stories of war and tragedy? Spiritual books with messages of hope and inspiration? What energy messages do the contents carry? What I am asking you to do is become more aware of things that at first may seem benign, but upon further exploration are not. I am aware that many people enjoy a good read before they go to bed, but if you are working on your health or trying to sustain or fix a relationship, you might want to reconsider the things that happen in the bedroom that are outside of the rest-and-lovemaking menu.

Remember that books bring many different energies, including the energy of everyone from the author to the clerks who may have handled it in the bookshop. Make sure you truly know whom you are "taking to bed with you," because their energy will remain with you long after the book is finished!

Relocate Towering, Dark Furniture

It's not uncommon for people to purchase large, beautiful armoires and other such furniture pieces for the bedroom. Although stylish, it's important that they are used in rooms that can accommodate them and give them the breathing room that they require. Make sure that the closet, armoire, or bookcase is positioned away from the bed and doesn't close it in or appear to be leaning over the bed in any way. Second, watch for headboards that are high and can be used for bookcases. This creates an energetic pressure that can cause headaches, unclear thinking, insomnia, and anxiety.

This especially holds true for furniture that is dark and heavy, because the darker the furniture is, the more absorbent it will be. It will be prone to absorb energy that is in the bedroom, including energy that is out of balance and unsteady. Although the weight might actually be a good thing for individuals who are not able to stabilize their health (or relationships), the darkness, without some contrasting colors, may be serving to hold on to the illness, sadness, and emotional pain that are in need of being discharged.

In general, lighter woods and other natural materials for beds and bedroom furniture are preferred. If possible, metal beds should be avoided because they can conduct and amplify problematic EMFs.

If the furniture has been given to you by an undesirable source, or is left over from a previous relationship, you should think about the energy it is carrying and how that energy is contributing or not contributing to your health and/or recovery process.

Space Clearing and Clutter Reduction

As discussed in chapters 1 and 4, one of the most influential factors governing your health today is the clutter that surrounds you, especially in your bedroom. It will slow down your healing and recovery process, and depending on how big the problem is, it could bring your healing to a complete standstill. Energy rises, so the clutter or dirt under your bed is rising up into your being while you are in that all-vulnerable reparative sleep state.

Review the things you might have collected or stored under your bed. Old clothes you wore when you were ten pounds lighter, letters and photos that depict old times. (Former relationships and past memories may be okay to keep elsewhere, but not in your bedroom and definitely not under your bed.) These kinds of collectibles have very strong energy fields around them because they were imprinted with emotional energy; they can retain their original charge for a lifetime. Very often the pains of the past and all the issues we consciously and unconsciously hold on to become emotional factors that can contribute to developing illnesses and diseases. Clear it out, and reduce an energetic aspect of your illness. Remember, when clutter is hidden in closets or drawers, locate the gua that it is in. Something about the issue of that gua is attracting the clutter and holding it in place.

Energetic clutter, discussed in chapter 4, is equally devastating, if not more so, and warrants particular attention in the bedroom. These are still life-force-depleting energy fields that are created by emotions, traumas, deaths, illness, and other events that are not properly cleared away. If just passing through these fields is enough to alter your energy, health, and outlook on life, imagine what sleeping in them must do to your soul. The energy in the bedroom should be cleared periodically, but if you are sick, even if it's just with a cold, you should clear the bedroom every few days. Change the sheets, turn the mattress over, open the windows, play music, ring some bells, and learn to work with therapeutic-grade aromatherapy oils (see chapter 10). Besides aromatherapy, you can use several excellent methods and substances for conducting a space-clearing session. These include, but are not limited to, sage, incense, Jusha, realgar, alcohol and Epsom salts, and sound. For further instruction, see chapters 9 and 10 on various space-clearing methods.

The Four Conditions of Proper Bed Positioning

The most important interior factor affecting your health in your bedroom and in your home is the positioning of your bed. If at all possible, always try to position your bed so that you face and see the bedroom door, the "mouth of the ch'i," which brings with it a powerful life force that also carries to you all of life's opportunities, all its ups and downs. By positioning the bed to face the door, you are also positioning yourself to face your life directly, to be in command and to receive the energy of the ch'i.

The four main conditions for proper bed positioning are: (1) Whenever possible, have the bed face the door; (2) Place the bed so when you're in it you have the widest view of the room; (3) Positioning of the bed is relative, which means that its proper placement is contingent on where the door is located in the room; and finally, (4) *Never* place the bed in direct alignment with, or in a position that has it overlapping, the door.

When given a choice, place the bed on a solid interior, non-window wall. The body's energy will be stronger that way, and more likely to heal with solid support behind it. Although I sometimes place beds on a window wall, I use this as a last resort when all other interior walls are not an option, especially when an individual is sick or in a weakened state. If the window is directly behind or directly in front of the bed, it may dissipate the energy flow and further weaken or slow down recovery. If the bed can't be moved, try putting plants in the window or behind the headboard to keep energy in the room. If it is by the window, also make sure that the bed has a solid headboard, preferably made of natural wood. Feel free to hang some curtains and place 40-mm crystals or brass wind chimes in each window in question and in the Health gua in the bedroom.

Fig. 13. Proper Bed Positioning

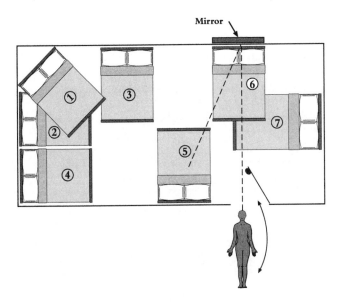

Mirror

Bed Position 1 is the ideal spot for a bed with the doorway location shown. The bed satisfies all the four conditions listed above for proper bed placement.

Bed Position 2 is also very good. Although it does not have the widest view of the room, it still fulfills the other very important conditions.

Bed Position 3 is also okay. Although it has a wider view of the room than bed position 2, its head-on view of the bedroom door is reduced. Try to move the bed to position 1 or 2, or place a mirror on an angle in the corner of the room clearly reflecting the entryway.

Bed Position 4 is not the worst but also not the best, because its view is further reduced by being in the corner and not having a head-on view of the door. Because one side of the bed is flush against the wall, it impairs the ability to establish supportive, equal relationships with your partner. In the relationship, whoever sleeps on the wall side of the bed will be even more affected, feeling more oppressed and limited. Treatments that are not working, illnesses that affect only one side of the body, imbalances in your hormonal, endocrine, and nervous systems, and chemical imbalances can all be affected by this bed position. Move the bed to a more auspicious position, such as 1 or 2. If you cannot, then hang a 40-mm clear crystal (on a nine-inch red string) from the ceiling in the middle of the bedroom, in the Health area. This will raise the ch'i for both partners and enhance the healing or one's recovery process. In addition, you can hang a picture with depth of field on the bedside wall. It can be a meandering river, a sunset, or anything that imparts a vibrant feeling of expansion. You may also hang a mirror on the opposite wall to the open side of the bed and visualize that the mirror is pulling the bed off the oppressive wall.

Bed Position 5 does not have the occupants facing the door at all, and, in turn, not facing their lives. This is stressful for the immune system and for one's healing process. It creates an energetic atmosphere in which opportunities are missed and the healing is spun around. It weakens your position in the world as well as your overall physical constitution, and makes you more vulnerable and susceptible. Move the bed, or place a mirror on the opposite-wall to the door.

Bed Position 6, although it faces the door, places the sleeper in a dangerous direct line with the door. When you are in direct line with it, the ch'i force is too strong and potentially very disruptive. If you really can't move the bed, hang a 40-mm clear crystal, on a nine-inch red string, from the ceiling in the middle area between the foot of the bed and the doorway. In addition, you can try to decrease the impact of the ch'i by placing a bookcase, a row of tall plants, floor-to-ceiling curtains, etc., at the foot of the bed to diffuse the ch'i being directed at the body.

Bed Position 7 is also in a very stressful and energetically compromised space. It's not only crossing a direct line with the doorway, but half of it falls behind the door itself! It creates all the same problems as position 6, *and* it generates an energetic split, placing half of the sleeper's body in direct line with the doorway and the other half tucked away. Be aware that the areas and organs of the body that actually cross the doorway will be much more susceptible to disease and accidents. The solution is to move the bed immediately. If this is not possible, hang a 40-mm clear crystal on a nine-inch red string between the door and the crossover part of the bed. Hang two bamboo flutes on an angle on the wall against which the headboard rests. Make sure that mouthpieces are at the bottom unless the bamboo is growing upward in larger and larger gradations, and then you would place the mouthpiece at the top.

Fig. 14. Proper Use of Bamboo Flutes

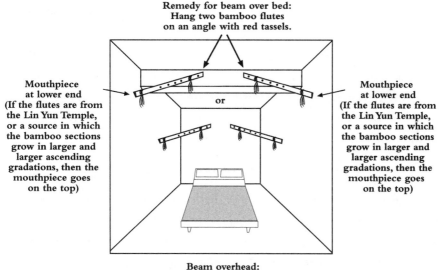

Remedy for beam over bed:
Hang two bamboo flutes
on an angle with red tassels.

Mouthpiece
at lower end
(If the flutes are from
the Lin Yun Temple,
or a source in which
the bamboo sections
grow in larger and
larger ascending
gradations, then the
mouthpiece goes
on the top)

or

Mouthpiece
at lower end
(If the flutes are from
the Lin Yun Temple,
or a source in which
the bamboo sections
grow in larger and
larger ascending
gradations, then the
mouthpiece goes
on the top)

Beam overhead:
Remedy: Move furniture out from under beam;
if not possible, try to position furniture parallel to
direction of beam, then use Bamboo Flute Remedy.

The Proper Bed Positioning diagram is based on the positioning of the doorway into the bedroom. If your bedroom doorway is in the Career gua, then the proper bed positioning would be determined by the swing of the door. If the door opens from left to right, the better positioning of the bed would be in the upper left-hand corner. If the door opens from right to left, then the better positioning of the bed would be in the upper right-hand corner. This means that if the doorway to your bedroom is located in the Self-Knowledge gua (on the left side of the entranceway wall), the proper bed positions would be reversed. For example, bed position 1 would be in the upper right-hand corner of the room where bed positions 6 and 7 are indicated.

When we begin to work with Feng Shui, and a suggestion is made that involves moving a piece of furniture, it is not uncommon that we will look for other, easier things to do as an adjustment, rather than moving the more difficult object. But remember that the best solution to most of these interior problems is usually the actual moving of the furniture itself. The remedies and cures offered throughout this book serve as backup for situations in which objects cannot be moved. So if you're thinking, "It's going to be a major pain to move this bed, I'll have to repaint, find new pictures, and so forth," then probably that's exactly what you need to do! The bigger the resistance, the greater the gain! Just make sure you aren't letting the "very convincing problematic energy" talk you out of the exact thing you need to do. If you are sick and are unable to make the major changes, especially the ones that require moving things, then go ahead and use all the backup solutions. But as soon as you're able to get some assistance or acquire some extra money or are feeling better, pick up where you left off and continue your health consultation.

Adjust the *Center/Health Gua*

Although we always augment the gua that is specifically related to the health problem in question (method 2, chapter 4, page 111), it is also very important to shore up the process by adjusting the Center gua that oversees all health and health-related issues. The *Ming Tang,* or T'ai Chi, is just another way of saying the center of the Bagua or the center of the room (method 3, chapter 4, page 112). The *Ming Tang* of the bedroom is extremely important to one's health because it represents the Health gua, which is the gua that's closest to you during the all-important reparative sleep state. It's the gua that acts as the main energy feed to the body and all its energy and energy systems. It works very closely with the Chakra Energy System (see chapters 7 and 8), and assists it in its healing process. It is crucial that all these systems be in alignment in order to reinforce your healing process.

You can adjust and strengthen the Health area by adding many of the Nine Basic Cures outlined in chapter 3. The best and simplest adjustments to this Center gua are 40- or 50-mm round faceted clear crystals and clear-sounding brass wind chimes. Remember, all crystals and wind chimes (when appropriate) should be hung on a red string, cord, or ribbon in multiple of nine (9, 18, 27, or 36 inches).

Specific Adjustment Items for the Health Gua

Round Faceted Glass Crystals
40- or 50-mm clear or AB (Aurora Borealis) crystal for an adult's bedroom

30- or 40-mm amber yellow crystal for an adult's bedroom

30- or 40-mm clear, AB, or amber crystal for an adolescent's bedroom

20- or 30-mm green, clear, or clear AB crystal for a toddler's bedroom

20- or 30-mm green crystal for a newborn's bedroom

Wind Chimes

Make sure all your wind chimes, especially ones that are used for healing adjustments and Transcendental Cures, are made of brass or have brass as their main metal. Copper is also good, as it conducts ch'i well. Avoid wind chimes that are made of ceramic or glass. Although they can be very beautiful, the materials connote a sense of fragility and precariousness. This doesn't mean you can never use them, but don't use them as a cure, especially for a health-related issue.

Very often we place wind chimes where there is no wind to activate them. Although it's better if the wind chimes can be activated (by natural wind or a tap of the hand), it's okay if they can't be, because we are using them as a Transcendental Cure (see chapter 9). However, it is also very important to enjoy the sound that the chimes make; let it be soothing to your ears whenever they ring.

Life-Force Quotient

When you are making your assessments, it is very important that you carefully try to interpret the life-force quotient of the overall bedroom. This is a crucial aspect that too often gets overlooked. When we are healthy, one of the main contributing factors is that we are living in an environment that has good Feng Shui that supports our life force and, in turn, our health. When we get sick or develop an illness, our natural flow of healthy ch'i, or life force, is diminished. During those times the body relies more on the life force from the environment to draw on when it is not able to produce its own. During the sleep state the body will seek to gain energy and life force from its surroundings. That's why it's important to assess and then enhance life-force elements inside the bedroom. These adjustments strengthen your physical as well as your etheric body, especially during times of change, illness, or fear. The life-force elements, as noted previously, are plants, flowing water, fish and birds, sunlight and full-spectrum lighting, rainbows (crystals), color, artwork, and natural elements, materials, and products.

Other Interior Factors

As you can see, the bedroom is a crucial component in one's healing process. When designing a room for healing or for maintaining your well-being, many factors need to be considered. Although I am not able to list all of them here, below are a few of the most significant ones. I will elaborate on others in subsequent chapters.

Pointed Arrows This is a common concern in Feng Shui Design. When you are assessing for pointed arrows or poison arrows (see Fig. 29), you are actually looking for furniture pieces or structural corners that jut out and form a point that meets at a 90-degree angle. This angle creates a powerful energy force that shoots the ch'i out rapidly and sharply. Although most of them need to be adjusted, the ones to be most concerned with, and that cause the most damage, are angles whose points go right through a main piece of furniture or an area in which the occupant(s) of the space spend a lot of time, such as the bed, stove, desk, entranceway, or favorite chair. Pointed arrows deplete our ch'i and create an energy field around us that makes us feel as if we are always under attack, being accused, or aggressed upon. Constant exposure to this type of energy pattern can create a very stressed immune system, anxiety, or high blood pressure, and emotionally leave us feeling untrustworthy, under attack, and unable to trust others.

SOLUTION: Mirror the two sides that are jutting out, to make the point go away, or place a tapestry, nine red ribbons, or a 40-mm clear or AB crystal on a nine-inch red string hung in front of the point to offset its negative energy pattern. Furniture pieces such as square or rectangular dressers or end tables also have pointed corners and cutting ch'i. Try to turn or place them in a way that does not allow the point to cross through the area of the bed where the individual is sleeping. If the furniture cannot be moved, place some material or a scarf over the top to soften the point and make it disappear. You can also place or hang a small plant that cascades down over the offending point or jutting corner.

Mirrors The appropriate use of mirrors in the Feng Shui community has always been controversial, especially when it comes to the bedroom. Some say that mirrors are okay in the bedroom; others disagree. From a Black Hat Sect perspective, Professor Lin says that if the mirror is in front of your bed, it is good for your career or future; if the mirror is behind your bed, issues of the past can be released and resolved. I agree with using one or two mirrors in the bedroom, but only if they are properly placed and not hung in a way that cuts off anyone's head as they walk past them. This can create headaches of the physical and situational kind. If the mirror cuts you off at the throat, you may experience throat- and neck-related problems.

If you have trouble speaking up for yourself in life, work, or relationships, or in talking with your doctors about your treatment plan, check your mirrors. Also make sure, whenever possible, they do not directly reflect the bed, especially during sleep time. This is because the bedroom is a Yin room. Mirrors tend to amplify and double a space, creating a very Yang energy in the bedroom. This can increase anxiety and insomnia. Mirrors can also contribute to magnifying and multiplying weakening and ch'i-depleting EMFs that may exist in your bedroom. Mirrors don't discriminate; they reflect what they see. If they are reflecting a very sick person who has tons of medication on his or her night table, or is hooked up to an IV, it's going to double that image *and that energy.* So be very mindful of how, why, and where you are using mirrors, and check very carefully what they are reflecting.

SOLUTION: Move the mirror and instead hang on the wall or over the dresser a piece of artwork that has color and depth. If you cannot move a particular mirror, one way to work around this is to have some motif or design actually painted onto parts of the mirror, or to drape some fabric around the frame of the mirror to cut down on the actual amount of mirror that shows. In addition, hang a brass wind chime on the ceiling at the midpoint between the mirror and the bed it is reflecting; this will transcendentally disperse some of the amplified energy, if needed.

Color This is a very important factor when we are assessing a bedroom. It affects what we do both consciously and unconsciously, because it directly influences the choices we make in life, and the people, places, things, and opportunities to which we are drawn. It also makes us more susceptible to certain types of illnesses, and can play a critical role in our healing process. Color affects us wherever it is and in whatever form it comes to us in, but the color of our bedroom has a profound impact on our health because we sleep in the vibration of its color frequency all night. Color not only shapes our vibration but interpenetrates our internal energy system. This will be discussed in detail in chapters 7 and 8 and, along with it, the many ways to work with color as a tool for healing.

Here are a few quick tips to get you started thinking about color in general, and the color of your bedroom in particular. First, and most important, the color of your bedroom should not be white (or shades thereof). White gets its noncolor by deflecting all other colors, and doesn't allow ch'i to adhere to it, causing it to ricochet and inadvertently create a very hectic energy field. This isn't a good pattern in any room, but especially not in the bedroom during the sleep state. It can result in insomnia, anxiety, and interrupted and restless sleep. It can also exacerbate depression and slow down the recovery process.

It is all right to use white for trim, borders, and ceilings. Just make sure that no matter what color you are painting the walls, use a different color for the ceiling. When you paint the ceiling and walls the same color, you actually box the energy into a room, creating an energetic pattern that limits growth and stifles opportunities. If the bedroom is the same color as the rest of the house, it will create boundary issues and a lack of focus and definition in your life.

Soft pastel colors do well in the bedroom, such as light greens, lavenders, pinks, and dusty roses. Pink is great if the bedroom happens to fall into the area of the home that oversees the Relationship corner, because the color pink resonates to the same vibration as the Relationship gua. Peach is also a great bedroom color if you are looking to date more often or find a marriage partner. *But there is one important caveat about this suggestion:* If you do find someone and want to settle down with him or her, it's very important that you repaint the room, because this color also promotes philandering and infidelity. Peach works well for the search, but not for the long haul.

Try to stay away from muddy colors like brownish blacks, mustards, dull grays, and other colors that have no life force. Incorporate what you learn about the Chakras in chapters 7 and 8 to customize your colors based on what your energy system needs to heal or transform—especially if you are being challenged by a particular illness. Feel free to add a touch of red if you feel the room needs a boost or your healing process needs a catalyst to jump-start it a bit. Because red can be quite overstimulating, test your tolerance by using small amounts at a time; otherwise it can create a very active ch'i flow, great for a few nights of passionate lovemaking, but horrible for sleep afterward.

After all is said and done, the final decision regarding color has to be left to you. No matter what you read in this book or any other that makes reference to color—*you* have to like it. "A good Feng Shui color" that doesn't appeal to you is not good Feng Shui. Remember, color is only one way of adjusting your space. If color does not work for you, use some of the other Nine Basic Cures referred to in chapter 3.

Aesthetics and Decor No steadfast rule dictates what type of furniture will create the best Feng Shui. What's most important is that you like the furniture you have, and that it gives you a good feeling. If the furniture is old and run-down but you love it, well, that's good Feng Shui; if the furniture is old and run-down and you hate it, that's not good Feng Shui! The energy that it elicits from the object and from you is what your body and vibration responds to. Better for you to keep the old, ratty, comfortable chair that you love in your bedroom than the brand-new bedroom set your ex–in-laws gave you as a wedding present.

Feng Shui Design is more about placement and energy flow than about traditional design and aesthetics. Even if you do not have a large budget for refurbishing, once you understand the principles behind the remedies I've suggested, you will be able to design spaces based on the principles of energy versus aesthetics. Ask yourself these questions as you begin to create a healthy and healing bedroom: What is the history of the furniture and gifts that surround you when you are sleeping? What are your hidden feelings and issues regarding the gift and the person it came from? What is in your sight line? Hang your artwork or pictures and strive for balance, not symmetry. What are the messages your furnishings bring to your conscious and subconscious mind? After all that information is compiled, then decide accordingly what you want to keep and what you need to change. Remember, objects in your bedroom should give you both a direct *and* an indirect message of calm, peace, hope, and healing throughout the night.

In addition, the more you can create a nontoxic bedroom filled with natural materials and nonsynthetic fabrics, the healthier your room will be, and the more support you will get in your recovery process. We are just starting to understand the impact a toxic home has on the health of the individuals who reside there. We are learning how to use silks, natural cottons, full-spectrum lighting, floors and beds made of natural materials, and nontoxic paints as a way of creating a truly healthy environment.[7] As our level of awareness grows, so does our innate need for gravitating toward wholeness and a better, healthier way.

Analyzing Bedroom Layouts

Another important factor is the overall bedroom layout and the structural arrangement of the room. When houses or apartments are designed, the intention is to create good function and form. Now we are finding that some of these layouts, however aesthetically beautiful, harbor energy patterns that suppress health and exacerbate illness. Listed below are twelve different bedroom layouts that can make you ill, and solutions that can be applied to offset their negative effects and rebalance the energy.

Fig. 15. Bathrooms Inside Bedrooms

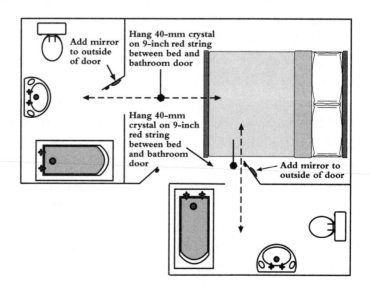

1. ***Bathroom Inside Bedroom*** This is a convenient and increasingly common arrangement in many master-bedroom suites. Having this arrangement doesn't automatically mean that there is going to be a problem. The two things that you first have to assess are (a) the positioning of the bed in relation to the bathroom door and (b) if any side of the bed or headboard is sharing a wall with the bathroom (see number 2, below).

Make sure that no part of your bed crosses paths with the bathroom opening or door (see Fig. 15). This is because the bathroom is considered unstable, due to all the constant water movement and drainage. The energy that the bathroom emits can destabilize the surrounding environments. The bedroom is a very Yin room, designed to create a space for sleep and healing. The bathroom creates an energy vortex that causes a suction effect (flushing) on the softer, more stable energy of the bedroom. This is particularly disruptive to health, sleeping, and pregnancies. When the ch'i is disrupted in that manner, it weakens the surrounding energy fields and, in turn, one's immune system, causing a host of unpredictable illnesses. So make sure your bed is not in a direct line with the doorway that leads to the bathroom. If the bathroom does not have a door, it can make matters even worse.

SOLUTION: Move the bed to another, more auspicious location or wall. If that is not possible, then keep the bathroom door shut and the toilet seat down, and hang a full-length mirror on the outside of the bathroom door, facing the bedroom. If the bathroom doesn't have a door, add one or hang a curtain of bamboo, beads, or, least preferable, cloth. In addition, hang a 40-mm clear crystal on a nine- or 18-inch red string from the ceiling between the bathroom door and the bed (see Fig. 15). Reinforce these cures with the Three Secrets Reinforcement Blessing (see chapter 9), visualizing that the mirror is deflecting the bathroom and all its unstable energy away, keeping your body, mind, and soul safe and clear. The crystal should be blessed also, visualizing its dispersing the unbalanced energy coming from the bathroom, before it affects the bedroom and your health.

2. ***Bedroom Shares an Outside Bathroom Wall*** This is a bathroom that

is not located directly inside the bedroom, but is a separate room on the same floor. It has a separate entranceway, but what makes it inauspicious is that it still shares a common wall with the bedroom. Of greatest concern is if the headboard or the bed is directly up against the shared wall. The headboard against the shared bathroom wall causes the most concern because the head area, the pituitary gland, and other body functions are weakened and made more susceptible to various illnesses.

Check to see if the wall behind the headboard shares a wall with a bathroom. If a bathroom is not directly behind the headboard, check to see if it is anywhere, right or left, along the opposite side of the shared bedroom wall. Because the body is made up mostly of water, during the sleep state it becomes highly susceptible and will resonate to the erratic flow of the unstable water in the bathroom. All flushing and draining of water add to the instability, throwing off the sensitive chemistry of the body. As the chemistry is altered, the different systems of the body are weakened, especially the circulatory, endocrine, and lymph systems, as well as overall biochemistry and all of the systems that carry waste. When these systems are compromised, they fall prey to a host of chronic, acute, and rare illnesses. This layout can also produce water-related illnesses such as sinusitis, allergies, edema, and the like.

SOLUTION: Move the bed immediately to another, safer wall. If the bed cannot be moved, place a securely fastened mirror on the wall above the bed or on the shared wall on the bathroom side. Reinforce with the Three Secrets Reinforcement Blessing (see chapter 9), visualizing that the bathroom and all its waste and erratic water flow will have no impact on you or anyone who occupies the bed. In addition, if the shared wall contains the toilet, also pour a mixture of Jusha and high-proof alcohol down the toilet to seal the toilet and the drain (see chapter 9).

3. **Bedroom Door Is Directly Opposite Bathroom Door** In this layout, the bedroom is directly opposite an exterior bathroom, with both the bedroom and bathroom doors facing each other. The instability from the bathroom ch'i will vibrationally spill over into the more balanced, stable Yin energy of the bedroom. This will throw off the healing energy that

needs to occur during the nighttime, and result in imbalances ranging from insomnia to frequent urination. Other dormant illnesses also may be triggered.

SOLUTION: Keep bathroom and bedroom doors closed. Hang a brass wind chime from the ceiling between the doors, and place a full-length mirror on the outside of the bathroom door (facing the bedroom) to deflect the energy from the bathroom away from the bedroom.

4. ***Bathroom Over Bedroom*** If you are living in a house or a duplex apartment that has several floors, check your floor plan to see if any of the bedrooms has a bathroom located directly above it. This arrangement can also be problematic because the instability of the bathroom energy is directly on top of the area where you are sleeping. During the sleep state the etheric body (the energy field that surrounds the physical body) rises upward as it replenishes and recharges itself. As it rises, in this particularly sensitive state it also moves closer to the bathroom's energy field above. That energy field, unstable and erratic, can adversely shape and alter the etheric realm around the body, weakening it as it slowly returns to the physical body. This weakens the strength and constitution of the physical body, making it more susceptible to illness and disease, resulting in a slower recovery process. In addition, the downward movement of the flushing and draining adds to the problem, as it moves waste in the direction of your physical body.

SOLUTION: Add four three- or four-inch rocks to the four corners of the bathroom, applying the Three Secrets Reinforcement Blessing (see chapter 9) while visualizing that all the movement energy is stabilized and not affecting the occupants in the bedroom below. Then apply a Jusha cure, mixing red cinnabar powder with strong alcohol and rice and pouring it down the toilet, flushing away all negativity and sickness ch'i (see chapter 9). Add one small, round three-inch mirror on the floor in each corner of the bedroom, with the mirror side facing up toward the bathroom above, and add a 50-mm crystal on a nine-inch red string to the center Health gua of the bedroom. Apply the Three Secrets

Reinforcement Blessing (see chapter 9), visualizing that the mirrors are reversing the impact of the bathroom above.

5. ***Bedroom Shares Wall with Kitchen*** This is another inauspicious arrangement, particularly if the headboard is up against the shared kitchen wall. The kitchen is a Fire-element room; i.e., a room with excessive Yang energy that has the elemental tendency to draw on the passive energy of the Yin bedroom, throwing it off balance and creating a weakened energy field in which to sleep and heal. With the stove at your back or at your head, this type of layout can also create various illnesses such as blood disorders, high blood pressure, heart disease, and strokes, and have you constantly feeling as though you are being attacked by others and you may find that you have many enemies at your back. This layout can also trigger bouts of anger and mood swings.

Any major appliances—stove, refrigerator, dishwasher, trash compactor, washer, or dryer—along the shared headboard wall are of special concern because of the high EMFs. Also, these appliances, which use water and discard waste, create a very similar energy field to the bedroom/bathroom layout described above. EMFs are not stopped or altered by divisive walls, unless they are lead-lined, and even that is not totally successful. Even if it isn't the headboard wall that is shared, estimate how far away the bed is from the back of the kitchen wall, and check whether that wall has any major appliances on it. If it is at least three yards away and there are no EMFs present, you are probably okay. Still, be sure to check for insomnia, anxiety, heart disease, rashes, temper flare-ups, arguments, and odd types of illness, as you are susceptible to them with this layout.

SOLUTION: Move the bed immediately! If you absolutely cannot do so, then paint the shared wall on the bedroom side blue or black. Add large pictures of water, waves, a swimming pond, or a snowy day. These colors and images can help offset, neutralize, and add cooling water to the Fire energy coming from the kitchen. Do not use mirrors over the bed on the shared wall, because mirrors can exacerbate and fan the Fire of the kitchen. Add a brass wind chime over the area where the head lies at night, and bless the offending wall and the bed with a mixture of cinnabar powder (Jusha) and alcohol (see chapter 9). Place a mirror on the opposite wall of the bed, symbolically pulling the bed off the shared kitchen wall. Apply the Three Secrets Reinforcement Blessing (see chapter 9) and visualize the water images cooling the Fire energies, or the mirror moving the bed away from harm. Test the EMF levels with a gauss meter and place the bed a safe distance away from higher readings (0–1.0 milligrams is the acceptable range for the bedroom).

6. ***Stove Is Directly Aligned Opposite a Bedroom Door*** If you have a kitchen that is directly opposite your bedroom, and both of the doors are facing each other and directly aligned, or you are in a position that allows you to see the stove, this layout can cause strange accidents and illnesses that are related to the blood.

SOLUTION: Move the bed out of alignment with the stove, hang a brass wind chime between the entranceways, and place a mirror on the outside of the bedroom door, blessing it with the Three Secrets Reinforcement Blessing (see chapter 9), visualizing that the stove and kitchen are being reflected away from the bedroom. You can also paint the bedroom door blue and hang pictures of cooling water scenes facing the kitchen and the stove. Keep the bedroom door closed; or, even better, if the kitchen has a door, keep that shut also. If it doesn't have a door, hang a bamboo curtain in the kitchen doorway.

7. ***Bedroom Door Opens to the Small End of the Room*** If the door into the bedroom opens to the *small end of the room* (see Fig. 16), the occupants of that space will feel psychologically limited, oppressed, and restricted. On a physical level, this door arrangement can contribute to neck and back problems, infertility, overall lethargy, depression, breathing problems, and difficult births. These problems can be exacerbated even further because it is also a bedroom.

SOLUTION: Switch the hinges to the other side of the door and its frame so that it opens to face the bigger part of the room. If you are not able to change the door's swing, then place a full-sized mirror on the wall you first see upon entering the room, at the head, throat, and upper-torso level. Although an octagonal mirror is considered the most auspicious, the mirror can be any type or shape you prefer. The mirror will reflect the larger side of the room, which the individual will immediately see upon entering the space. Also place a brass wind chime inside the entranceway to raise the ch'i and disperse any negative energy.

Fig. 16. Door Opens to the Small of a Room

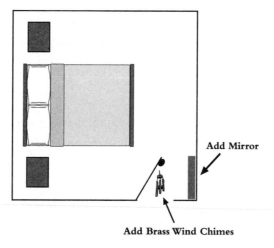

Add Mirror

Add Brass Wind Chimes

8. ***Bedroom Directly at End of Hallway*** Hallways or long corridors can pose a health risk in Feng Shui, because long tunnel-like structures tend to accelerate the ch'i. If your bedroom is at the long end of a hallway, with the ch'i directly facing the door to the bedroom, then you and your bedroom are being bombarded by this constant force of powerful ch'i. This type of arrangement can result in elevated anxiety levels, heart disease, high blood pressure, and problems with pregnancy and the reproductive organs. The hallway structure re-creates the fallopian tubes and can wear away at the delicate balance of the hormonal system, causing imbalances, mood swings, and difficult menopause. For women who are already pregnant, it can weaken the pregnancy and create difficult births, since the hallway also replicates the birth canal during deliveries. I've found that hallways ten feet or more in length tend to aggravate this

energetic dynamic more aggressively, but use your own judgment. If the hallway is shorter but it feels like a concern to you, adjust it anyway.

SOLUTION: Hang two brass wind chimes from the ceiling a couple of feet from either end of the hallway to break up the fast ch'i flow. Add bright lighting or raise the wattage in the hallway. Use several small throw rugs instead of one long runner on the floor to break up the ch'i; do the same with pictures and art on the walls, staggering them several feet apart. If the hallway has the space, place a statue or a heavy vase at the end of the hallway near the bedroom door. Most important, keep the bedroom door closed and hang a full-length mirror on the side of the door that faces the hallway. Bless all the adjustments with the Three Secrets Reinforcement Blessing (see chapter 9), and visualize all your intentions behind the cures. Remember that the mirror is being used to deflect all the quick-moving ch'i that is coming toward it.

Fig. 17. Bedroom Outside Main Door to House

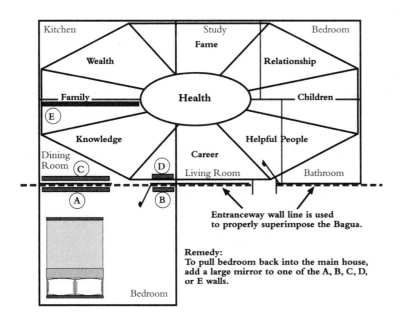

Entranceway wall line is used
to properly superimpose the Bagua.

Remedy:
To pull bedroom back into the main house, add a large mirror to one of the A, B, C, D, or E walls.

9. *Bedroom Outside Main Door to House* When your bedroom falls outside or behind the main door line of your house, the ch'i has a very difficult time reaching that room (see Fig. 17). In order to determine this, you need to look at your floor plan and superimpose the Bagua map over it. If you have a U- or L-shaped house, it's likely that certain rooms fall outside of the Bagua. If one of those rooms happens to be a bedroom, specifically a master bedroom, this can be a potential problem. First of all, if you are trying to heal or recover from an injury, operation, illness, or emotional setback, without a constant flow of healthy ch'i it will be much more difficult. Because the natural direction of ch'i is to move forward, it has a hard time circling around without being guided or prompted to do so. Another repercussion of having a bedroom outside the main door to the house is the increased possibility of infidelity, or being out of the house a lot, which can lead to separation and eventually divorce. This arrangement can also contribute to partners feeling distanced from each other, a loss of intimacy, or at least one partner not being available emotionally for the relationship. This bedroom layout can also lead to melancholy, depression, and lots of stressful marital problems. If you are single, it may make it very difficult to find a relationship or hold on to one.

SOLUTION: Find a symbolic way of connecting the bedroom with the other rooms of the house. Place matching vases in the bedroom and in a room outside the bedroom and in the main area of the house. Or, place one of two similar plants in the bedroom and the other in the room directly outside the bedroom. Then take a handful of soil from the bedroom plant and place it in the soil of the plant in the main area of the house, thereby symbolically "planting" the connection with the main house. Place a mirror on the shared internal wall (either side will do) and bless it with the Three Secrets Reinforcement Blessing (see chapter 9), visualizing that the mirror is reflecting the outside bedroom back into the main house. Augment the bedroom with appropriate adjustment items, adding a 40-mm clear crystal in the center Health gua of the room.

10. ***Bedroom in Basement or Below Entranceway Level*** In this type of
layout, we are assessing how the flow of ch'i is moving through the different areas where bedrooms and beds may be located. A layout that
places the bedroom below ground level is a situation where the ch'i has
to dip down to connect with the space. Air quality is poorer. Natural
light and life force are scarce. Windows are smaller and fewer, creating a
feeling that everything is pinched and happening "over your head and
out of reach." This constant reminder can create feelings of hopelessness
and ongoing frustration, and depress moods and immune systems. This
type of setup can also weaken constitutions and contribute to a host of
problems and illnesses.

SOLUTION: Design a bedroom that extensively increases life-force
energy. Add full-spectrum lightbulbs to all lamps. Grow live plants that
do not require much care (use plant lights). Hang pictures at eye level
that have depth of field, with scenes of nature and life-affirming art.
Install air purifiers with special HEPA filters that reduce 99.9 percent of
microorganisms, pollen, and dust particles. Add a large crystal in the center of the room, and use music, wind chimes, and uplifting essential aromatherapy oils (see chapter 10). Bring nature indoors as much as
possible. Place four three- or five-inch-round mirrors (using double-
stick tape) in all four corners of the ceiling, with the mirror side down
facing the bedroom. Bless the adjustment with the Three Secrets
Reinforcement Blessing (see chapter 9) while visualizing the bedroom
being lifted up above ground level, and all health and emotional challenges being lifted with it. Create a sensual, nurturing haven for you to
sleep and heal in.

11. ***Bedroom Over Garage*** When a house is built with an attached garage,
often the space above it is made into an extra room or a bedroom. A
room such as a bathroom or an occasional guest room is fine, but a bedroom that people sleep in regularly can be a problem and potentially a
hazard to their health. From a Feng Shui perspective, the garage is a very
unstable space, with cars moving in and out of it, putting the ch'i in con-

stant motion. This in itself is neither a good nor a bad thing, but because of the constant motion, the energy inside the garage has a hard time stabilizing. Combining an open space with constant movement creates a foundation that is weak and changeable. The garage is a very Yang space with much activity under a very Yin space, the bedroom. At night, when the body repairs itself, it needs stability and calm. It is hard to ground yourself when the foundation below you offers no support. From a health perspective, this instability can weaken one's core constitution, leading to a host of health-related problems. The instability can also affect aspects of your career, finances, and relationships.

More seriously, cars parked in the garage can also emit carbon monoxide and other fumes. Caution needs to be taken to avoid noxious fumes and poisoning. Even if the levels aren't dangerous, they aren't something you want to be breathing in, especially during your restful sleep state. In addition to that concern, parked cars also create a huge magnetic energy field. Magnetic (as well as electric) fields have been associated with certain types of cancers, nervous and sleep disorders, lethargy, and headaches.

SOLUTION: Move your bedroom from above the garage. If you can't do this, try to park your cars outside the garage and away from the bedrooms. Install a carbon monoxide detector in your bedroom for a quick alert of any leakage. Place a flat dielectric resonator (an EMF-reduction device) to offset some of the EMF impact from the magnetic field of the cars below. Hang a 50-mm crystal in the center of the room and use the Three Secrets Reinforcement Blessing (see chapter 9), visualizing that the crystal will create a protective field around the bodies of the individuals who sleep in that room, protecting them from any harm or health consequence. Add nine potted plants to the bedroom. In addition, hang a large brass wind chime in the Center Health gua of the garage and paint the garage brown and the bedroom green, with additional colors and objects that represent fruits and flowers. Together the colors will stabilize the environment, creating an image of a solid tree trunk below and a big, beautiful green tree above. Add colors, objects, or decals that represent fruit and flowers. Add four heavy weights, vases, rocks, or quartz crystals, one in each corner of the bedroom, to give weight to the bedroom and its energy field. Reinforce all cures with the Three Secrets Reinforcement Blessing (see chapter 9).

12. *Bed Crosses Bedroom Door* This is a *very* problematic layout leading to all types of financial, emotional, family, work, and health problems.

SOLUTION: See chapter 6, pages 191–92 for cures.

Remove or Reduce All Electrical Items from Bedroom Area

Electromagnetic "smog" is basically the out-gaussing of AC and DC electric and magnetic fields emitted by certain appliances and faulty wiring that leak into the environment.[8] These items range from home appliances like microwave ovens, TVs, clock radios, electric blankets, and the like to high-tension electrical wires and transformer boxes outdoors. EMFs are becoming a worldwide health concern, with studies showing that they can contribute to various types of cancers, tumor growths, blood disorders, and a host of autoimmune diseases. Countries like Germany and Switzerland have put the United States to shame with their truthful and progressive data on the effects of EMFs on our health today. Although we still know very little, what we do know now is that improving your Feng Shui in your home and your bedroom is *not* enough to ensure good health. To complete a thorough assessment of the health quotient of your home, we now need to include testing for levels of problematic EMFs.

Without knowing very much about EMFs, how to detect them, test for them, and what to do with them once you find them, you can still take several steps to reduce them. EMFs in your bedroom will have the greatest impact on your health, because it is during our sleep state that we are vibrationally most vulnerable to unhealthy energy patterns.

A good way of creating the healthiest space possible is to remove from the bedroom all plug-in clock radios, TVs, answering machines, and any electrical appliances that have AC/DC transformer boxes attached to the plug. If you can't do this, for whatever reason, at least try to move these things eight to twelve feet away from your body while lying in bed. Other EMF no-no's are electric blankets and water beds (in the case of the latter, the type with the heater attached underneath the bed itself). All these devices produce extremely high readings of EMFs and can have a dire impact on health and especially on the immune system, reproductive organs, heart, and pregnancies. Using a wind-up clock or walking to the other side of the room to shut off your radio may be somewhat inconvenient, but cancer and its ravaging effects can be a lot more inconvenient.

Closing Client Story

Here is a story told in the words of one of my clients:

Fifteen years ago I discovered a fairly large, hard swelling in my neck. A biopsy showed the lump to be benign, and for the next ten years I visited an acupuncturist on a regular basis, and under his care the lump softened and stabilized as a soft, invisible mass on my neck.

A little over five years ago the lump increased in size, and my acupuncturist recommended that I see a traditional doctor. Although a biopsy again showed it to be benign, the swelling had grown considerably, so I underwent a partial thyroidectomy in 1995. The next biopsy of the removed thyroid showed that in fact the lump was malignant, and I was put on a permanent dose of thyroid medication.

During this time I divorced and moved into my own house with my two children, who are both attending college. I loved my new house and especially my bedroom. My life and health had been going well, until a situation came along that was cause for concern.

As a follow-up to my past health situation, each year I have a full-body scan. These recent X rays showed a slight abnormality (a suspicious lump), and I had another follow-up ultrasound on September 7, 2000. The ultrasound confirmed the lump, and a biopsy was scheduled for September 18, 2000. On September 10, 2000, I began Week 1 of The Accelerated Path™ Feng Shui Consultant Training Program course with Nancy SantoPietro. On the third day of the course, Nancy introduced the class to the Chakra Color Breathing Meditation, in which we breathed in white light, visualizing it washing the insides of our bodies and carrying the impurities and imbalances out of our bodies through our fingertips and toes. She suggested we think of the colors associated with the specific Chakra colors. Because of my thyroid, I imagined that my throat was washed with light blue, which is the color of the fifth Chakra, also referred to as the Throat Chakra. I imagined pieces of concrete in my thyroid area were being broken up and washed out through my fingers. I also did this meditation in my hotel room each morning and night of the six-day class. In the middle of the week Nancy asked me if I had a lot of color in my home, because she felt that my energy field needed more color. On the last day of class I mentioned that I had been doing the color meditation throughout the week, and Nancy observed that my throat seemed to look energetically more open.

We also had a chance to work on our own floor plans in class. Nancy and another student, while reviewing my floor plan, noticed that in the layout of my bedroom, directly above my bed, there was a pipe jutting out from the wall that carried the sewage from my children's bathroom above. It went through not only the Health gua of my overall floor, but through the Children section of my bedroom. The Children section corresponds to the Throat Chakra and oversees the functioning of the thyroid. The pipe mimicked the exact shape of the esophagus and throat.

Besides many other changes that were recommended, the main suggestions to off-set this problem (the bed couldn't be moved) were to place two small lights on the floor, at the sides of the bed, shining up at the drain; then to place three-inch circular mirrors on the floor behind the bed, also facing up, reversing the flow and direction of the drain. It was also recommended that I perform the Jusha-and-liquor cure, dotting the drain three times while using the Ousting Mudra [see chapter 9], visualizing that my health would not be affected by the positioning of the drain. I also needed to place an EMF-reduction device underneath my bed and on the fuse box in my basement, which was directly under the head of my bed, to offset some of the negative effects of the electromagnetic energy being emitted from the fuse box.

On September 18, 2000, I went to the hospital for the scheduled biopsy. The first step was to repeat the ultrasound so that they could see the area of concern, but neither the doctor nor the technician could find anything abnormal. A second doctor who was called in for a consultation couldn't find anything, either. My lump was gone, and I left the hospital without even having to undergo the biopsy.

Almost ten months later, in July 2001, I returned to the hospital for another thyroid ultrasound. The results were again another clean slate! My doctors are still perplexed that they didn't find anything abnormal.

CHAPTER SIX

COMMON LAYOUTS

Floor Plans That Can Make You Sick

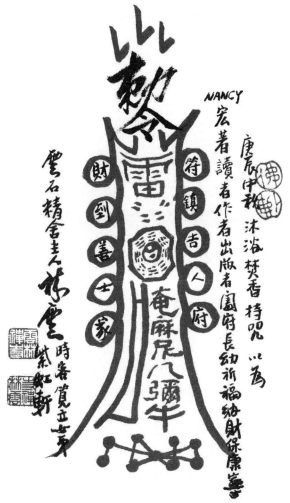

"Talisman."

CALLIGRAPHY BY H. H. PROFESSOR THOMAS LIN YUN RINPOCHE

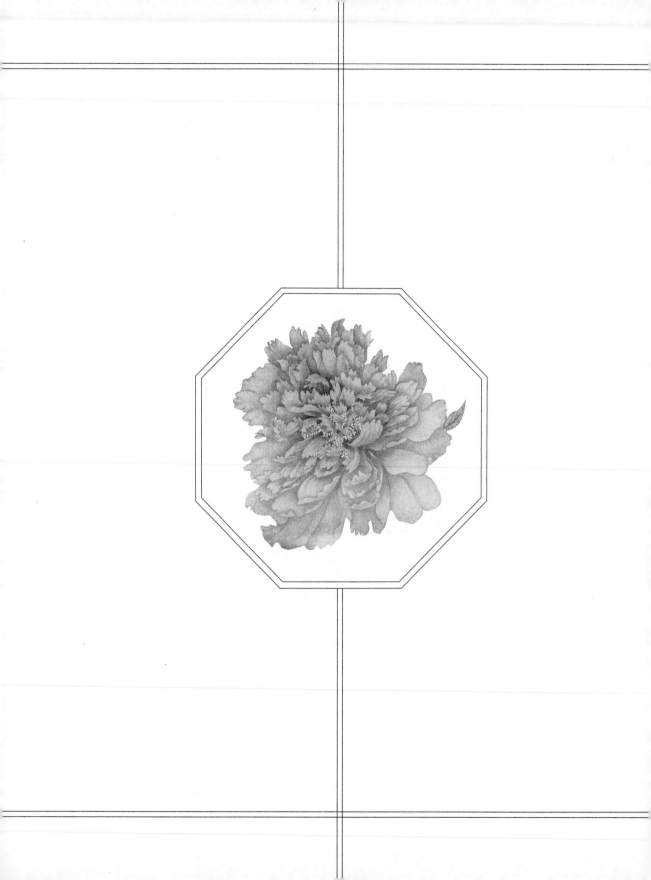

THE NEXT STEP on your home health journey is to revisit your floor plan and begin to work with it from a different angle. As you once again review it, see yourself this time, now switching from the wide-angle lens to the close-up lens, taking one more look at another set of details that may be contributing to the impact your home will have on your health.

Unless you can afford the luxury of designing and building your own home from scratch, the layouts of most homes are usually created and constructed long before we move in to the space. Even the most beautiful designs can come with a host of Feng Shui problems that can weaken immune systems or activate dormant miasms (energetic factors that can trigger illnesses and hereditary diseases). Analyzing our floor plans and hand-sketched drawings gives us the ability to interpret our Feng Shui and inner conflicts from another angle, a subconscious one.

Our subconscious mind plays a very big role in the Feng Shui of our spaces because of one simple fact: *Anything that has ever been created in our environment, and in the world around us, first had to exist inside someone's mind.* Whatever issues are happening in our lives, both the joys and the fears, are energetically embedded in our whole being and, over time, are transmitted by our DNA. Whatever we conceive or create, from a child to an architectural plan for a 30-story apartment building, is imbued with all of our energy patterns. Coded in all those various energy patterns are the emotional, spiritual, and physical undercurrents of our lives, and our experiences that were present during the act of creation.

When I am on a consultation and I see a recurring Feng Shui Design problem in the original design of the building, I can't help wondering what was happening in the architect's life during the time that he or she was creating the designs for the project! If this sounds somewhat far-fetched to you, I urge you to think again. Even at this stage of your introduction to Feng Shui principles, do you really think, knowing all you now know about energy, that we can separate our personal lives and thoughts from our work life? Most of us, including myself, would like to believe that we can, but the truth is, we can only really do it to a certain degree. And yes, I know being able to do your job well, over and over again, in spite of what's happening or not happening in your life, is the mark of a true professional, but from an energetic point of view, even if you are able to do a great job in spite of tremendous stress, you will still carry with you the vibrations of your experiences, especially the most current ones.

This double-sided sword is also what makes us good at what we do, because in bringing our whole self to a job, we also bring the qualities that make us special and unique.

From a Feng Shui perspective, we are greatly affected by the issues or state of mind that the architect, the designer, the painters, and even the Feng Shui consultant bring to their daily work. It is important to know and feel good about the people you allow to work in your home, because the impact of their energy will affect you and whoever lives there long after they are gone. A vibrational pattern is formed by the original blueprint and design that was created, and in turn this design sets into motion an energy that for years to come will be attracting tenants and owners who energetically resonate to some aspect of the original frequency. Your input and part in this equation is that you then get pulled karmically into the Feng Shui vibration of the space, and together you create your life and its circumstances.

The following are design layouts that are quite common and exist in everyday homes. Get your floor plan out (you have one by now, right?), and again, don't fret if some of these situations appear in your home, because there is a cure for everything that is listed. The solutions listed will empower you and give you the tools from a Feng Shui perspective to take action and assist your own cause.

Discovering these design problems places you among a very small percentage of people who now have this very valuable cutting-edge information. So try not to be alarmed by your discoveries, but instead be grateful for your blessed finds.

1. Entranceways

Let's imagine that you exercise regularly, eat healthily, and take really good care of your body. If you have a very small or obstructed windpipe, it doesn't matter how strong or beautiful your body is, because you won't be able to get enough air into it, which means you will not be able to live very long. The same thing applies to the entranceways of your home. If you cannot get the ch'i in, it doesn't matter how big your place is, or how beautifully it is designed. So it is very important to assess the type of entranceway that you have, and correct any limitations or imbalances.

The foyer or the entranceway into your home is also very important because it serves as a significant place of transition where you switch from your social persona to your private life. Its space helps you change hats and let your hair down at the end of a long day.

A. ***Ideal Entranceway*** With an ideal entranceway, the door opens to the largest part of the room, is expansive, well lit, and colorful, has life force, no clutter, reflects the individuals who live there (books, artwork, etc.), and is welcoming. A combination of these variables will help keep the energy flowing and the ch'i abundant and healthy.

B. ***Entranceways with Contrary Doors That Open to the Small of a Room*** These are entranceways that have doors contrary to the flow of the room. Instead of opening to the larger part of the space or foyer, they open onto the closest wall on its side. This type of entranceway squeezes the ch'i flow, causing neck, shoulder, spine, and back problems. Headaches and other head-related ailments, both physical and emotional, are also common with this type of entranceway. It can also make you feel like you are swimming against the current or that life is an uphill battle (see Fig. 16).

SOLUTION: Reverse the door by switching the hinges to the other side of the door and its frame, so that it opens to face the largest part of the room or foyer. If this cannot be done, place a full-size mirror on the wall closest to the door swing. Make sure that the mirror is as close to the door as you can get it, and that it does not cut off the top of the head or the throat of anyone who lives there. Add a brass wind chime with a wind tag that can be activated by the opening of the door, over the entranceway. Bless with the Three Secrets Reinforcement Blessing (see chapter 9).

C. **_Entranceways with Contrary Doors That Open Out Instead of In_**
Doors that open out toward you, or open inside out toward the house or a room, siphon off the ch'i of a space (see Fig. 18). When a door opens out, it pulls the energy away from the space, keeping the ch'i from coming inside. This is commonly found with doors that are either screened or that lead to a porch. When you see this layout, quite often a solid internal door immediately follows that opens inward, helping the situation tremendously (but not curing it) by counteracting the ch'i and pulling it back in. When you don't have this type of built-in semi-remedy, the entranceway can affect your overall health, energy level, and breathing, and leave you feeling emotionally overwhelmed. It will also slow down business and romantic endeavors.

Fig. 18. Doors That Open Out

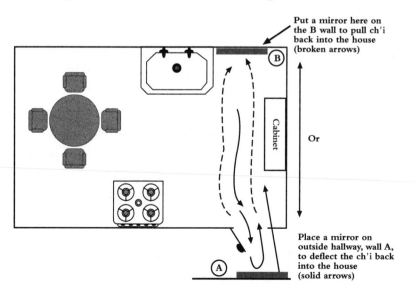

Put a mirror here on the B wall to pull ch'i back into the house (broken arrows)

Or

Place a mirror on outside hallway, wall A, to deflect the ch'i back into the house (solid arrows)

SOLUTION: Change the door and its hinges to the other side of the door frame so the ch'i can flow directly into the space. If this is impossible, hang a brass wind chime or brass bells between the two doors, and then place a brass wind chime overhead outside the first door to help contain the energy. Also, hang a Bagua or a circular mirror outside the apartment, house, or room directly opposite the door that opens out, with the mirror side facing into the house to deflect the ch'i back inside. Bless with the Three Secrets Reinforcement Blessing (see chapter 9).

D. ***Long, Narrow Entranceways, Foyers, and Hallways*** When the entranceway, hallway, or foyer is longer than approximately 12 feet, it can accelerate the ch'i, causing it to be forceful. This narrow layout can also constrict the flow of energy, triggering medical problems such as respiratory ailments, heart-related problems, anxiety-related feelings and ailments, and spine discomforts. In addition, from a Feng Shui perspective, entranceways that are long and narrow can replicate the birth canal. If you are trying to get pregnant, have a history of miscarriages, or are already pregnant, make sure that the area is clear and ch'i is moving freely, otherwise pregnancy- and delivery-related problems could result.

SOLUTION: Hang a brass wind chime overhead inside the doorway, positioning the chimes so that the opening of the door rings them upon entering the space. Add bright lighting and uplifting colors to raise the overall vibration of the ch'i. In addition, place decorative mirrors at head level along the length of the wall to double the small space. Place at least one mirror directly on the wall the occupant first sees upon entering the space. This should be a large mirror (e.g., approximately two feet across) that is placed as close to the door as possible without cutting off anyone's head or throat. *Three or more doors in close proximity to the hallway or foyer* create an arrangement that can be weakening to the bladder, kidneys, or intestines. If this layout appears in your space, add an additional brass wind chime from the ceiling at the midpoint where all the doors converge; if the hallway is very long, add two brass wind chimes, evenly spaced. Bless with the Three Secrets Reinforcement Blessing (see chapter 9).

E. ***Split-View Entranceway*** If, immediately upon entering a space, your view is split in half by a vertical wall that divides your line of sight, you have a split-view entranceway (see Fig. 19). This layout literally splits your vertical vision in half. One eye's view stops at the wall you are facing, and the other eye's view extends beyond into the open space. The effect is similar to having one eye nearsighted and the other farsighted. It creates an imbalance of the optic nerves and throws off the delicate neurochemical balance of the body. This dynamic, repeated every day over time, can cause emotional vertigo, problems with equilibrium, melancholia, and other anxiety- and health-related ailments.

Fig. 19. Entranceway with a Split View

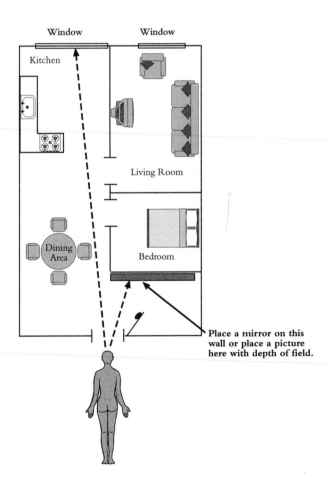

Place a mirror on this wall or place a picture here with depth of field.

SOLUTION: Hang a brass wind chime inside the door to disperse negative ch'i. Place a mirror or picture with depth of field on the obstructing wall to extend and rebalance the vision.

F. ***Brick-Wall Entranceway*** Upon entering this type of entranceway, the occupant faces a full wall that is relatively close to the front door, limiting and oppressing the ch'i flow (see Fig. 20). The ch'i is stopped and constricted in the most crucial of all mouths of the ch'i, the main entranceway. This sets the tone for the ch'i of the house, the occupants, and all the guests. If the layout is dark, dreary, or cluttered, the situation is compounded by a sense of hopelessness, defeat, and overall depression. Physically it can affect the head and neck area, causing confusion, headaches, and head-related health issues. Pregnancies are strained, and the ability to speak out and advocate for oneself is greatly diminished.

Fig. 20. "Brick Wall" Entranceway

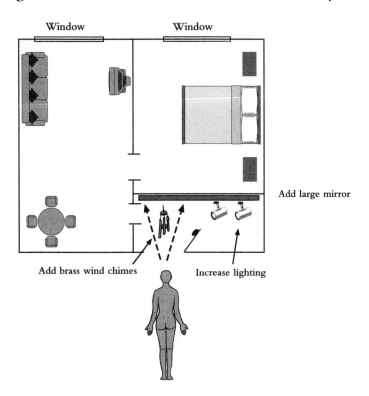

SOLUTION: Same as in situation E, above. Place a full-length mirror on the wall that is directly in front of you. Make sure the entryway is uplifting and well lit, and that it has color, life force (plants, fish tank), and a brass wind chime hanging from the ceiling directly inside the entranceway to help circulate the oppressive and stagnant ch'i. Reinforce with the Three Secrets Reinforcement Blessing (see chapter 9).

Please note that although all the entranceways listed above are referred to as the main entrances into a space, the same principles apply to all interior doors and entranceways.

2. The First Room That You See

After evaluating all the entranceways, the next very important aspect to consider while doing your home health assessment is the impact of the energy pattern elicited by the *first room* that you see upon entering. This room is a very important factor in how your ch'i is shaped and conditioned, because it is the first room that your being comes in contact with, every time you walk through that door, seven days a week, 365 days a year. By understanding the conditioning process that takes place over time, it is easy to see how the ch'i of that specific room can impact your personal ch'i and shape your life and your health.

There are two different ways in which the vibrational pattern of these rooms can influence ch'i. The pattern itself can either be ch'i-enriching or ch'i-depleting to the occupants of that space, resulting in various outcomes.

Ch'i-Enriching Rooms: Living Room, Den, Study, Foyer If the first room you see is a foyer, living room, study, or den, the ch'i will be uplifted and positive. The living room and den encourage relaxation. The study encourages reading, learning, and education. The foyer can be a wonderful place of transition, especially if it is uncluttered and welcoming, and reflects different pieces of the occupants' interests and personality (plaques on the wall, needlepoint pictures, a bookcase with favorite books displayed). This is where the occupants move from their social/work persona to their more personal and intimate home persona.

SOLUTION: No specific remedy is needed if these rooms are unclut-tered, bright, and pleasant to enter. Maintaining these rooms is crucial to keeping the ch'i strong and positive. Feel free to augment these spaces with Feng Shui crystals, wind chimes, fish tanks, plants, and your per-sonal, special touches that make you feel even better about being in the space. Remember to include the Three Secrets Reinforcement Blessing (see chapter 9).

Ch'i-Depleting Rooms: Bathroom, Kitchen, Bedroom, Game Room, Office These rooms create various vibrational patterns that deplete, nega-tively condition, and alter the occupant's ch'i, contributing to a variety of health issues.

If the bathroom is the first room you see upon entering your space, this may cause a general weakening of the bladder, kidneys, and urinary tract, possibly manifesting in infections, difficult or excessive urination, and prob-lems with the bowels (diarrhea or constipation). In addition to weakening the water elements in the body, this layout can also create problems with finances, wealth, and other abundance-related issues.

If the kitchen is the first room you see upon entering your home, you may be prone to digestive problems, stomach ulcers, and eating disorders such as obesity, anorexia, and bulimia. This type of layout shapes children's eating habits significantly. Emotionally this constant confrontation with the kitchen and all its Fire energy can elicit fits of anger and rage, especially if you are able to see the stove at first glance upon entering your home. In addi-tion, seeing the stove can cause fighting in the family, disharmony, and money-related problems. Physically, the visibility of the stove upon entering can also contribute to the occupants' developing a host of different blood disorders and heart disease.

If the bedroom is the first room you see, it can contribute to lethargy, depression, malaise, melancholy, a preoccupation with sex, and either hav-ing or not having a relationship.

If a game room or cardplaying room is the first room you see (this is usu-ally more common if the occupants enter through the basement), one's per-ception of life becomes more risky, filled with ups and downs in business and relationships. The occupants can experience financial and business successes and failures that fluctuate, creating periods of time when money is made, then lost. These inconsistencies can heighten anxiety levels that can trigger fluctuating conditions such as high blood pressure and high blood sugar levels, weight struggles, and the like. For children who spend lots of time in the game room during their formative years, their concepts of money are easily influenced and shaped by these energy patterns.

If you have a home office and it is the first room you see or have to walk past upon entering your house, your work ch'i will always be triggered. If you are a workaholic, your attention to your work will be constantly tugged at, with little or no separation of the rest of your life from business. Depending on the level of success or organization of your business, this trip past it every day can bring a host of stress-related illnesses.

SOLUTION: If any of these rooms have physical doors, close them immediately and place a full-length mirror on the outside of the door facing you. If the room does not have a door, add a beaded or bamboo curtain to the open entranceway, and a brass wind chime at the entranceway to the problematic room. Reinforce all adjustments and cures with the Three Secrets Reinforcement Blessing.

3. Room Positioning

Besides where a room is in the house and which interior factors it possesses, the positioning of that room in relation to other rooms in the house is crucial. Certain rooms, when positioned side by side or when sharing a common wall, can complement one another, creating mutually supportive energy. Other rooms, energetically speaking, when standing on their own are not problematic, but these same rooms, when positioned in a certain way next to one another, can factor in to a variety of serious health and personal problems.

In chapter 5 I listed eleven different combinations of bedroom/ bathroom, bedroom/kitchen, and other various bedroom layouts and how their room positioning can contribute to poor health and illness. The following list is of other problematic room positionings, specifically kitchen- and bathroom-connected layouts.

A. *Kitchen Runs Through the Center Meridian of Your Floor Plan*
The kitchen, by nature, is associated with the element of Fire. When the kitchen is located in the center of the house or apartment, it symbolically passes through the center of the body (see the Mystical Being material in chapter 4), which crosses the stomach, intestines, heart, and all related organs (see Fig. 21). In addition, that area overlaps with the Center gua, which represents Health on the Bagua. From an elemental perspective, this activates the Fire energy further, because the Center area element is Earth, and in the Five Element Theory, Earth is created by Fire. Fire in this gua can be too aggressive.

Fig. 21. Kitchen or Bathroom That Is Located in the Middle of the Floor Plan

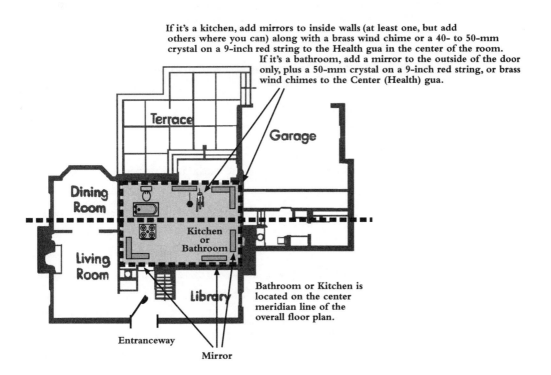

If it's a kitchen, add mirrors to inside walls (at least one, but add others where you can) along with a brass wind chime or a 40- to 50-mm crystal on a 9-inch red string to the Health gua in the center of the room.

If it's a bathroom, add a mirror to the outside of the door only, plus a 50-mm crystal on a 9-inch red string, or brass wind chimes to the Center (Health) gua.

Terrace

Garage

Dining Room

Living Room

Kitchen or Bathroom

Library

Bathroom or Kitchen is located on the center meridian line of the overall floor plan.

Entranceway

Mirror

SOLUTION: Hang in the center of the room a 40- or 50-mm clear crystal on a nine-inch red string, or a large brass wind chime, and add mirrors to as many walls as you can to diffuse the Fire energy. Bless with the Three Secrets Reinforcement Blessing (see chapter 9).

B. ***Bathroom Inside a Kitchen*** It is not uncommon in large older homes to see a kitchen contain a bathroom. Historically, plumbing often had to be confined to one area. And this also meant that the cooks and servants could confine their personal needs to one area. Nowadays we see this arrangement in smaller studio apartments where a bathroom door opens into the kitchen space itself, or very close to it. This layout is not problematic if the bathroom is simply next to or close by the kitchen, but is not directly in contact with it, or sharing a wall.

The kitchen and the bathroom have two distinctly different functions. The kitchen helps you to take in nourishment and food; the bathroom is a room of renewal, cleansing, and elimination. The vibrational patterns emitted by both rooms should not be placed in juxtaposition. Disagreements and disharmony within the family and personal relationships can be a result. Also, water-associated health problems can occur, such as bladder and digestive disorders and urinary tract infections.

SOLUTION: Keep the bathroom door closed at all times and the lid to the toilet shut, especially during flushing. In addition, secure a full-length mirror on the outside of the bathroom door, facing the kitchen. Place a brass wind chime between the bathroom door and the kitchen, and hang a 40- or 50-mm crystal on a nine-inch red string in the Health gua in the kitchen. Bless with the Three Secrets Reinforcement Blessing (see chapter 9).

C. ***Kitchen Shares a Wall with a Bathroom*** In this layout the bathroom and its entranceway are not in the kitchen but next to it. Problems arise when one of the bathroom walls is shared with one of the kitchen walls. Although this is a different arrangement from layout B, above, it still follows some of the same cure principles. What you are assessing for are the types of appliances against both sides of the shared wall. If you have a stove on one side of the wall and a bathtub or toilet on the other, that can become a big health problem, because these appliances have very different functions. Water puts out Fire, and the mix of elements will result in many health problems, as mentioned above.

In addition, this layout puts these two rooms into an aggressive elemental cycle in which the Water element of the bathroom will constantly be attacking and trying to put out the Fire element of the kitchen. This layout is very bad for health but excellent for creating anxiety, stress, friction, and digestive-tract disorders. It is also very weakening to one's finances.

SOLUTION: Paint the shared wall green (green is the color of the element of wood, which, when added, puts the Water and Fire elements in more conducive, nonaggressive order), hang a mirror on either side of the common wall, and hang a brass wind chime over the stove. Bless with the Three Secrets Reinforcement Blessing (see chapter 9).

D. **Kitchen Shares the Headboard Wall with the Bedroom** See chapter 5, pages 154–55, for details and cures.

E. **Bathroom Is Located in the Center of the Overall Floor Plan** The unstable energy of the bathroom superimposed over the Health gua of the overall floor plan can cause much instability regarding Wealth- and Health-related issues (see Fig. 21). In addition, having the bathroom in this gua can be disastrous to all things connected with finances, employment, and wealth. Water vibrates to the same frequency as money; therefore, when the water is unstable, so are the finances. Financial stress is often the underpinning to many health-related issues. The bathroom is the room where we do our eliminating, and in this layout it sits directly in the Health gua.

SOLUTION: Place a brass wind chime in the center of the bathroom ceiling, and place four heavily weighted objects, such as a terra-cotta vase, a large quartz crystal, or a four- or five-inch garden stone in each corner of the bathroom to offset the instability. Traditional Black Hat Sect teachings also recommend that you place a full-length mirror on the outside of the bathroom door. Bless with the Three Secrets Reinforcement Blessing (see chapter 9).

F. **Bathroom Is Over a Front Door or Entryway** Since the front-door entryway is the mouth of the ch'i, it needs to be as unobstructed—physically as well as energetically—as possible. When a bathroom is above that entryway in a two-story house, it can alter and disrupt otherwise healthy ch'i when it enters a space. The instability of the moving water also compromises everyone's energy field that passes under it. This inconsistent flow can upset good health and lead to missed opportunities and money loss. The risk of diseases of the blood and lymphatic system can also be increased.

SOLUTION: Place a brass wind chime in the center of the bathroom, and four heavy rocks or weights, one in each corner of the room. Add a three-inch circular mirror to the ceiling directly above the toilet or on the inside of the toilet lid, with the mirror side facing the water. (Keep the lid closed.) In the entryway under the bathroom, hang a brass wind chime or two bamboo flutes (see Fig. 14 for proper positioning of flutes) in the area of the ceiling that would be under the bathroom floor. Apply the Blessed Rice Cure (see chapter 9). Bless all adjustments with the Three Secrets Reinforcement Blessing (see chaper 9).

G. **Bathroom in Any Gua** Check all the bathrooms in your home and identify which guas they are located in. Although the bathroom obviously has to go somewhere, certain bathroom placements will create more life- and health-related problems than others. Bathrooms that fall in the Center, Relationship, Fame, Wealth, and Career guas need to be adjusted. If you are building or reconstructing a house, try to have the bathroom out of the above areas and, if possible, in between guas.

- **Bathroom in Center Gua of a Room.** See section E, above.

- **Bathroom in Relationship Gua.** Since water resonates to the emotions, this placement creates an unstable environment for emotional relationships and issues. The Relationship gua also oversees all of the body's organs, especially the stomach. A weakened flow of the unstable ch'i in this area will affect all health issues pertaining to these areas in the body.

SOLUTION: Add four weights to the corners and a 40-mm pink or clear faceted crystal to the center of the room. Augment the Relationship corner of the bathroom with wind chimes or, preferably, with a healthy, growing plant. Bless with the Three Secrets Reinforcement Blessing (see chapter 9).

- **Bathroom in Fame Gua.** This can create a lot of chaos because Fire is the main element in the Fame area, and Water puts out Fire. Fame, reputation, and one's overall ability to maintain and sustain success will be thwarted. In addition, the Fame gua oversees the eyes and our ability to see things clearly. Having unstable water in that area is like having water constantly thrown in one's eyes. This can lead to a lot of crying and feelings of disempowerment and failure.

SOLUTION: Paint the bathroom green or blue (this adds the mitigating color and Wood element to help put both the Fire and Water elements in a conducive order). Add a 40-mm clear crystal in the center of the room and four weights in the corners, and augment the Fame gua in the room with brighter lights, nine red candles (remember to light them), nine potted plants, or a large mirror. Bless with the Three Secrets Reinforcement Blessing (see chapter 9).

- **Bathroom in Wealth Gua.** This can create major financial drains and problems. This placement can also weaken all aspects related to the bones, spine, and pelvic area.

SOLUTION: Paint the bathroom purple or in shades of lavender. Add four weights to the corners and a 50-mm crystal to the center on a nine-inch red string. Augment the Wealth area of the room with a brass wind chime. Place a small, round five-inch mirror on the ceiling directly over the toilet, mirror side down. Place a long mirror on the outside of the bathroom door. Bless with the Three Secrets Reinforcement Blessing (see chapter 9).

- *Bathroom in Career Gua.* The corresponding element in the Career gua is Water. Again, water resonates to the same vibration as money, causing a major destabilization in the area of Career. The Career gua oversees all issues having to do with the ear, both physically and metaphorically. Any imbalances in this area can affect any or all of these concerns.

    SOLUTION: Place a rock in each corner and a brass wind chime in the center of the ceiling. Add nine small potted plants to the inside of the bathroom, preferably in white-colored pots. Bless with the Three Secrets Reinforcement Blessing (see chapter 9).

H. *Bathroom at End of a Long Hallway* Hallways in Feng Shui are like the veins and arteries in our bodies, connecting rooms and locations as well as different aspects of our lives. The same hallways can also replicate the passageway into the bladder, and the fallopian tubes, which lead to the uterus. If the hallway is longer than 12 feet, it will automatically pick up speed and accelerate the ch'i as it travels down the corridor. If there is a door at the end of that corridor that leads directly into a bedroom or a bathroom, certain health problems can arise from this layout. (The bedroom/long hallway layout has already been discussed in chapter 5.) When the bathroom is at the end of the corridor, problems with the bladder, kidneys, pregnancy, the labor process, and overall health can erupt.

    SOLUTION: Keep the bathroom door closed, and hang a convex mirror at eye level to disperse the force of the ch'i and to symbolically widen the walls of the corridor, expanding the hallway. Hang a brass wind chime in the center of the hallway. If the hallway is very long, hang two brass wind chimes, one at either end. Bless with the Three Secrets Reinforcement Blessing (see chapter 9).

4. Analyze the Shape of the Floor Plan

To begin the next step in assessing the Feng Shui health quotient of your home, you need to first take out your floor plan, take a step back, and switch your eye's camera to the wide-angle lens. In previous chapters I discussed the psychological importance of drawing your own floor plan, and how a trained eye can interpret its hidden unexpressed meaning. Here we begin to learn the connection between health problems and the shapes of floor plans. Six of the most common and problematic floor plans are discussed below.

A. ***The L-Shaped Floor Plan.*** In an L-shaped floor plan, one or more guas are missing, throwing some aspect of the occupant's life out of balance. First, find the entrance door, which will automatically give you the wall of the entranceway. This will help you determine what is missing and what adjustment to make.

  When placed correctly on this floor plan the Bagua indicates that the entire Relationship gua is missing, meaning the pocket of ch'i energy that supports relationships is weakened. This layout also weakens all issues having to do with marriage, mother, and all the organs of the body. In addition, part of the Fame, Center, and children guas are missing (see shaded areas in Fig. 22).

Fig. 22. L-Shaped Floor Plan

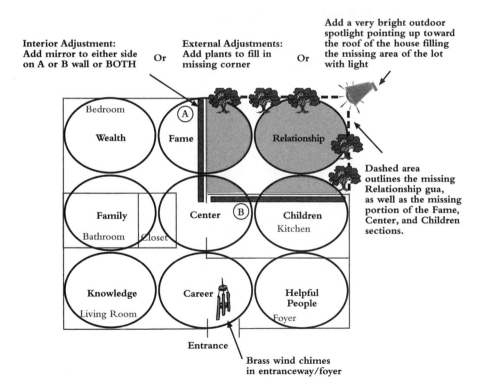

Interior Adjustment: Add mirror to either side on A or B wall or BOTH — Or — External Adjustments: Add plants to fill in missing corner — Or — Add a very bright outdoor spotlight pointing up toward the roof of the house filling the missing area of the lot with light

Dashed area outlines the missing Relationship gua, as well as the missing portion of the Fame, Center, and Children sections.

Brass wind chimes in entranceway/foyer

SOLUTION: Hang a brass wind chime over the entranceway. Then place a mirror indoors on either side of the L to fill out the missing piece, or, if possible, install a spotlight outside pointing up at the house, filling in the missing area with bright lights. Bless with the Three Secrets Reinforcement Blessing (see chapter 9).

Fig. 23. Rooms That Fall Outside of the Bagua (U-Shaped Floor Plan #1)

Add mirror to *either* the A, B, C, D, or E walls to pull the master bedroom back into the Bagua.

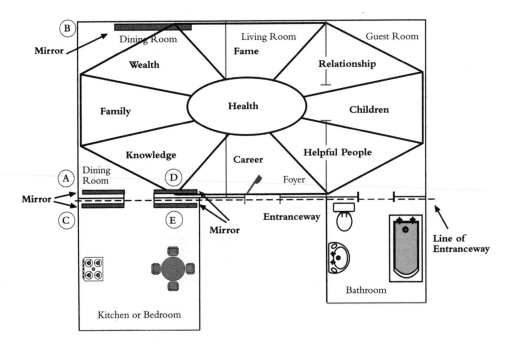

Fig. 23 shows another door location, which is creating a different set of concerns. The Bagua is superimposed over the floor plan based on the entryway door line. Notice that some rooms fall outside the Bagua.

SOLUTION: Add a mirror (to the indicated walls) to pull in the room outside the Bagua, especially if it is a kitchen or bedroom. Bless with the Three Secrets Reinforcement Blessing (see chapter 9). If the room happens to be a bathroom, office, or closet, leave it outside the Bagua unadjusted.

B. **Boot-Shaped Floor Plan.** Although the boot shape looks similar to the L-shaped floor plan, if you look closely at Fig. 24 you'll see that the ankle part is much thinner, and the shoe part much thicker, than in Fig. 22. This type of layout also contains missing guas. In this case the missing section falls in two guas—Fame and Relationship, which affect the eyes and organs and Fire element respectively. With a boot-shaped floor plan, you must first determine what area of the boot contains the toes. It's very

Fig. 24. Boot-Shaped Floor Plan

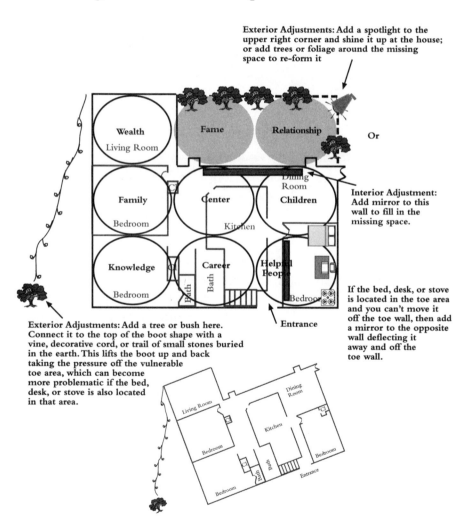

Exterior Adjustments: Add a spotlight to the upper right corner and shine it up at the house; or add trees or foliage around the missing space to re-form it

Or

Interior Adjustment: Add mirror to this wall to fill in the missing space.

If the bed, desk, or stove is located in the toe area and you can't move it off the toe wall, then add a mirror to the opposite wall deflecting it away and off the toe wall.

Exterior Adjustments: Add a tree or bush here. Connect it to the top of the boot shape with a vine, decorative cord, or trail of small stones buried in the earth. This lifts the boot up and back taking the pressure off the vulnerable toe area, which can become more problematic if the bed, desk, or stove is also located in that area.

Wealth — Living Room
Fame
Relationship
Family — Bedroom
Center — Kitchen
Children — Dining Room
Knowledge — Bedroom
Career — Bath
Helpful People — Bedroom
Entrance

Living Room
Dining Room
Kitchen
Bedroom
Bedroom
Bath
Bedroom
Entrance

important that you do not have a *bed, desk, or stove* placed against that wall if it happens to fall in the toe area of the boot. These three objects are the most important interior factors that you have in your home, in that they can affect your health, relationships, finances, and work opportunities. Having these objects in the toe areas can cause you to trip up in these different areas of your life. Problems can and will ensue.

SOLUTION: Move the bed, desk, or stove to another wall that is away from the toes. If you can't do this, place a mirror on an opposite wall to deflect the objects away from the offending "toe" wall. Also, if you have access to the outside grounds, connect a vine or a row of 108 stones from the top left-hand corner of the foot and connect to a large tree or bush at the lower left-hand corner of the foot. This adjustment symbolically tips the foot back and takes the pressure off the toe area. Bless with the Three Secrets Reinforcement Blessing (see chapter 9).

C. **Cleaver-Shaped Floor Plan.** This floor-plan shape can appear in individual rooms as well as in apartment buildings. There are different variations of the cleaver-shaped floor plan, but basically they all have a noticeable area that looks like a cleaver handle and another obvious part that looks like the blade. Again, it's important to identify where the blade side is, and make sure that the *bed, desk, and stove* are not up against that wall. Having those very crucial interior factors on the blade can cause serious health problems, including unexpected surgeries, relationship heartaches, and separations. In addition, the bed on the blade can cause various illnesses; the desk on the blade can cause firings, demotions, and declines in success; and the stove on the blade can cause financial losses.

SOLUTION: Move the furniture piece in question off the wall of the blade. If you cannot, then position a mirror so that it reflects the furniture piece and pulls it away from the blade wall. Add two bamboo flutes (see Fig. 14) on the blade wall over the bed, desk, or stove. Add a brass wind chime to the room, and bless all adjustments with the Three Secrets Reinforcement Blessing (see chapter 9).

Fig. 25. Cleaver-Shaped Floor Plan

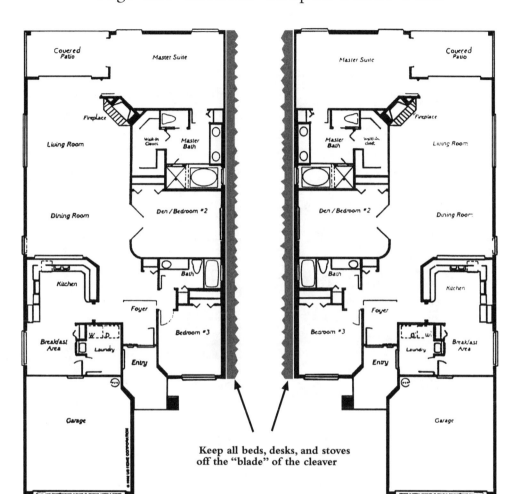

Keep all beds, desks, and stoves
off the "blade" of the cleaver

D. **Small Nose Floor Plan** This is also a very common layout in many
homes—even in big, beautiful ones. If the mouth of the ch'i is pinched,
obstructed, or narrow, it will choke off the energy going into a space.
This type of layout creates health problems related to the head, breathing, pregnancy, and the delivery process, resulting in problems connected
with the heart, blood pressure, and various illnesses.

Fig. 26. Small Nose Floor Plan

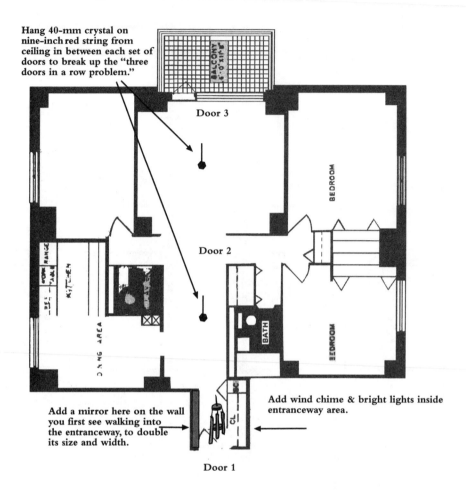

Hang 40-mm crystal on nine-inch red string from ceiling in between each set of doors to break up the "three doors in a row problem."

Door 3

BEDROOM

Door 2

KITCHEN

WORK TABLE

RANGE

OVEN

DINING AREA

BATH

BEDROOM

CL

Add a mirror here on the wall you first see walking into the entranceway, to double its size and width.

Add wind chime & bright lights inside entranceway area.

Door 1

SOLUTION: Make the entranceway as cheery and bright as possible. Add color, life force, and a brass wind chime to the area above the door to circulate the ch'i, and, most important, add a large mirror to double the size of the space. If the layout permits, place the mirror on the wall closest to the doorway upon entering to reflect the occupants as soon as they enter into the space. Reinforce with the Three Secrets Reinforcement Blessing (see chapter 9).

E. ***U-Shaped Floor Plan.*** Because the Bagua gets placed along the wall of the entryway, this type of layout creates a division of the floor plan that places two key sections of the house outside the Bagua (given that the entranceway is located in the inside of the U of the layout). Based on their size, those outside sections can contain more than one room. The types of rooms they are, and what functions they serve, will determine the severity of the impact on your life and health.

The two rooms that cause the most concern if they fall outside the Bagua in a U-shaped plan are the bedroom (especially the master bedroom) and the kitchen (see Fig. 23). Having the bedroom outside the main Bagua not only cuts it off from the rest of the house, but also creates energy patterns that can lead to one partner traveling a lot, one partner being emotionally absent, or to separation, divorce, or widowhood. If the kitchen is the room outside the Bagua, that design layout can discourage the occupants from coming together as a family, and can eventually contribute to a lot of family disharmony and fighting. Both of these situations are detrimental to one's emotional and spiritual well-being, and are common underpinnings to many stress-related illnesses and diseases.

Fig. 27. U-Shaped Floor Plan #2

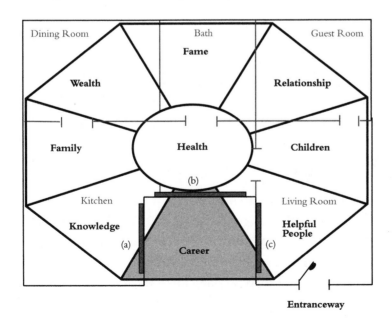

SOLUTION: Place a large mirror on either the A, B, or C wall to fill in the missing Career gua (see Fig. 27). In addition, add plants or bushes to the outside area in front of the missing Career gua to help fill the missing space. Bless the cures with the Three Secrets Reinforcement Blessing.

F. ***Missing Guas.*** When you are assessing the shape of your overall floor plan, check for negative space or missing guas (see Fig. 22). Complete shapes connote a sense of completion. That's why in Feng Shui we are always striving toward rounding off corners and squaring away choppy floor plans. If you have a floor plan that has negative space or missing guas, first determine which guas are missing, then check your Bagua map and see what the corresponding emotional and physical issues are. For example, if the Family section is missing, then all issues regarding the family or your creating a family may be energetically vulnerable. Since the Family gua also oversees the feet, all health-related concerns in that region might be compromised too.

SOLUTION: Augment the missing gua by filling in the missing space with mirrors on the connective wall, hanging a 40-mm crystal on a nine-inch red string in the window located in the missing area, or filling in missing sections of the space from the outside area with lights. Then go to all the smaller related areas in the individual rooms and raise the percentages by augmenting the smaller guas in the individual rooms to make up for the missing gua in the larger layout. Bless all intentions with the Three Secrets Reinforcement Blessing (see chapter 9).

5. Interior Factors of Major Concern

The most important factors to influence your well-being are the interior factors in your home. The Circle of Life chart in chapter 1 illustrates that although all aspects and elements of ch'i flow affect your life, the energy flow that has the most influence in shaping your everyday experiences is the one that is physically closest to you. The closest environment to you is the one in your home, and it is created mainly by the way you place your furniture and by the interior factors influencing your Feng Shui.

The number of interior factors in one's home (or office) can be enormous, ranging from obvious things such as the position of the bed to more obscure factors such as the type of artwork hanging over one's desk. It would be nearly impossible to name all possibilities here. The interior factors listed below are the ones I feel are common to many homes and that wreak the most havoc on one's health.

As you read the descriptions, you may notice that some are labeled simply "problematic to health or health-related issues," and do not state the specific health problems to which they contribute. The reason for this is that although Feng Shui has been around for thousands of years, we in the West are just now starting to understand its hidden influence on health and life issues. We are learning as we go along. Nothing has been carved in stone; all the data we need for a final conclusion is not in yet. Some things need to be left open-ended and fine-tuned to your personal interpretations. This is really true for much of the information given in this book. If you find that certain interior factors produce results different from those mentioned here, by all means follow your own findings. You have the final word on all you see and do.

A. *Bed, Desk, and Stove Placement.* As I have said before, the bed, desk, and stove are the three most important interior factors in your home. The bed oversees all issues regarding relationships and health; the desk oversees all issues pertaining to work, creativity, and opportunities; and the stove oversees matters related to finances, health, and wealth. All these issues may create the emotional underpinnings of a variety of stress-related health problems. **It's important that the bed, desk, and stove are in good condition, and that they are positioned to face the entryway of the room but are not in a direct line with it.**

Fig. 28. Proper Bed, Desk, and Stove Positioning

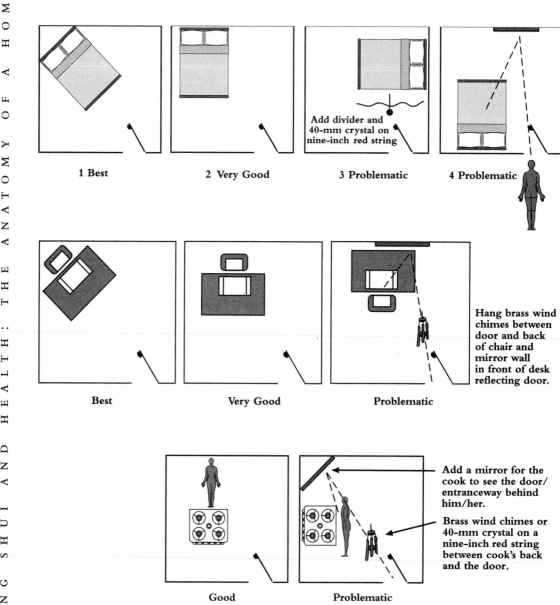

1 Best

2 Very Good

3 Problematic

Add divider and 40-mm crystal on nine-inch red string

4 Problematic

Best

Very Good

Problematic

Hang brass wind chimes between door and back of chair and mirror wall in front of desk reflecting door.

Good

Problematic

Add a mirror for the cook to see the door/entranceway behind him/her.

Brass wind chimes or 40-mm crystal on a nine-inch red string between cook's back and the door.

Chapter 5 discusses the importance of bed positioning, and illustrates the correct bed position in detail. Desk and stove placement follow the same basic principles. The most important thing is that when you are at your desk, you should be sitting in a position that has you facing the door.

The stove needs to follow the same logic and rules as those for the bed. The stove oversees the finances, different aspects of our health, and the time we allow ourselves for self-nurturing. It's important that when you are working at the stove that you are able to see the door into the room easily and clearly, without being in direct line with it. The orientation and location of the stove are also very crucial to one's health. Incorrect positioning can cause fires, heart disease, strange ailments, and illnesses of the blood.

If the stove is in the Fame area of the kitchen (example A), it can cause fires. If you can see the stove directly through and from the door to the kitchen or house, diseases of the blood could develop (example B). If your stove is located between two doors, it can compromise your health and may lead to arguments in the family and possible loss of money (example C).

SOLUTION FOR STOVE (A): Place a Bagua mirror across from the stove, in the Career area. The Career area oversees the element of Water, and water puts out Fire. Hang a brass wind chime in the cook's station where one stands, just in front of the cooking area of the stove. Place a mirror (regular or convex) in front of the stove or off to the side of it, so that while you are cooking you can effortlessly glance up and see what's going on behind you. Make sure when you place the mirror over the stove that the space is large enough to hold a mirror that, when hung, will not cut off any part of the cook's or the adult members of the household's heads. If the space is too small to accommodate the correct size mirror, use a convex mirror, instead. Do the Three Secrets Reinforcement Blessings (see chapter 9) on either mirror cures and, in particular, visualize that the mirror in the Career gua is pulling the stove off the Fame wall and into the Career/Water gua, and that the wind chime is breaking down any negative energies that may be affecting you from behind.

SOLUTION FOR STOVE (B): Try to create a visual divider between your vision and the stove. Add a bamboo curtain in the entranceway and hang a brass wind chime between the door and stove. Use the mirror cure from example A over the stove as indicated above. You do not have to put the mirror in the Career gua if the stove is not in the Fame gua.

REMEDY FOR STOVE (C): Place a brass wind chime in or over each entryway. Try to position two convex mirrors, one on either side of the stove area, so that at a glance the cook can see who is coming into the kitchen through either door. *Make sure you are able to see the door without being in direct line with it.* If you are in line with the door and you absolutely cannot move the stove, hang a brass wind chime over your head in front of the stove in between the door and the stove. The mirror should not cut off any of the cook's head. If it does, reposition the mirror elsewhere. Apply the Three Secrets Reinforcement Blessing (see chapter 9).

B. ***Staircases (too close to front door, spiral, and "mandarin duck").*** Staircases are the veins that carry the ch'i to different places in your house, so it's very important that they be well lit and free of obstructions. When you are assessing the impact of the staircases in your home, the two significant things that you want to look for are how close a staircase is to the front door, and if you have any spiral staircases.

Staircases (close to front door). If a staircase opening is facing or very close to the front door, the ch'i will be pulled in and siphoned up to the second floor, creating an imbalanced rush of ch'i moving toward the second floor and a lack of much-needed, softly flowing, meandering ch'i on the first floor. In addition, it will reverse the flow of ch'i and pull the energy out toward the front door, carrying along with it one's finances, energy, and any stable health. This layout throws off the natural flow of ch'i and creates a range of problems from money losses to neck, spine, back problems, and overall health problems.

SOLUTION: Place a 40- or 50-mm crystal on a nine-inch red string, or a brass wind chime, between the door and the staircase. If space allows, place a live plant at the bottom of the stairs and a large mirror at the first wall you face at the top of the steps to pull the ch'i back up. Apply the Three Secrets Reinforcement Blessing (see chapter 9).

Spiral staircases. Although a spiral staircase in your home may be quite charming and aesthetically pleasing, it can damage your health, especially if it is in the center of the house or in the Fame gua. If it is located in either place, a spiral staircase can contribute greatly to developing heart, circulatory, and coronary disease. Wherever they are, they act like corkscrews boring through your home.

If a spiral staircase already existed in your home before you moved in, that's a slightly better situation than if you installed one after you moved in, because the construction the space has to go through in order for the staircase to be installed also adds to the health and life-related upheaval issue.

SOLUTION: Place a bright light on the ceiling above the staircase, and hang a 40- or 50-mm crystal on a nine-inch red string next to it. Wrap something around the handrail to create energetic continuity, such as a string of white lights or artificial vines. If space allows, you can also set up several live plants at the bottom, with a light under the steps. Apply the Three Secrets Reinforcement Blessing (see chapter 9).

"Mandarin Duck" Stairs. "Mandarin duck" stairs are stairs that split and go in two different directions. One leads upstairs to a second floor, while the other leads to a lower level or basement. This layout is problematic because it splits the ch'i, dividing it in half as it enters the space and confusing its natural tendency to flow forward. This can cause discord among family members, between boss and employees, and among tenants. Separation, lots of fighting, and divorces are also common. Scattered thinking, fragmented energy, and a lack of focus can also occur.

SOLUTION: Hang a 40- or 50-mm crystal on a nine-inch red string and hang it halfway between the door and where the stairs begin. Place an adjustment item on the railing that somehow connects the handrail symbolically as it goes in two different directions, creating an energy field that's aligned and harmonious. Try winding silk vines or small white lights along the railing, or painting a design on it. If the length between the door and the steps is longer than the height of the tallest person in the house, then add a potted plant on the inside of the doorway. Bless with the Three Secrets Reinforcement Blessing (see chapter 9).

C. **Pillars, Posts, Columns, and Structural Corners.** These are the various structures that jut out, poke through, and take up little corners and pockets of space in your home or apartment. Their impact depends on what gua they show up in. Check your floor plan, then the Bagua map for detailed information.

Fig. 29. Structural Corners

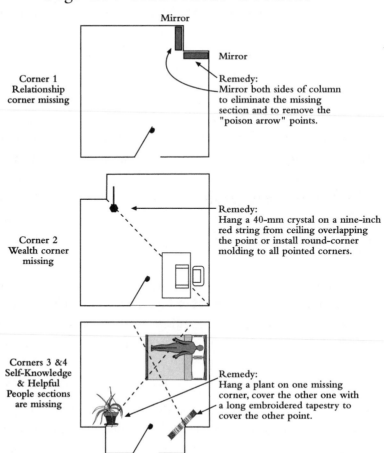

Corner 1
Relationship
corner missing

Mirror

Mirror

Remedy:
Mirror both sides of column to eliminate the missing section and to remove the "poison arrow" points.

Corner 2
Wealth corner
missing

Remedy:
Hang a 40-mm crystal on a nine-inch red string from ceiling overlapping the point or install round-corner molding to all pointed corners.

Corners 3 & 4
Self-Knowledge
& Helpful
People sections
are missing

Remedy:
Hang a plant on one missing corner, cover the other one with a long embroidered tapestry to cover the other point.

Pillars, posts, and columns create blocks and missing areas in a part of your home that is also connected to a part of your life and your body. If the column shows up in the Children area, then it is reducing the amount of ch'i and/or creating a block in that area that is not allowing the ch'i to flow through. This placement can negatively affect the children in the house, new creative ideas, and all issues having to do with the mouth. This means possible problems with the teeth, gums, throat, neck, and the ability to speak up for oneself.

SOLUTION: If the columns are square, round them out by wrapping them with sheets of non-image-distorting Mylar. Round out the 90-degree corners because they create "poison arrows," sharp corner points that send offending and attacking lines of energy (Fig. 29, Corner 3). Hang a plant and let the vines cover the points, or purchase round-corner molding from a lumberyard and nail it over the points. Use your own imagination and creativity to figure out a way to do this.

In addition, hang mirrors on all sides at eye level to create an opening through the solid mass, allowing the ch'i to flow through again. In addition to cutting out a piece of the gua and reducing energy flow, structural corners also create "poison arrows." Adjust them the same way as the posts and columns with mirrors that offset the cutting ch'i. Bless with the Three Secrets Reinforcement Blessing (see chapter 9).

D. ***Exposed Beams and Structural Overhangs.*** Energy moves by way of walls, around furniture, and over ceilings. The placement of these interior factors determines what the ch'i must navigate. When you have an exposed beam or a structural overhang of some sort, the ch'i will have to follow its shape and form. If the beam itself protrudes and drops down, so must the ch'i. As a result, the energy drops beneath the overhang and compresses the ch'i below. The energy of whoever spends a substantial amount of time under it will be affected.

If your bed, desk, or stove is under an exposed beam or structural overhang, the compressed energy will affect all things related to your health, relationships, finances, creativity, and work opportunities. In addition, if it is over the bed, the area of the body lying below the beam

FENG SHUI AND HEALTH: THE ANATOMY OF A HOME

will be affected. If the beam crosses over the foot of the bed, then the feet will be weakened and health problems affecting your feet, such as gout, sprained ankles, and the like, will be heightened. Symbolically, the ability to move forward in life will be thwarted too.

SOLUTION: Hang two bamboo flutes with red tassels on the beams in a diagonal position, with the mouthpieces facing down (see Fig. 14). It's most important that the flutes be made of bamboo, because the bamboo itself is actually part of the cure. The bamboo plant symbolizes strength as well as flexibility, enduring all types of weather. The knuckles on the bamboo actually serve to pump the ch'i upward, reversing the process of the compressed energy.

E. **Doors.** The doors are the main entryways through which the ch'i enters your home. They also reflect the mouths of the adults and the head area of the body. The combination of what they oversee makes them a very crucial interior factor. It is important that they are in good working order and that the areas around them are kept well lit and uncluttered. In addition, the way that they are positioned next to each other will dictate how they impact your health and your health-related issues.

"Bad bite" doors are doors that are in a hallway and are in juxtaposition. Although they are positioned opposite one another, *their door frames are not aligned with each other.* The more misaligned they are, the more problems you will have with your teeth, mouth, gums, temporomandibular joint (TMJ), back of neck, head, and your ability to speak up and voice your authority, especially where children are concerned. Fighting, separations, and divorces are also common results from the offenders

SOLUTION: Place a brass wind chime between the two doors, and hang a mirror on the wall side of each door that is cut off by the misaligned doors. You can identify this by standing in each doorway, facing the opposite door. Bless with the Three Secrets Reinforcement Blessing (see chapter 9).

"Big eats little" doors. This energetic pattern occurs when you have two doors facing each other and one of the doors is much larger than the other. Assess what rooms or areas in your home the doors lead to. Energetically speaking, the bigger door will always overpower the smaller door, so it is important that the smaller door doesn't lead to a master bedroom or a room with more significance than the room with the bigger door. This causes imbalances, and can choke off the ch'i just as it is entering the bedroom. Additional health problems can result if the smaller door is to a bedroom and the larger door is to a bathroom.

SOLUTION: Place a brass wind chime or hang a 40-mm crystal on a nine-inch red string on the ceiling between the doors. Hang a full-length mirror on the outside of the smaller door, which reflects the larger door, thus restoring a sense of balance, as now both doors are the same width. Bless with the Three Secrets Reinforcement Blessing (see chapter 9).

Too many doors. Too many doors in the same area causes energy leaks that can weaken the bladder and the kidneys. An excessiveness of doors (adult mouths) can also create a lot of adult fighting and difference of opinions among family members or co-workers.

SOLUTION: Hang a brass wind chime from the hallway ceiling in an approximate midpoint section where all the doors converge. If the hallway is rather long, hang two or more brass wind chimes accordingly.

Three or more doors in a row. This design layout occurs when you have three or more entranceways in succession. Each entryway may have a physical door or just an arched opening, but either way they are lined up so you can see directly through each of the doorways. This arrangement can be very weakening down the center line of the body, affecting the heart, circulatory system, digestion, and the like.

Fig. 30. Three or More Doors in a Row

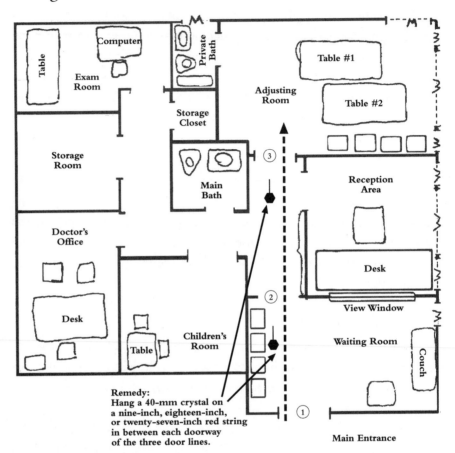

Remedy:
Hang a 40-mm crystal on a nine-inch, eighteen-inch, or twenty-seven-inch red string in between each doorway of the three door lines.

SOLUTION: From the ceiling of each room, hang one 40-mm crystal on a nine-inch, or a multiple of nine-inch (18, 27, or 36 inches), red string between each set of doors (two crystals in total). Bless with the Three Secrets Reinforcement Blessing (see chapter 9).

"Fighting" doors. This energetic dynamic occurs when you have two doors in your house that, if opened at the same time, could possibly bang against each other. Doors positioned this close to each other can create volatile situations, constant arguing with partners, bosses, employees, family members, children, and oneself. Life irrita-

tions and conflicts can prevail. Tooth, gum, and other mouth-related problems could also manifest, along with the inability to speak up for oneself.

SOLUTION: Cut a red ribbon or cord in multiplies of nine inches (18, 27, 36, 45, etc.) closest to the length that would allow you to tie each end to each opposing doorknob. Then take the ribbon and place it between your mattress and box spring under where you sleep. Before you place it under your mattress, apply the Three Secrets Reinforcement Blessing (see chapter 9) and visualize all the clashing problems being lifted and resolved for the higher good of all involved. Then sleep on it for nine nights. Take it out and tie each end to opposite doorknobs and repeat the Three Secrets, cutting the string in the middle. (Even better, leave the string hanging from each doorknob for the following 9, 18, or 27 days.)

Blocked or broken doors, or doors that no longer open. These types of doors can cause everything from breathing problems and headaches to depression and missed opportunities. The gua in which it is located will further determine which life and health issues it will affect.

SOLUTION: Unclutter and fix all blocked or broken doors. For doors that don't open and at one time did, place a three-inch circular mirror just above eye level on the inoperable door. Dot the door three times with a solution of Jusha and liquor (see chapter 9). Apply the Three Secrets Reinforcement Blessing (see chapter 9).

Entranceways and Doorways Without a Physical Door. These types of doorways are very common to kitchens, dining rooms, and living rooms. Not all rooms that are missing a physical door are problematic. The rooms that you need to be concerned about are the kitchen, bathroom, and bedrooms, especially the master suite.

Entranceways are the very important mouth of the ch'i and represent the adult voices. When a significant room does not have a physical door, in essence it's like having a mouth without a tongue. These rooms without a tongue can create financial- and health-related problems, with the bedroom being the greatest offender. In addition, a doorless bedroom can create separations, infidelities, and losses.

SOLUTION: Add a physical door, when practical. Otherwise, help the door grow a tongue and a voice by adding a brass wind chime, a 40-mm clear crystal on a nine-inch red string, and a bamboo curtain. You can also fix this problem by painting the door frame a vibrant contrasting color to give it visability and definition. Bless with the Three Secrets Reinforcement Blessing (see chapter 9).

Contrary doors are doors that open out instead of in, or doors that open opposite into a side wall instead of to the largest part of the room. Please refer to the section on entranceways at the beginning of this chapter for symptoms and remedies (see Fig. 18).

F. **Windows.** Windows are the secondary way that ch'i enters a space. Just as doors oversee the mouths of the adults, windows oversee the voices of children (or employees). Windows enable children to have a voice and develop their own healthy identity, separate from their parents. If the house has a ratio of three windows (or fewer) to every one door, this is a good balance of adult mouth to child voice and no major parent-child power struggles will emerge. The higher the ratio, the more potential for problems.

The windows also oversee the physical eyes and our ability to see things clearly. If the windows are broken or do not work properly, our eyes will suffer, and our need to see the truth in all situations will be hindered. Broken panes will trigger many little personal and business pains.

SOLUTION: Fix all broken panes and reopen jammed, old, or painted-shut windows. If windows cannot be repaired, place a circular three-inch mirror on the window, slightly above your eye level. If the window-to-door ratio is higher than optimal, add a 30-mm crystal on an 18- or 36-inch red string to several of the windows to rebalance the energy. If you really need to become clear on an important situation or truth in your life, take out the paper towels and glass cleaner and clean your windows. This can be an incredible Feng Shui ritual for clarity. Bless with the Three Secrets Reinforcement Blessing (see chapter 9).

G. *Skylights.* Although beautiful and often providing much-needed light, skylights can be problematic from a Feng Shui perspective, especially if they are installed after you have already moved into your house. In order for a skylight to be installed after the original roof has been completed, contractors have to create an opening in the ceiling. Any type of construction is considered surgery in Feng Shui because you are opening up a part of the house that oversees a life situation and a body area. Skylights are in the top portion of your home, so they also correspond with the head on the body.

SOLUTION: Caution has to be taken, auspicious days have to be picked, and a blessing and ritual of some sort performed in order to ensure a safe construction transformation. If a skylight has already been installed, hang from its center a 40- or 50-mm crystal from an 18- or 36-inch red string or, if wind is available, hang a brass wind chime. Bless with the Three Secrets Reinforcement Blessing (see chapter 9).

H. *Lighting, Color, and Life Force.* How much natural or incandescent light does your house or apartment have? Very often my clients tell me that they bought or rented their apartments during the evening, and never realized until after they moved in that there was no natural light! Lighting, along with plants, pets, fish tanks, and the like, create a life-force energy that permeates a space and supports its occupants when they are well, and also carries and feeds them when they are ill. A home with a rich life force offsets potential illness and nurtures and accelerates the recovery process.

Color is another type of energy and life force that can either increase an energy field or drain it and help create illness. Generally speaking, when a home is devoid of a certain amount of color, you will often find that the energy field is either erratic, creating high levels of anxiety, or without life force, contributing to occasional bouts of melancholy or frequent cycles of depression.

SOLUTION: Increase wattage on all bulbs, and add extra lamps and lighting fixtures. Use full-spectrum lightbulbs, which produce the closest light spectrum to natural sunlight. Try to avoid all usage of fluorescent and halogen lighting—both create very high EMFs and can alter the alpha-beta brain waves, affecting moods, concentration, and one's biochemistry. Add plants and plant lighting to keep your plants alive and flourishing. Depending on what gua they are placed in, they can increase and circulate the ch'i of that particular health and life area as well. Add color, soft, bold, or energizing. See chapters 7 and 8 on color and the Chakras for more specifics.

Closing Client Story

Kirstie's Story

Nancy was my therapist for five years, but we lost touch when she made Feng Shui her full-time practice. We reconnected when she started doing private sessions again, which she called Therapeutic Feng Shui. These sessions focused on specific issues and combined talk therapy, Chakra Psychology, color breathing and meditations, childhood processing, and past-life regression, coupled with Feng Shui adjustments and Transcendental Cures. We began working on issues around career and finances, adult ADD, and some long-standing health issues.

I have battled with interstitial cystitis for years; it's a chronic bladder irritation, or erosion of the bladder lining, that manifests in a very similar way to an ulcer. After so many years of suffering with it, I had pretty much resigned myself to the disease. The symptoms would come and go, but in recent years the symptoms had been somewhat subdued, although I had had a few recent bouts of discomfort. I was on various medications to control the pain, but I couldn't tell whether they were helping the condition or not. I was anxious to get off them because of their many side effects, which included fatigue and blurred vision.

At the time, Nancy and I had already had several weekly sessions where we were working on everything from my finances to my painful health conditions. It was then that I decided to schedule another Feng Shui consultation with her, in which she would come over and visit my loft apartment once again. The focus for this appointment was to review and change some of the original adjustments we had made a few years pre-

viously, before we lost touch, and to support the current issues we were now working on through the Chakras.

She recommended specific things that really helped with ADD, as well as making my space more pleasing to the eye. One part of her recommendations involved my dining room table, which was not only sitting in the center of my Health gua; but when she superimposed the Mystical Being, the table also fell into the area that oversaw my bladder. We moved the table slightly on a diagonal. Then, to break up the preponderance of wood that I had in that same area (a wooden floor and a wooden table), she suggested placing a rug under the table. Having an excessive amount of the Wood element in the Health and Bladder area can cause a lot of disruption because, in the Five Element cycle, Wood destroys Earth, and Earth is the ruling element of the Health gua. From a Feng Shui perspective, it could easily have created additional friction and pain to that area. Having the rug placed there was much easier on the eye, and created a sense of separation and division from the wood floor. The rug also broke up the visual field and created more visual serenity, a big advantage for persons with ADD.

We adjusted my candelabra so that it hung centered over the dining room table and created symmetry; the prior location had it off center from the table, further irritating that area. That table area was constantly cluttered with tons of mail, paper, and bills. Nancy pointed out that the area oversaw my bladder, and that the clutter only exacerbated the symptoms. The clutter also contributed to my scatteredness and my ADD, so part of my Feng Shui assignment was to clean it up and keep it cleared. We moved my desk and turned it around so that when I worked I was facing the entrance of my space. We also angled my small computer table so that it ran parallel to the dining room table, again to assist in reducing some of the environmental triggers of my ADD.

A few weeks after the consultation, I had a severe bladder attack that landed me in the emergency room. I had been working on a special assignment at work that had aggravated my medical condition, and I was eating and drinking things that I knew weren't good for me. My bladder felt constantly irritated, and the pain was becoming excruciating. Once again my search for relief intensified, but the pain remained relentless—it was constant and chronic. I had been working with a nutritionist who put me on a very strict diet specifically for the condition. It helped keep the pain at bay, but it was very hard to maintain.

In our next therapy session, Nancy drew a body over my floor plan and again I saw that my dining room table that we had angled was directly over the area that rep-

resented my pelvis and bladder. She said she wasn't surprised I was having problems in that area. She suggested that all the changes we had made in that area might have caused the symptoms to come to the surface. She then made some additional recommendations and reminded me to keep the table free of clutter when it wasn't being used. She also suggested that I create an altar of sorts, to keep on the table as we were working with the disease and the pain it brought.

I had several structural columns in my bedroom, and my bureau had a sharp edge that jutted out and cut across the pelvic area of my body when I slept. So I hot-glued eucalyptus leaves to soften all the edges and diffuse the cutting ch'i.

When I related my story to a friend, she looked up my symptoms in a book and suggested that part of the trouble might be fibroids, so I decided to check it out. Not only did I have six fibroids, but one of them was the size of a baseball and was sitting on top of my bladder! I scheduled an operation as soon as I could, had the fibroids removed, and have felt much better since. The most amazing thing now is that after all the Feng Shui adjustments and Chakra work I did that focused on my second center (where my fibroids were), I now respond positively to medication that previously I wasn't able to tolerate and that never really seemed to help.

It took three months from the time Nancy visited my loft to the time that I felt great relief. Since the fibroids were removed, my general health has improved greatly. Stress and bad eating habits cause my symptoms to flare up, but now I can control and manage them. I wish the symptoms would disappear altogether, but this is the next best thing.

THE CHAKRAS AND FENG SHUI

The Colors of Medicine

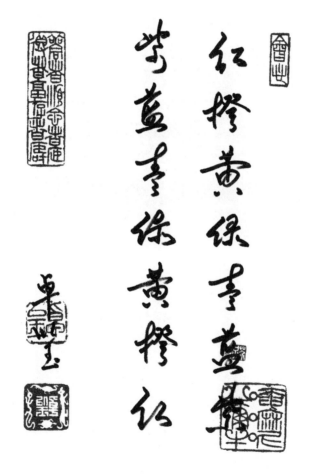

"The Seven Colors of the Rainbow/Chakras."

CALLIGRAPHY BY DR. CATHERINE YI-YU CHO WOO

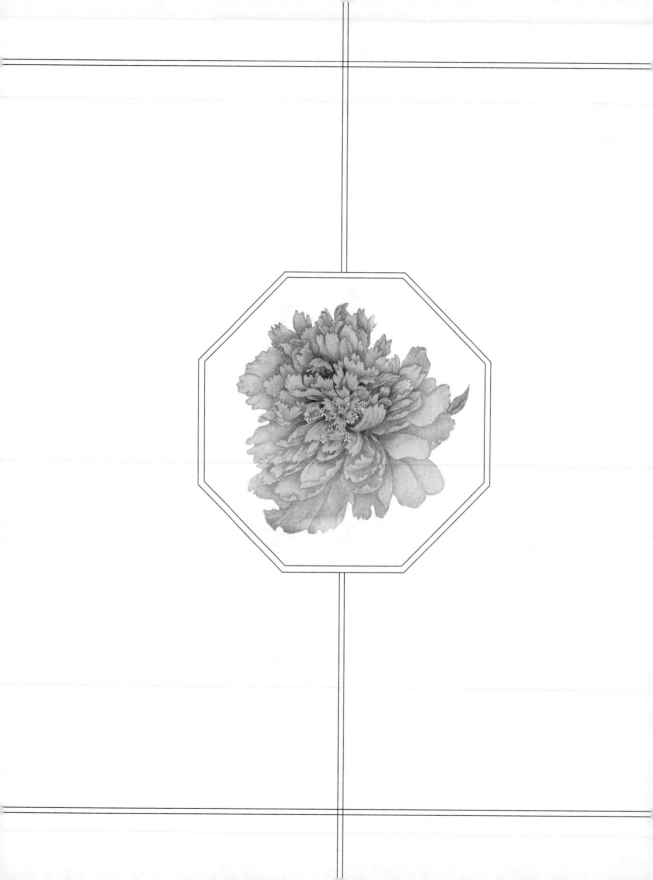

WHAT ARE THE CHAKRAS?

THE WORD *CHAKRA* is from Sanskrit, and means "spinning wheels" or "wheels of light." The Chakras are spiritual energy centers in the body and around it, and they act like little invisible computer centers, each storing various information and an energy force that relate specifically to the individual and the different areas of his or her life. Also very important, each Chakra resonates to a different color, vibration, and musical note. Although there are seven main Chakras, plus one above the top of the head, some sources say we have up to 144. For our purposes, and as they relate to my experience and teachings, we will be addressing the eight major Chakras and their four minor ones, twelve in all. Although all of the Chakras interpenetrate both the physical and ethereal bodies, seven technically exist in the body, one exists six inches above the top of your head, and one exists in the palm of each hand and on the sole of each foot. These energy centers are invisible to the untrained eye, but carry the spiritual DNA that will first shape, then determine, the type of people, places, lessons, and health-related issues you will draw to you in your life. When used in tandem with Feng Shui Design, they can create good health, accelerate your spiritual growth, and expedite one's healing process.

As I mentioned in the Introduction to this book, in the mid-1980s, years before I became a Feng Shui consultant, I was a psychotherapist in private practice. Although I was trained as a social worker, my area of expertise was the Chakra Energy System, and I practiced a form of therapy that I referred

Fig. 31. The Chakra Energy System

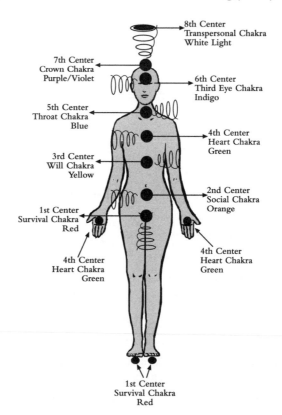

8th Center
Transpersonal Chakra
White Light

7th Center
Crown Chakra
Purple/Violet

6th Center
Third Eye Chakra
Indigo

5th Center
Throat Chakra
Blue

4th Center
Heart Chakra
Green

3rd Center
Will Chakra
Yellow

2nd Center
Social Chakra
Orange

1st Center
Survival Chakra
Red

4th Center
Heart Chakra
Green

4th Center
Heart Chakra
Green

1st Center
Survival Chakra
Red

to as Chakra Psychology. This approach allowed me to analyze my client's personal issues and challenges from the perspective of energy flow and where in the body that flow was blocked. It was a tremendous tool for assisting them in navigating through past life, childhood, and adult issues. Each Chakra holds certain corresponding links to emotional events and various life events. Zooming in on related Chakras helped me focus on what formed the underpinnings of certain current-day events.

I started practicing as a Feng Shui consultant in 1990, and after several years of doing both things, I decided to close my psychotherapy practice and work full-time as a Feng Shui consultant. In 1994, after thinking that my work in the field of Chakra Energy and psychotherapy was behind me, I had a very interesting experience during a Feng Shui consultation.

I was standing in the Wealth area in a client's home, discussing with her some of her issues that were related to her money concerns. As she was talking, I started to think to myself, "These sound just like Base Chakra issues to me." I didn't give it much more thought until a few weeks later when I was with another client. We were standing in the Fame gua of his home, discussing issues related to fears and energy blocks around visibility and success, and I thought, "This sounds just like the issues I used to work on with my therapy clients regarding their Crown Chakra issues."

After several months, much contemplation and meditation, and a little help from my guides, little by little I started to develop a system that combined both Feng Shui Design and the Chakra Energy System. Over the years I began referring to this system as Therapeutic Feng Shui™ and believe it to be spiritual technology at its best, for when I used the two systems in tandem, I saw it accelerate my clients' healing process. By addressing and approaching their health or personal problems from both the internal and external energy systems, I was watching them experience an accelerated healing. This approach focuses simultaneously on the ways a problem can manifest in the internal vibrational programming system, the Chakras, and on the ways that the problem has energetically been re-created in the external energy system, the Feng Shui of one's environment. I have found that when both systems are used together, it significantly increases the chances that the health problem or issue of concern will be transformed and a healing will occur. These two systems helped my clients to approach their issues or problems from both ends and to work toward permanently shifting the energy matrix that was holding the vibrational pattern of the issue in place.

Through my experience, I found that using just one system wasn't enough to ensure that the challenge, problem, or health issue wouldn't surface again, or re-create itself elsewhere. Many of my clients were very committed to their healing and worked very, very hard on their lives, only to find that changes happened slowly and in small increments. For all the years I was in psychotherapy practice and didn't know about Feng Shui, patients came into my office for 50 minutes per week to work on their lives, only to return to their homes and offices, where they spent most of their time. In not considering as a serious factor the impact that the Feng Shui of an environment may have had on their situations, they inadvertently short-circuited many of their efforts. In addition, many of my hardworking clients' recovery and healing processes were slowed down, if not thwarted altogether. And for the first few years of my Feng Shui practice, because we didn't address the Chakra-related issues, I discovered, in retrospect, that although my clients were making major shifts in their homes and their lives, they found that on occasion their unresolved or unaddressed emotional or spiritual underpinnings would resurface, or manifest in just another form.

As you begin to use these two systems together to address illness, keep in mind that energy shifts and that sometimes things get worse before they get better, especially during the "reordering" period. I developed this combined system to assist individuals who were experiencing life changes, difficulties, and unpredictable illnesses, and who were having a hard time understanding what might be happening to them energetically. Many of the personal changes we encounter can and will create various problems with our health. Along with the general anxiety that health challenges bring, in addition many people are experiencing job, relationship, identity, and residential upheavals. I have found that the two systems, when used in tandem, are powerful tools that are now a current-day necessity for facilitating smoother transitions in our accelerated and often chaotic new world.

Every Soul Has Two Main Responsibilities During Each Incarnation

Soul's purpose: The Soul's Purpose is the part of the incarnation that focuses on both the personal and karmic issues that the individual wants to work on and address during their lifetime. It consists of the more private issues that are about their own soul's growth, spirituality, unresolved hurts, unfinished business, former issues of the heart, and resolution of prior relationships, to name a few. These are also the circumstances that, once experienced, will move the soul farther along on its path toward enlightenment, helping to clear up any old karma or wrongdoings from prior lives. This is also the piece of the soul's existence that experiences new skills, genders, and people; it focuses on us having our own personal, emotional, spiritual, and physical esperiences.

Destiny: The other very important reason for the soul to incarnate is that it allows the individual to carry out a certain set of responsibilities and contribute some personal gifts to the evolutionary process, while he or she is here on the planet. These are the things that are preprogrammed into the vibration that constitutes the type of work the person will contribute or a particular role or mission he or she is here to see through and complete. This might be to become a schoolteacher, a mother of three, an artist, a politician, a massage therapist, or a lightworker, to name a few. Often some of the highest souls are the ones who come to the planet and quietly and humbly do service. Take a moment and think about the jobs that you could never see yourself doing in a hundred years. What comes to mind? Secretary? Garbage collector? Mortician? Token-booth clerk? Soldier? Some of the strongest and most spiritually evolved souls are the ones who chose to incarnate and take on work that most of us, somewhere, would never want to do. For, without those courageous souls, our lives would truly be unmanageable and in shambles. Imagine trying to get on a train without a ticket or living around garbage that has piled up since the beginning of time! These are the souls that come down without ego, willing to do the job that needs to be done so all the rest of us can tend to the business of what we came here to be.

Keep in mind that *preprogrammed* does not mean *absolute*. It just means that you've incarnated with a basic game plan, a life map to follow. But we live in a universe with its most important rule being that of *free will!* We start off with a structure and, depending on circumstance, timing, and various karmic influences that can and will change things, the initial plan often has to be modified and revised. In addition, the universal law of free will most times leave you with the final say on most things but not with absolute control.

The Body Is the Temple Where the Soul Resides While Here on Earth

Before your vibration incarnates into a human body it is basically a beam of white light in an ethereal state where it floats around and exists without any need for gravity. Once it is programmed and ready to incarnate and do service, it needs to energetically move into the vibration of the Earth's atmosphere and be weighted down, so it doesn't just float away. The way the universe helps ground the vibration or the white light is by giving it a physical body. The physical body houses the soul so that it can manifest all the things that were programmed into its vibration or white light before you incarnated.

All White Light Breaks Down into the Seven Colors of the Rainbow

When our individual strands of white light break down, they refract into the seven colors of the rainbow. You may recall in fifth-grade science class when your teacher placed a glass prism on the windowsill and let the sun pass through it. Do you remember what happened? The prism broke the light down into the seven colors of the visible light spectrum, or the rainbow.

When our soul's white-light vibration is placed inside a denser container such as our physical bodies, the surrounding structure breaks down the white light's molecular structure. As it scrambles to reorder itself, it naturally breaks down into its individual components or separate pockets of ch'i. These smaller pockets of energy vibrate to different frequencies, which also resonate to the seven main colors of the rainbow. Each pocket of color energy is a Chakra, and each Chakra oversees a grouping of specific issues that the soul is here to manifest.

THERE ARE MANY DIFFERENT COLOR SYSTEMS

As you start to explore the world of energy, you will begin to notice that many healing methods available to us utilize corresponding color systems. Each of these systems have their own specific approach to healing and can be utilized, depending on the need of the individual and the chosen treatment approach. Knowing that these various color systems work independently and interdependently gives you a much wider range of choices to work with. In addition, using two or more color systems at once (e.g., Feng Shui and the Chakras) for the same objective raises the odds that the combined color approaches will render a successful outcome. By learning how to use color not only aesthetically but also as a Transcendental Cure, you will be able to apply its healing abilities to help transform illness also.

Color and light therapy is now being utilized extensively as a "new" form of treatment for everything from seasonal affective disorder to vision and vision-related problems. Dr. Ray Lieberman, in his groundbreaking video, *Healing with Light and Color,* states that "we are just beginning to see the incredible healing powers of color." Studies have shown that color profoundly affects physiological systems. Dr. Lieberman suggests that the quickest way for the body to absorb most forms of color is through the visual cortex of the brain. The amazing thing about this is that although blood is constantly flowing through the body, only the passageway through the visual cortex in the back of the brain has all the blood in the body pass through its blood vessels regularly at approximately every two hours. So, approximately every two hours, this biological process exposes visual color to every cell, muscle, organ, and bone in your body! What we see in the form of color every day, through our eyes, influences and vibrationally shapes our physical bodies as well as our energetic bodies. This process, if used correctly, and as an adjunct medicine, can greatly affect how we understand, diagnose, and treat illness.

Each shade of color, or hue, like everything else has a unique vibrational pattern that it vibrates and resonates to. When the energetics of an environment are out of sync or the delicate balance of an individual's homeostasis is off, specific color can be applied as a "vibrational medicine" to help restore the vibrational imbalance in question. This is how the interplay between color and healing occurs. By applying the correct color combinations to the environment and through various color breathing methods, painting, and other color-cure techniques, you can help heal many aspects of your life and transform many illnesses.

Although there are many systems of color available for us to work with within Feng Shui and through other healing modalities, in this book we focus on the two main color systems that I work with extensively, the Chakra Energy System and Black Hat Sect Feng Shui Bagua. As you begin to work with the Chakra and Feng Shui color systems (as well as others), keep in mind that it is perfectly okay to work with the different color systems simultaneously. Each system has its own frequency module, and just the way FM radio waves and TV radio waves can both simultaneously exist in your home at the same time, so can various color frequencies and vibrational systems. So, feel free to use as many different color systems that appropriately apply to the illness or health concern you are addressing. The important thing to keep in mind is that you have a clear and conscious intention as to why you are using it, and for what reason. Make sure that every time you use color as a vibrational or transcendental cure, you bless it with the Three Secrets Reinforcement Blessings (see chapter 9) to enhance its effect; otherwise the color application would just act as aesthetic complement, and not necessarily a cure. Below is a chart of my exclusive energy color system that I use for diagnostic and treatment purposes. I have created this twofold combined system over the past several years after working with various clients, color applications, and energy systems. It has passed through many incarnations of my work, from psychotherapist to Feng Shui consultant, especially for you to receive its wisdom and gifts.

Fig. 32. Feng Shui and The Chakras©

Developed by Nancy SantoPietro

Connecting the Internal and External Energy Systems

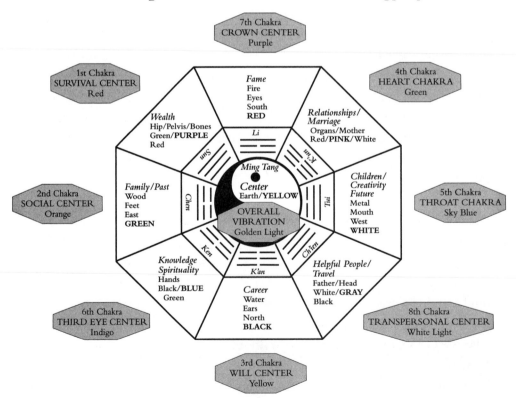

THE ANATOMY OF A CHAKRA

The Chakras are chock-full of valuable information and details that, once decoded, will provide you with a slew of data to help you assess the specific emotional, spiritual, and physical condition of the Chakra. The unveiled information will help you to navigate through the lesson, situation, or illness by working with the higher systems of energy that hold it in place.

We work with the Chakras as a tool for guidance and insight because the Chakras, through their matrix of energetic patterning, symbols, and color, bypass logical thought. Logical thought, although an important function of the rational mind, keeps us out of our heart-and-soul's inner wisdom and guidance.

Keep in mind that as you begin to develop your own style of interpreting symbolism, you will be enhancing your inner knowing and sharpening your intuitive skills. Besides the various attributes listed in the chart below, the

The Chakra Energy System, Feng Shui Guas, and Their Corresponding Factors

CHAKRA ENERGY CENTER	BODY LOCATION	FENG SHUI GUA	CHAKRA/FENG SHUI COLORS
Survival Center	base of spine	Wealth	red/purple
Social Center	2 inches below the navel	Family	orange/green
Will Center	solar plexus	Career	yellow/black
Heart Center	center of chest	Relationship	green/pink
Throat Center	throat	Children/Creativity	sky blue/white
Third Eye Center	between eyebrows	Knowledge	indigo/blue
Crown Center	top of head	Fame	purple/red
Transpersonal Center	6 inches above head	Helpful People/Travel	white light/gray
Overall Vibration	throughout body	Health	golden light/yellow

Chakras will also try to communicate information to you in many other ways. The ways that they will try to convey information to you will depend on your own particular style and language of intuition. The more ways that you get to know yourself, become authentic, and cultivate your ch'i, the more heightened your level of sensitivity will become and the clearer and more accurate the information you'll receive. As you learn to work more with the power of color, you are actually learning to interpret ch'i as it manifests in the form of color. Color as a metaphysical and/or transcendental cure provides objective, diagnostic information to help accelerate the healing process.

Remember, intuition and the Chakras go hand in hand; both are types of "spiritual muscles" and like all other muscles, if not used or exercised they will become flabby and eventually atrophy. But, the more you work with them over time (through meditation and Feng Shui), the more you will come to trust your insights and be comfortable with interpreting their messages.

The information that follows lists some of the main attributes of the Chakras and the many ways that you can interpret their message to you. In addition, the more you practice different Chakra meditations (especially the ones listed at the end of this chapter) the more you will clear out your blocks, strengthen your overall constitution, and help yourself create a life worth living.

EVERYTHING THAT EXISTS IN YOUR LIFE MUST FIRST PASS THROUGH YOUR CHAKRAS

In order for anything that has been programmed into your vibration to manifest while you are here on Earth, it must somehow pass or move through your Chakras. Your Chakras act as an energy conduit pulling information from the prelife plan, then creating a magnetic field around what needs to be pulled into your life, in order for specific manifestations to occur. This is a crucial step because anything, including an idea, inspiration, emotion, thought, or a physical ailment, must move from the etheric into the physical in order to manifest. All these things are processed through the Chakras because the Chakras turn spirit into matter, ideas into reality, and thoughts into action.

Each Chakra Has Its Own Set
of Characteristics

Each of the eight main Chakras (seven in the body, one above the top of your head) has a corresponding tone, rhythm, spirit guide, and its own style of intuition. Each one oversees certain body areas, organs, and gland functioning, as well as psychological, emotional, and health-related issues. The main characteristic that is so significant to your ability to live and transform illness is that each Chakra vibrates to the frequency of a color! As this chapter unfolds you will learn how to work with the power of color as a tool for healing.

By learning to work with the Chakras through awareness, meditation, and the Feng Shui Design system, we help them open up to their subtle energy fields. This keeps them flexible, loose, and responsive so the energy can flow through them, bringing with it all the life experiences that we are here to process. This helps them to further magnetize the people, places, and things that support the Soul's Purpose and Destiny, our two main reasons for incarnating. When we are ill or have a disease it is usually a sure indicator that the corresponding Chakra to that illness is blocked, overactive, under-active, or in need of some type of assistance.

ANCIENT WISDOM COMBINED: THE FENG SHUI GUAS AND THE CHAKRA ENERGY SYSTEM

1. The Survival Chakra/Wealth Gua

Your Birthright: A Life Filled with Abundance
When these centers are balanced, all flows well in your life, and you get to experience abundance as a natural birthright, because having the correct energy alignment places you in attunement with the universal flow of abundance. In that connection you make contact with the vibration and nurturing of Mother Earth, drawing on her energetic sustenance, and all that you need for a comfortable stay while here on the planet will be provided for.

The Survival Center The First Chakra is located at the base of your spine, and its energy pattern resonates to the color red. This center also has two smaller Chakra vortexes located in the soles of each foot. It oversees all issues that have to do with survival, such as your ability to take care of yourself, secure proper housing, and attend to your basic needs regarding food, work, and emergency situations. It oversees issues regarding money and your ability to follow through on projects and complete them. It's also our root center that provides the grounding energy needed to stay clear and focused in life. This center oversees all physical and health-related aspects of the genitals, blood, legs, knees, feet, and sexuality in relation to procreation. It also oversees all issues having to do with your mother and with you as a mother. When this center is *balanced,* you will feel rooted, able to follow through and complete simple tasks such as doing the laundry or cleaning the kitchen with relative ease. When balanced, it increases your confidence and helps you to feel secure in the way life needs to unfold. You are able to accept and generate abundance and feel at peace with your entitlement rights and issues. When this center is *underactive,* it can cause you to be overly dependent on others, to the point of codependency, and it creates a vulnerability that affects your ability to earn money and take care of yourself. When this center is *overactive,* you can easily fall into patterns of caring for everyone else's life but your own. This energy dynamic is common to individuals who have a lot of responsibilities and/or children to care for.

The Wealth Gua. This gua oversees finances and all the things that we perceive as connoting wealth, abundance, luck, and power. Shoring up this area will help strengthen your ability to draw on the power source that connects us with the abundant universal supply. The bones, hips, and pelvic area of the body are represented here, and its corresponding color is purple.

2. The Social Chakra/Family Gua

You Have Chosen Your Life and All the Players in It
As you start to understand the bigger picture of why you are here and why your soul chose to incarnate in your body, you can fully embrace the universal law that governs all of us, which is known as the law of free will. The spiritual law of free will states that you not only made the choice and had the

final say to incarnate, but you handpicked your parents, gender, race, religion, socioeconomic status, hair color, bone structure, sexual orientation, and birth location. You've also chosen your family of origin and many of the significant events in your life. With this in mind, you are gently reminded that you wrote the initial script, did the casting, and had the starring role in your own life story. It's a reminder that you are always in your own movie, and although sometimes your film gets spliced with pieces of film from the movies of others, your friends, your parents, and your partners all are in their own movies, too! This simple truth about your life can empower you and help you own all your important decisions, not so you can blame yourself for painful situations or unwanted illnesses, but to give you the opportunity to make choices, come to understand, heal, and transmute whatever you created. Life's circumstances bring lessons for your own soul's growth while here, helping you to fulfill your soul's purpose.

The Social Center. The Second Chakra is located approximately two inches below the navel, and its energy pattern resonates to the color orange. The energy in this center is very absorbent and collects information regarding your culture, family dynamics, and sense of who you are in the world. It oversees all issues related to how you feel about yourself and how you came to understand who you are through your early life's experiences. The Social Center is the Chakra where we come to define ourselves in relation to others. The way that this center eventually evolves results in the development of either clear and healthy personal boundaries or ones that are distorted and do not honor who we are and what we really need. This is the "feeling center" and stores most of our emotions and all things related to them. Because of the high level of sensitivity of this center, it often tends to be the area where we hold on to all our childhood issues and traumas ranging from abandonment to incest. All addictive behavior is stored here. Sexual energy, intimacy, and raw creative energy are activated from this Chakra. It is the Chakra that stores and relates to all sexual and intimacy issues regarding our adult partners. (The Survival Center oversees sexual issues related to procreation and self-care.) It oversees all physical and health issues related to the spleen, kidneys, lower intestines, ovaries, reproductive organs, and lower back. Issues, memories, and blocks related to the father are addressed and retained here.

When this Chakra is in *balance,* you will feel balanced emotionally and comfortable with who you are in the world with your partners, creativity, and emotions. When this center is *underactive,* you will tend to be shut down emotionally, cut off from your own feelings, or depressed; you might often feel lonely and have a difficult time accessing your creative energy or personal fire. You may be cut off from your sexual feelings and not desire intimacy or lovemaking. When this center is *overactive,* you might tend to overcompensate, trying to control the energy through behaviors like excessive eating or frequent sex. Although you may see yourself as extremely empathetic, you might often find that you inappropriately take on the emotional states of others. With an *overactive second center,* you might use your sense of passion and creativity for pleasing others rather than for self-benefit or self-gratification.

The Family Gua. This section overseas all issues related to your ancestors, family history, support groups, religious congregations, co-workers, and inner circle of friends that you consider to be like family to you. Because it represents the past, all family secrets and childhood issues are stored here. Physically it oversees the feet and the ability to move forward in life and away from the past. Its corresponding color is green.

3. The Will Chakra/Career Gua
Taking Action, Moving Forward

The Will Center oversees all the energy and inner drive you need to move forward and take control of your life. It's the energetic motivator that provides the impetus and the fuel to move you constantly forward toward your highest good and help keep you on the road of your path and life's work. It's the vehicle, but not the driver (you are), that keeps you going and keeps you from stagnating.

The Will Center. The Third Chakra is located in the solar plexus area, in the front of your torso where the rib cage parts, and its energy pattern resonates to the color yellow. This center oversees the energy force behind our will and our ability to focus our energy on a specific direction or purpose. This is the center where our intellectual mind and our ability to reason is stored: where we can step back and take an objective look at a situation using rational thinking. From this center we analyze, process, and distribute our thoughts, form new ideas, and tap in to our own willpower. It is this center that activates our drive and moves us through our goals, getting us over inertia and stagnant energy or through challenging times. Although most emotions are stored in the Second Center, this is the center that holds on to all our fears, anger, and guilt. This center also oversees health issues related to our stomach, intestines, liver, gallbladder, pancreas, adrenals, and middle back.

When this center is in *balance,* you will feel focused and able to move forward with your life's goals, plans, and challenges. When this center is *overactive,* you can find yourself very willful, controlling, and manipulative, always trying to get your way by misusing your powerful will to force things to happen. When this center is *underactive,* you will tend not to have much energy and to lack the ability to get going on projects, follow through on goals, and think clearly. It will feel like you have lost your sense of personal power and your sense of having presence in the world. Fear and guilt will dictate your actions and nonactions. When this energetic drop-off occurs, you will often find yourself acting powerless, feeling like a victim without any sense of healthy discipline or willpower.

The Career Gua. This section of the Bagua oversees all matters concerning your career, hobbies, or personal skills that are unique to your work and journey during this incarnation. This section addresses the type of work you do, or that you aspire to do. This can range from raising a family to volunteering at a local hospital. This gua oversees the ears on the body, and corresponds to the color black.

4. The Heart Chakra/Relationship Gua

Opening to Unconditional Love

The energy shift of the Heart Chakra is probably the most important and pivotal one on the planet, and for most individuals who are trying to heal their lives, because, in a genuine effort toward healing illness, we first have to open our hearts and explore the core wounds and pains we have stored in there so deeply. By doing this, we begin to move into the healing process of forgiveness, releasing others and ourselves from the prison of blame. This crucial piece of our healing process gently moves us, and society, away from our learned sense of conditional love to our newfound understanding of compassion and unconditional love for self and others.

The Heart Center. The Fourth Chakra is located in the center of the chest, and its energy pattern resonates to the color green. This is the center from which we are able to feel love for ourselves and unconditional love for others. From this center we connect with the oneness that unites us with all living things, including other people, nature, the animal and mineral kingdoms, the Universe, and God. This is the center from which we derive our true personal power, security, confidence, and trust. This Chakra is also the energy center from which all healing is generated, for it connects directly to the two minor Chakras located in the palms of the hands. In health, it oversees the upper back, chest, shoulders, arms, hands, lungs, and all physical and emotional issues of the heart.

When this center is in **balance,** you will have a strong sense of who you are and what your connection is to the bigger picture of humankind. When you are connected in this center, you will be able to be more empathetic, kind, and unconditionally loving. You will have a healthy, well-balanced sense of your personal power and will be able to use it to empower others and create good, instead of misusing it. When this center becomes **underactive,** it becomes harder for you to connect with yourself, others, a higher power, and with the world as a whole. An underactive Heart Chakra can create a feeling of insecurity, a lack of confidence, and a void regarding a sense of spirituality in your life. You will also have a hard time connecting with a family system or community. When this center is **overactive,** you can lose a sense of yourself and merge with others, overidentifying with other people's problems and life situations. This can scatter you and create a feeling that you are "all over the place," with no "personal center" to return home to. You can find yourself taking others in, in the name of love, saving all the stray animals, and bypassing loving yourself.

The Relationship/Marriage Gua. The Relationship/Marriage area on the Bagua represents the marriage ch'i in your life, and your ability to draw on a successful, loving partnership. It also oversees other types of intimate relationships including dating, living together, and nontraditional unions such as gay and lesbian partnerships. This section also oversees all issues related to all the organs of the body, and to mother issues. It resonates to the color pink.

5. The Throat Chakra/Children-Creativity Gua

The Inner Child and the Outer Adult

This energy combination creates an ongoing mirror for us throughout our lives, as we bob in and out of our unresolved adolescent issues and watch how we re-create them over and over again in our adult lives and our adult relationships. This dynamic is a constant reminder that we are always pieces of who we were, but transformed into higher levels of energy and light. Honor and bless every stage of life, for we will keep re-creating all our lessons until our adult self finally resolves them or eventually gets them right.

The Throat Center. The Fifth Chakra is located in the center of the throat and resonates to the color sky blue. This is the center of our identity, and oversees our sense of who we are as individuals. This Chakra's issues of identity differ from the "Who am I?" issues of the Second Chakra (the Social Center). This energy center is considered to be an active one, and it doesn't collect information as the Social Center (which is a passive center) does, but instead shows the world who we are by acting it out through our worldly outward identity. This center is the higher vibration of the Second Center; it oversees communication and all aspects and types of creativity, from artwork to writing. All issues related to authority, teaching, leadership, and organizational and managerial skills are generated from this center. Anything having to do with the voice, whether singing or speaking, also comes from here. This center oversees adolescence (the Second Chakra, our Social Center, stores our earlier childhood issues), because it is during that period in our lives that we form our identity and show it to the world. This energy center oversees all physical and health-related issues regarding the thyroid throat, neck, mouth, teeth, jaw, and gums.

When this Chakra is in **balance,** you are able to assert comfortably and advocate for yourself—express your creative skills, oversee projects and responsibilities with ease, and have a healthy sense of who you are in the world. When in balance you are fully able to access your "inner authority" and seek it less from outside sources. When this center is **underactive,** you will find difficulty expressing your feelings, creativity, or sense of identity. You may withhold and repress your adult self, while feeling stuck in issues and respond to life in ways that still reflect your adolescence. When this center is **overactive,** you may find yourself very rigid and responding to situations in an authoritative way, trying to control other people and situations by being demanding and bossy and by giving orders. You may find yourself acting like everyone's parent, wanting all things your way.

The Children / Creativity Gua. This section of the Bagua represents the future and all the life-affirming things that we give birth to. It represents all your future ascendants, your children, issues regarding fertility and all aspects of creativity, including new thoughts, ideas, projects, art, writing, and inspirations. The area of Children also represents physical issues related to the mouth, teeth, gums, throat, and ability to speak up and advocate for yourself. This gua resonates to the corresponding color of white and shades thereof.

6. The Third Eye Chakra/Knowledge Gua
Honoring Your Truth: Knowledge That Empowers

This energetic combination holds the space for us to look at life, using truth as our knowledge base. It's the vibrational pattern that encourages us to see all people, situations, and realities for what they are and not for what our minds and feelings want them to be. It reminds us that honesty connects us to the pristine knowledge of the soul, which will continually set us free as it reminds us to seek, live, and come to know our own truth.

The Third Eye Center. The Sixth Chakra is located on the forehead, directly between the eyebrows, and its energy pattern resonates to the color indigo. This center is called the "third eye" because it is the vertical eye in your mind that oversees all aspects of your intuition. Your intuition is the part of you that is your sacred sense of inner knowing and is sometimes referred to as having a "hunch" or a "gut feeling" about something. It's the part of you that knows something without fully understanding why or how you know. The Third Eye is the center of truth, because it is from this center that you can intuitively see an outcome or a particular situation for what it's worth, without attaching your emotional needs or wants to it (the emotional center is the Second Chakra). This center oversees all physical or health issues relating to the eyes, ears, and nose.

When this center is *balanced,* you become more open to receiving intuitive information and trust your gut feelings about people, places, and things. When this center is *underactive,* you can often mistrust your own feelings and seek out other people's opinions as truth for your own life. Oftentimes you'll play down or block your own self-knowing, so that you don't have to deal with the truth of a situation. When this center is too *overactive,* you may find yourself trying to deal with everything through the use of your intuition only, relying on your intuition often inappropriately as a means of avoiding the real world. Although you may find yourself to be very insightful, you tend not to function very well in the physical realm. Often this type of excessive Sixth Center energy creates problematic behavior such as chronic lateness, or spacy and unfocused energy. In addition, you might find that you will have a difficult time maintaining and staying connected with your physical body and may become distracted from certain responsibilities.

Knowledge/Spirituality Gua. This area oversees all types of self-knowledge and the ways that we are able to enrich our understanding of who we are. This gua brings us our opportunities and lessons for spiritual growth, our energy force for meditation, self-reflection, and prayer. It supports all aspects of educational pursuits ranging from academic to informal and non-traditional types of study. It represents the hands on the body, and it resonates to the color blue.

7. The Crown Chakra/Fame Gua

Embracing Your Life

This combination helps you to stay on track energetically and encourages you to strive constantly to find your life's work and follow through on what you want to accomplish and contribute to the planet during your incarnation and stay on Earth. These energy forces serve to pull in the people, places, and things that make up your life and provide for you the opportunities that will serve your soul and support you in all your life's endeavors.

The Crown Center. The Seventh Chakra is located at the top of the head, and its energy pattern resonates to the color purple/violet. This center oversees your connection to your destiny and to your specific path here on Earth. The Crown Center acts as your own personal compass, directing and pointing you toward the next part of your journey here. The energy emitted from this Chakra acts as a transmitter, drawing and repelling people and situations that will serve and guide you along your path. In the esoteric realm, this center connects you to your "higher wisdom" and provides you with the energy source that is used for creative visualization and your ability to envision your future. This Chakra also connects you with the gifts that your soul is here to contribute to the world. It oversees all physical and health-related aspects of your skull, brain, pituitary functioning, nervous system, and many systemic-type illnesses.

When this center is **balanced** properly, you will feel a clear sense of being on the right path regarding work, relationships, and self-actualization. It is through this energy center that you will also easily be able to use your powerful gift of creative visualization that, when activated, can help you to establish and achieve success, money, happiness, and the ability to heal yourself. When this center is **underactive,** you can feel not in control of your life or your destiny, and may feel disconnected from any sense of God or spirituality. When the Crown Chakra is **overactive,** you may feel all-powerful and misinterpret your life's path, believing that it is your destiny to control other people's lives. A chronically overactive Seventh Center can create a delusional person, a megalomaniac, an oppressor, or a tyrantlike personality. When this center is out of balance it can also contribute to all types of mental illness and personality disorders, including schizophrenia and all other psychoses and neuroses.

The Fame Gua. The Fame area represents your success, the way the public acknowledges you, who you would like to be known as, and what you would like to accomplish in this lifetime. This gua also oversees all issues relating to the eyes; it is ruled by the Fire element and resonates to the color red.

8. The Transpersonal Chakra/The Helpful People-Travel Gua

You Are of Spirit, You Are of Matter

"You are of spirit, you are of matter." This is the mantra that will constantly serve to remind you that we are basically etheric spirits living in a physical body during this incarnation, so that we can provide service to the planet and help bring all our personal issues into consciousness and transmute and heal them. Because we are made of equal parts spirit and matter, we will be faced constantly with living in the duality of both the spirit and the flesh. This gua/Chakra combination serves as your personal oversoul, housing your guides and spiritual help, so you can freely turn to them as often as you need to. This combination holds the energy space for all the helpful people needed in your life, both embodied and in spirit.

The Transpersonal Center. The Eighth Chakra is located approximately six inches above the top of your head, and its energy pattern resonates to a white or golden light. This is the center that connects you to your higher self, spirit guides, and other realms of assistance and guidance. It is the center where the core of your vibration is at its strongest before it splits off into the physical body. This center acts as a conduit, sending light, channeling energy and information back and forth from the Chakras in your body to the spirit world. The Eighth Center also acts as a lighthouse, sending out a beam of light to illuminate your path and help direct your journey. This Chakra is your vibration's safe, natural resting place where all meditation should begin and end. It also oversees the spiritual counterpart to all the same illnesses located in the Seventh Center, the Crown Chakra, which houses the physical components of the same illness (see chapter 8).

The Helpful People/Travel Gua. This section oversees two main categories in your life: the first being the helpful people in your life, ranging from friends and doctors to new opportunities and additional clients. The other category this section oversees is the area of all types of travel and transportation. It also oversees the Head area of the body and all father-related issues. It resonates to the color gray.

9. Overall Vibration/The Health–Center Gua

Good Health: A Result of Doing What You Love and Loving What You Do

When you look at the bigger picture of your life, it's important to note that what you are really looking at is the totality of all your experiences, for this is what collectively creates a happy and content life, versus a sad and an empty one. As you have come to realize, it's the quality of your life in all its components, Chakras, and guas, that make up good health. As you strive to bring all aspects of your life into balance, you create optimal health and a life worth living as a healthy person. **The more you are in line with your truth and your work here while on the planet, the more you raise the percentages that you will have a healthy life, *even if that life happens to include an illness.*** For illness alone should never be the only measure you use to determine if your life and health are good versus not good.

Your Overall Vibration. Your Overall Vibration is the compilation of individual Chakras and preprogrammed experiences, opportunities, lessons, and circumstances that you are here to address during this lifetime. The more life force and ch'i that enter the overall vibration and the physical body, the stronger your health becomes and the more aligned you are with your life's path. This combination resonates to a vibration of white or golden light.

The Health/Center Gua. This gua is located in the middle of the Bagua map, and it is the hub that connects all the eight other sections. It is represented by the Yin/Yang symbol. Although it oversees all the other issues and life situations that are not represented in the eight other guas, its main focus is on health-related issues. We interpret good health as a result of balance among all the different areas (guas) in your life.

This center space also oversees all other health areas that are not represented in the other eight guas. Its ruling element is Earth, and it corresponds mainly to the color yellow, but other Earth-based colors such as browns, peaches, and terra-cottas can be used also.

HOW THE CHAKRAS FUNCTION

The Chakras are units of energy that function through four main systems. The first two systems react internally to people, places, and things through their Chakra counterparts, referred to as Corresponding Chakras and Parallel Chakras. The third way the Chakras respond is in an outward motion connecting outside of themselves to other people's and places' Chakras through an extended line of energy that moves externally. The fourth way the Chakras react is through various energetic motions such as deflecting, absorbing, or polarizing the energies that surround them and come into their energy fields. For our purposes, regarding the material in this book, we will be focusing only on the first two systems of how the Chakra Energy System works.

1. *Complementary Chakras* These Chakra pairs are opposite by nature, but vibrationally have complementary energy fields that make them compatible. You will also see them appear as complementary colors on the color wheel. These two Chakras are energetically connected by an invisible cord of energy that acts like a pulley system. Often you will find that if one of the Chakras in the pair is overactive, the other will very typically be underactive. If one of the Chakras of the pair is underactive, the other one tends to be overactive. If you are having a health problem and you think you have found the Chakra that is the source of the problem, make sure you check with its complementary partner and see if the real source lies there instead.

   1. Survival Center (red) and 4. Heart Chakra (green)
   2. Social Center (orange) and 5. Throat Chakra (sky blue)
   3. Will Center (yellow) and 6. Third Eye (indigo)
   4. Heart Chakra (green) and 7. Crown Chakra (purple)
   8. Overall Vibration (white light)

2. ***Parallel Chakras*** These Chakra pairs vibrate to a similar frequency, the main difference being that the upper Chakra of the pair vibrates one energetic octave higher than its complementary Chakra above in System number 1. These pairs are on the same frequency module, just with one being a little farther up the resonance scale. If you are addressing an issue that is lodged in one of the Chakras of the pair, look at its Parallel Chakra to see if any of those issues are contributing to the issue you are working on. Also check whether the issue or Chakra that you are working on has thrown off the energetic balance of its higher or lower parallel Chakra.

1. Survival Center (red) and 5. Throat Center (sky blue)
2. Social Center (orange) and 6. Third Eye (indigo)
3. Will Center (yellow) and 7. Crown Center (purple)
4. Heart Chakra (green) and 8. Overall Vibration (white light)

So, for example, if you have an issue or an illness that is located in the base, Survival Center Chakra, you also need to check out its Complementary Chakra, the Heart, and also look into its Parallel Chakra, the Throat Center. By reviewing and working with all three aspects of the same energy line, you increase your chances of addressing, remedying, and transforming that issue or illness.

FENG SHUI, THE CHAKRAS, AND ILLNESS

Below is a quick reference list of the various Chakras, their matching Feng Shui guas, and some of their possible corresponding illnesses. You can utilize and apply this list in two different ways.

First Method. If you have a particular illness or disease, try to locate it on the chart below, and then find the corresponding Chakra and gua that the illness is associated with. Go back to the section titled "Ancient Wisdom Combined: The Feng Shui Guas and the Chakra Energy System," earlier in this chapter (see page 219), and reread the different issues and traumas associated with that Chakra and gua. Then make a list of the ESPs that you can identify and associate with your illness, and begin to address these issues. List

Chakra	Gua	Physical Area, Illness
9. Overall Vibration	Health Gua	all illnesses/miasms
8. Transpersonal Center★	Helpful People/Travel	central nervous system, systemic illnesses, top of head
7. Crown★	Fame	blood disorders, central nervous system, mental illness, muscular system, skin, circulatory system, head, brain, skull, immune system
6. Third Eye	Knowledge/Spirituality	eyes, ears, pineal gland, brain and neurological system, nose, hypothalamus, pituitary gland, nasal passage, forehead, hands
5. Throat	Children/Creativity	throat, thyroid gland, teeth, parathyroid, hypothalamus, mouth, gums, neck, jaw
4. Heart	Relationships	thymus gland, lungs, arms, shoulders, heart, upper back, circulatory system, ribs, chest, immune system, organs, breasts
3. Will	Career	adrenals, stomach, liver, pancreas, gallbladder, middle back, small intestine, ears, anxiety
2. Social	Family	reproductive organs, spleen, large intestine, kidney, appendix, urinary tract, bladder, lower back, feet, depression
1. Survival	Wealth	birthing canal, genitals, pelvis, bones, ankles, feet, legs, coccyx, rectum, hips, blood disorders

★Most of the illnesses that are listed separately in both the Seventh and Eighth Centers are actually located in *both* the Seventh and Eighth Chakras. In the Eighth Chakra, the illness is in its *nonphysical* manifestation, and in the Seventh Chakra the same illness is in its *physical* manifestation. Also, certain illnesses will manifest from several Chakras. To determine the one(s) that you need to address, reread the prior information that describes what each Chakra oversees and then connect to the one that makes the most sense regarding your personal issues.

the corresponding colors that are connected with those systems, and use those specific colors to adjust the corresponding Chakra and gua that are related to your illness. If you choose not to use the color system to adjust the correlating gua, then instead go to chapter 3 and review the Nine Basic Cures, and use one of them to augment the Feng Shui gua instead.

Next, begin a daily routine of "color breathing," to begin working with the Chakra-based part of your issues/illness, and do a specific color-breathing routine based on the corresponding Chakra color of your illness, as described in the summary at the end of this chapter.

Second Method. You can also use the chart on page 233 if you have had a particular illness in the past that is on the list, or a family predisposition to a particular illness. Then you can shore up the corresponding Chakra and gua as a preventive measure before the illness or recurrence develops. In addition, you should also review all your personal, emotional, and spiritual issues that are associated with that particular Chakra, and then check in with yourself on where you are in your life and assess how much more exploration and healing are needed regarding those issues.

Many diseases and illnesses are pervasive, and the only way you can connect them with a particular Chakra (for diagnostic purposes) is through identifying their location on the body. For example, if a cancerous tumor is found in a woman's left breast, then that tumor is a physical manifestation of issues that belong to the Heart Chakra or its complementary or parallel Chakra. If that same cancerous tumor is found in the lining of your stomach, then that tumor is a manifestation of issues having to do with the Will Chakra or its complementary or parallel Chakra. So, for starters, locate the area of the health problem first, and that will lead you back to the Chakra that you need to explore.

FENG SHUI, THE CHAKRAS, AND THE THEORY OF SYMPATHETIC RESONANCE

The musical theory referred to as Sympathetic Resonance states that when, for example, you have two identically tuned stringed musical instruments in

Fig. 33. The Influence of Environmental and Human Energy Fields

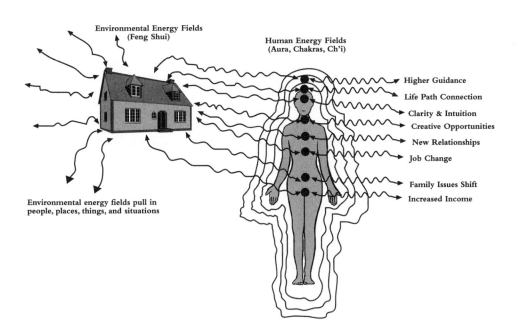

Environmental Energy Fields
(Feng Shui)

Human Energy Fields
(Aura, Chakras, Ch'i)

Higher Guidance
Life Path Connection
Clarity & Intuition
Creative Opportunities
New Relationships
Job Change
Family Issues Shift
Increased Income

Environmental energy fields pull in
people, places, things, and situations

the same room and you play a specific note on one instrument, the same note on the second instrument will react by vibrating also, even though it was never struck, because it resonates to a similar frequency. Similarly, if your physical energy field is vibrating to a certain illness frequency pattern, that illness can be triggered by a home or office environment that is resonating also to the same illness vibrational pattern. **The two vibrational systems become a mutually reinforcing "illness ecosystem" that activates the illness and then keeps it alive and thriving.**

In chapter 1 is the Circle of Life chart (see Fig. 1), which illustrates how the flow of ch'i from universal factors causes a trickle-down effect and helps shape and influence everything from the ch'i of a country to the ch'i in your home or office. The ch'i of your home and office, when intermingled with the ch'i in your body, helps shape and influence the vibrational patterns and energy signals that your Chakras send out. These energy signals act like little invisible Morse codes summoning to you the exact set of circumstances that creates your life and your health. In the same way that Sympathetic

Resonance works in the music example given on page 235, it also works energetically in creating the same vibrational magnetism, which connects the Chakras with the Feng Shui guas.

Vibrational patterns are composed of many different factors, but the three main components that create a specific or general frequency are *energy, placement,* and *intention.* These three things come together and formulate a certain vibration that resonates to a particular frequency. In turn, the frequency takes on a certain shape, size, thought, element, feeling, circumstance, relationship, or illness. The vibrational pattern then becomes the energetic counterpart to its physical or worldly manifestation, acting as its magnetic oversoul, pulling to it all the different aspects that it needs to sustain equilibrium and remain a living entity.

Every illness or predisposition to an illness that exists energetically in your body has a vibrational "bar code" that resonates to a specific frequency and is stored inside your Chakras, which is your internal energy system. Depending on the way certain houses are designed and decorated, they too create specific energy patterns and bar codes that, if weakened or left unbalanced, may also resonate to various patterns of disease and illness. When these two systems of energy come together and connect energetically, they can act as a catalyst, triggering the onset of certain illnesses that otherwise might have remained dormant. In addition, when these two separate energetic patterns dovetail, collectively they can also cause relapses or slow down one's recovery/healing process.

The physical body or realm is always the last place that disease surfaces, not the first. But physical manifestations or illnesses are often (not always) the only way your spirit can get your attention and force you to address your life issues. By addressing the ESPs of your illness, you then begin, issue by issue, to dismantle each energy and thought-form that is holding the consciousness of that illness in place. Unless the vibrational matrix of the illness is changed, the illness will continue to thrive, as the individual's thought-form feeds the bigger-picture energy system. Each thought-form consists of Emotional, Spiritual, and Physical (ESPs) components that you, as well as the society that the illness was developed in, will have to address if there will ever be a lasting cure or treatment for that particular disease. When you dismantle the underpinning issues, expose them, and disempower their logic, you alter the energetic environment that hosts the disease and, in turn, the matrix that the disease needs in order to exist.

The vibrational patterns of disease from an energy perspective come from two smaller systems (Chakras and Feng Shui) that together mirror the illness thought-forms that exist within the different levels of the individual's consciousness. The smaller vibrational patterns that exist in the individual and then get fed back again into the bigger vibrational patterns of illness that are part of our mass consciousness, which, in turn, again fuel the individual's smaller vibrational patterns of illness that exist within themselves. Again, from an energetic perspective, this is where all illness comes from and how it gets sustained energetically and globally.

As the ESPs, thoughts, and underlying belief systems change, first on an individual level, and then on a societal level, the core matrix of the illness begins to dissolve, reversing the need for that particular illness on the planet or within that particular individual. The illness then comes to its end, for it has served its individual and bigger-picture purpose, since its presence has forced individuals, as well as the collective in which the individual lives, to deal with issues that existed on the emotional and spiritual levels long before the disease manifested on the physical realm. Energetically speaking, when this happens, research breakthroughs occur and various cures are found. Once the emotional and spiritual underpinnings of an illness have been transmuted, some hardworking scientist somewhere in a lab discovers the antidote, or some layperson accidentally stumbles across the cure.

All the aspects of the ESPs of an illness, conscious and unconscious, are vibrationally encoded in the Chakra Energy System and equally reflected in the Feng Shui Design of the person's home. By learning to work with both systems in tandem, you aggressively approach the problem, conflict, illness, disease, or health challenge from both its external manifestation (Feng Shui) and its internal root causes (the Chakras).

Through the conscious application of color, various adjustment items, meditation, color breathing, Chakra work, Transcendental Cures, and Feng Shui Design principles, you can learn to adjust your "personal frequency waves" and shift the frequency of your illness, just as you do when your radio dial is not exactly tuned in to the station, or when your TV picture needs its horizontal and vertical controls adjusted.

HOW DO I USE THE CHAKRAS, COLOR, AND FENG SHUI DESIGN TO TREAT MY ILLNESS?

As all of these changes begin to take place, the vibrational patterns within the Chakras begin to change also, and in turn they send out a new set of signals that create new circumstances and magnetize to you new people, places, and things. These new aspects now in our lives will serve to re-create the exact core energy of the situation that we are trying to resolve or heal. Often these changes manifest by way of a significant shift in a person's illness. Sometimes it is evidenced by a change of doctors, medication, or treatment plan, or by an improvement or decrease in one's physical health. Sometimes these changes surface as an insight, disclosing or making peace with a childhood trauma, leaving a bad relationship, or releasing some memory or grief that had previously been embedded in the emotional or spiritual components of the illness. Each new situation becomes another opportunity presented by the universe to understand another part of self and some of the reasons for the specific disease and its manifestations.

Through learning how to work with the Chakras, Feng Shui, and color, you can help facilitate and accelerate the healing process. Illnesses that are born of imbalanced vibrational patterns, either internally or in the environment, heal best when they are treated with vibrational medicines "cut from the same cloth." These vibrational medicines work so well because they bypass conscious thought and work with the healing process through the use of symbols, sound, color, and the like.

If you are thinking to yourself, "I don't know if I can do this," keep in mind that *working* with these systems is a birthright, not something that some of us acquire in life while others do not. Most of our perceived and real psychological blocks to working with this form of vibrational energy come from fear, not from our inability to perceive energy. Try to keep in mind that you are able to work with the invisible vibrations of color and energy just as much as you are capable of changing the channel through your TV's remote. I know this for a fact. Why? Because if not, you would not have picked up this book and connected with these teachings. Trust that your soul knew what it was doing when it led you to read this. I do.

TEN WAYS TO APPLY COLOR TO SHIFT ILLNESS AND ALIGN ENERGY

1. *Food "Coloring."* Eat foods that correspond to the different colors of the Chakras. If you are working on the Heart Chakra or on Heart Chakra–related illnesses, eat more greens and green foods. If you are working with an illness whose corresponding Chakra colors appear excessive or overactive, then reduce food of that color from your diet until things settle down, or eat more of the color of foods that are connected to the Chakra's corresponding pair. Sometimes you just can't tell if you need more or less of a particular food color. Experiment and figure out what feels right.

2. *Clothing.* Clothing is our second skin. It is the potential color source that's closest to our body and energy field, which is the main conduit for carrying color energy to the body. On a daily basis, choose the colors you wear based on the colors that you intrinsically need to combat a specific issue, situation, challenge, or disease. Clothing color is a great tool for color medicine because you can change your clothes as often as you change your color needs. It's transient and flexible, and allows you to wear colors you wouldn't normally wear but vibrationally need.

3. *Body Color.* These are the colors of objects other than clothing that come in contact with your body, and can influence your vibrational composition via color. Jewelry is a powerful source of energy because it combines the power of color with metals and gemstones (see chapter 10). And natural stones have other healing properties as well. Hair color is also a powerful way of changing your vibration. One of my assistants needed a change in her life, so she changed the color of her hair to a darker shade of blond. As her life was changing, so was her vibration. She chose to adjust her frequency by adjusting her hair color to reflect her new life and vibration.

4. *Looking at Color.* Use the colors that you come across in your environment every day for what I call an "open-eye meditation." Look at the colors that surround you in pictures, artwork, furniture, cars, the sky, flowers, and plants, and make eye contact with them. Use your eyes to absorb the color directly into the visual cortex of your brain, allowing it to bring visual color to all areas of the body that are in need of that color adjustment.

5. *Objects of Color.* You can bring in the colors needed to adjust your energy and vibration by adding them as different objects to your home. For example, if you are dealing with an upper-respiratory infection and are in need of the color green because green corresponds to the Heart Chakra (which oversees the lungs and the respiratory system), you could purchase green sheets for your bed to bring in and reflect that color to stimulate the Heart Chakra; or hang a picture in the Relationship gua (corresponding to the Heart Chakra) of your bedroom with a green frame around pink flowers, since the Relationship gua corresponds to the color pink. You can use both color systems separately or in tandem to support your healing.

6. *Add Chakra Colors to Your Environment.* Depending upon the specific colors you may need to balance your underactive or overactive Chakras, you can add those corresponding colors via paint, furniture, or various fabrics to the interior of your home. If you're working on a Base Chakra issue or have developed problems with your knees (which is a Survival Center–related ailment), you would first find the corresponding Chakra color, which is red, and bring that color into your immediate environment so your energy field can absorb it and then nourish the Base Chakra (Survival Center). To make the application stronger and even more focused, locate the corresponding Feng Shui gua (in this example, it is the Wealth/Purple area) and make your color addition as an adjustment in that gua. For another example: if you are having problems with your kidneys, those organs are located in the Second Chakra, which resonates to the color orange, but parallels the Family gua in the Feng Shui external "energy" system. As an adjustment you can try bringing in the color orange to an area

in your home that oversees the Family gua. Remember, the Chakra colors are red, orange, yellow, green, light blue, indigo, and violet/purple.

7. *Paint Your Interior with the Feng Shui Bagua Colors.* Use the corresponding colors of the Feng Shui Bagua to bring in the colors that you are in need of for healing, and to adjust the color vibration from a Feng Shui perspective. These colors can be applied to the specific corresponding gua in each room (the bedroom would be the strongest) or in a specific room that corresponds with the gua of the overall floor plan area. The Bagua colors are red, pink, white, gray, black, blue, green, purple, and yellow.

8. *Interweave Both Color Systems.* Feel free to use both the Chakra and Feng Shui color systems in tandem, as you paint and explore ways to add finishes into the color schemes of your home or office. By using both systems, you energetically strengthen your objective, health challenge, and healing process. For example, if you are having an operation on your foot, you might want to augment the Family gua with something green, because the Family gua in Feng Shui oversees the feet and corresponds to the color green. You may also want to add some red to the Wealth area, because the Wealth area corresponds to the First Chakra (the Survival Center), and in the Chakra Energy System the first center oversees the feet and resonates to the color red.

9. *Color Breathing.* This is one of the quickest, easiest "color meditations" for daily color tune-ups and focused healings (see the meditation at the end of this chapter). Breathing in each color strengthens the Chakras and allows you to do a daily check-in to see what colors are weak, strong, or indifferent on that particular day, for that particular health issue or situation, and then adjust accordingly. Color breathing can also be used specifically on a focused Chakra color that is needed to assist your healing and recovery process. Breathe in nine breaths, with each breath consisting of both an inhale and exhale motion. Do this for 9, 18, or 27 consecutive days. (See the NSP&A website for CDs.)

10. ***BHS Transcendental Color Cures/Color Meditations.*** Black Hat Sect Feng Shui has a plethora of cures that focus on color and health-related issues (see chapter 9 for those regarding health). The cure given below is one that can be applied to a variety of heath-related illnesses and challenges. This cure is a call for help to your Higher Power(s) and connects Heaven (ceiling) and Earth (floor) with the middle, smaller string representing *you*. The way the smaller string hangs mimics Chinese calligraphy for the character "human." You are the human trying to access help from the heavens for your Earth-based problems. Leave this cure up indefinitely, or until the problem or health-related issue has been resolved.

Please note that all color cures, number 1 to number 10, need to be blessed with the Three Secrets Reinforcement Blessing (see chapter 9) to truly be effective as a vibrational transcendental cure.

MULTICOLORED CANOPY-TO-HEAVEN CURE

Fig. 34. Canopy Cure with Multicolored String

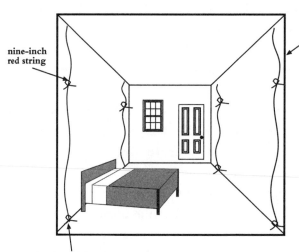

nine-inch
red string

Hang the four corner strings from the ceiling to the floor in the color of the particular Chakra/corresponding gua that you are working on and want to enhance; then add to each string a nine-inch piece of red string tied like a knot just above eye level. As a final touch to the cure, tie a nine-inch piece of yellow string, representing earth, to the bottom of each of the four strings.

nine-inch yellow string tied
to the bottom of each
of the four canopy strings

First, identify the Chakra that the problem or illness is lodged in. You'll need to have enough of that color string, ribbon, or yarn to run the distance from ceiling to floor four times over, because you will be hanging a string in each of the four corners of your bedroom.

Cut the string into an auspicious length, in multiples of nine (72 inches, 81 inches, etc.), that comes closest to the distance between ceiling and floor, allowing any additional string to lie on the floor.

Then cut four nine-inch pieces of yellow string (yellow represents the element Earth and the Health gua in Black Hat Feng Shui), and tie it to the end of the string that is resting on or nearest to the floor.

Next, you'll need 36 inches of red string, ribbon, or cord, so that you can cut four nine-inch pieces from it and tie them separately onto each of the four full-length color strings that are hanging from your ceiling in the four corners of your room. Tie these red strings just slightly above your eye level. The symbol the tied red string makes is the calligraphy character for "humans."

Don't forget to bless the string in each corner with the Three Secrets Reinforcement Blessing, visualizing the health problem being transformed and released; otherwise you will not get the transcendental effect and the desired outcome (see chapter 9).

USING FENG SHUI DESIGN AND THE CHAKRA ENERGY SYSTEM TO COMBAT ILLNESS

Now you can begin integrating all the teachings of the other chapters. First outline the illnesses or health issues that you would like to address, and then identify the Chakra and the Feng Shui gua that correspond with that illness. Make a list of all the ways that you can tackle the illness from the perspective of the Chakra Energy System, then make a list of all the things you can do with the Feng Shui of your space to help approach the illness from both the internal and external energy fields. Remember, the more methods you use to disempower the illness, the more you raise the percentages that the illness will transform, your perspectives will change, or your helpful people will come to the rescue. Don't forget to throw a little color into the plan.

All white spaces create an energy field that escalates anxiety and triggers depression. If you want a colorful life, you need to have color in it. Your energy systems depend on it, and your healing process requires it.

Closing Client Story

My partner persuaded me to get a Feng Shui consultation. I agreed, though quite skeptically. I had lived in my apartment for forty-two years, through one marriage, two children, and two relationships. At the time I was feeling completely stuck in my life. My health was poor, my relationship with my children was difficult, and I was unable to stop feeling responsible for everyone. Within five minutes into our first consultation, I was mobilized to get my life back on track. I felt as if she [Nancy] could see into my soul. She said the unspeakable—that I would die metaphorically and perhaps physically if I didn't begin to make some changes. My ulcerative colitis was chronic and pervasive.

During our consultation, Nancy pointed out how my personal issues of taking care of everyone (First Chakra, Survival Center) dovetailed with the inauspicious Feng Shui layout of the house that had contributed to my deteriorating health condition. Nancy pointed out that the shape of our apartment was re-creating the shape of a colon and that the main corresponding wall in our entranceway was painted red (Fire element). On one end of the hallway was the kitchen, which added even more explosive Fire energy to that area. To aggravate matters even further, the bathroom (Water element) was situated at the other end of the hallway and the red wall, dousing the fire with water.

In Five Element Theory, these elements (Fire and Water) create a very aggressive combination. She explained to us that although the Water element may have helped slightly to cool down the raging Fire element (colon), the aggressive nature of these two elements together helped to exacerbate my symptoms and escalate my diarrhea (fire and water). She also pointed out that the Children area was missing, and in fact I was experiencing some challenges with my sons at the time.

She suggested many remedies that we began to work on immediately. Ultimately they enabled us to move to our dream house in the country—something I'd wanted to do for over ten years. I found new doctors and my health began to improve.

Of course, we asked Nancy to Feng Shui our new home. At this consultation, Nancy suggested that I do a series of private Chakra Therapy sessions with her. The sessions were a series of guided meditations into the Chakras and their various fields of color. Initially we worked on clearing out the energy blocks through visualization and color breathing through the Chakras connected to my colon and to the issues with my younger son (Base Chakra/Survival Center) to help improve our relationship, which was very stuck. These sessions were equally helpful and challenging. Work with Nancy was not easy. It required daily color meditations and a commitment to action.

I have always felt a special affinity for color and felt its effect on my emotions. Nancy encouraged my use and expression of color. Two sessions in particular come to mind. In the first, we went into the center of the Base Chakra and she had me visualize breaking many of the unhealthy ties that I had with people, both living and dead, that were so binding for me. She asked me to visualize those ties and then cut them and let them fall away. I had trouble visualizing the ties falling away, so Nancy asked me to focus on seeing the cut ends. When I did focus on their ends, they first became spokelike, but afterwards developed into beautiful colors that eventually turned into butterflies that flew away. Through that meditation, I was introduced to the concept of power animals and animal guides. I now have spectacularly colored butterflies around me to help me through life.

In the other memorable session, I was guided into the door of my Heart Chakra and entered what appeared to be a university without walls. There were people of all sizes, colors, and nationalities—and even from other worlds—using a variety of different languages, and they were all able to understand one another. This universal imagery formed a metaphor for me, bringing me many lessons in letting go of many of my judgments and rigidity. It led to ways for my son and me to be together, and also to separate. It opened up so much space for us. With all that room, my other son has had the space to come into his brother's life as well.

Several years later, as I continue to work on my own with the Chakras, color breathing, and meditation, I continue to improve the quality of my life and my health. The new doctors I have been seeing have enabled me to get off some of the medications I had been using. Although the medications had helped reduce some of the worst symptoms of my colitis, they made me feel terrible, and had negative side effects. My yearly colonoscopies are reassuringly negative, and, given the odds of my body developing colon cancer, that's pretty great news!

Color has now become even more important to me. Often when I am frustrated, angry, hurt, or confused, I close my eyes and try to visualize a color. Then I think about the roots of my distress and the possibilities for resolution. This method of stress

THE CHAKRAS AND FENG SHUI

reduction is also great for my physical, mental, and spiritual health. I feel fortunate to have color, and Nancy's assistance, in my life.

Closing Chapter Exercise
Color-Breathing Meditations

One very effective way to infuse color into your Chakras and diagnose your health issues is through a meditation process called *color breathing*. This is a process that allows you to use the flow of your breath, along with Creative Visualization techniques, to bring the various colors of the Chakras into your body to fine-tune and strengthen your energy field.

Below is a simple Chakra Color Meditation that was designed to recharge and strengthen your energy system on a daily basis. You can use this meditation as a daily energy tune-up, bringing all the eight Chakras a daily infusion of color ch'i, or you can use the color breathing as a diagnostic tool for locating where the main energy block is in your illness.

1. Find a comfortable spot that is quiet and traffic-free. Close your eyes, relax, take a deep breath, and exhale. Take another breath in, and then out. Focus your awareness on your breath. Allow your breathing to naturally find a comfortable rhythm and pace.

2. With each inhalation, feel your body relaxing, and with each exhalation, feel yourself releasing all the tensions of the day and all the worries on your mind.

3. With your eyes closed, bring your attention to the open area approximately six inches above the top of your head. In your mind's eye, visualize a beautiful ball of pure white light circulating above the top of your head. As you continue to breathe, the light becomes brighter and brighter with a warm, luminescent glow.

4. Visualize yourself slowly breathing this beautiful light in through an imaginary opening in the top of your head. Slowly, using your breath, breathe this light through your eyes and ears, into your nose and mouth, contin-

uing to breathe the light down your throat, into your heart, lungs, down each arm, through each hand, and out each fingertip. Continue to breathe the light through the intestines, each organ, down the spine into the legs, past the knees, through the feet, and out the toes.

5. With each full inhalation, breathe the light in through the top of your head, and with each exhalation, release the white light through imaginary openings at your fingertips and toes. Inhale and exhale several times, circulating the light in, through, and out of your body.

6. Bring your attention back to the top of your head, to your Seventh Chakra, located at and referred to as the Crown. Slowly visualize the white light turning to a beautiful shade of violet, and breathe this color in and out of the top of your head, saturating it. If you have a difficult time visualizing the color violet (or any color), visualize any object you own or may have seen that contains that color (perhaps a purple dress, flower, or candle).

7. Watch the light move slowly down to your Sixth Chakra, between the eyebrows, called the "third eye." As you continue to breathe into that Chakra, watch the light slowly turn into the color indigo. Breathe indigo in and out of your eyes, ears, and nose.

8. As you continue to breathe, slowly watch the ball of light move downward into your Fifth Chakra, located in the center of your throat, called your Throat Chakra. Slowly it turns to the color sky blue, filling up your mouth, your throat, and the back of your neck. Continue to breathe sky-blue energy in and out of these areas several times.

9. Move your awareness down to your Fourth Chakra, the Heart Center, located in the center of your chest. Slowly breathe the light down into the center of your chest, watching the light turn to a beautiful shade of green energy. Continue to breathe the green Heart energy into your upper back, shoulders, lungs, down your arms and into your hands several times.

10. Continue to breathe the light downward into your Third Chakra, called the Will Chakra, located in your solar plexus, in the center of your ribs. Visualize the light turning into a beautiful shade of yellow. With each breath, imagine yourself breathing yellow energy into your solar plexus, stomach, liver, gallbladder, pancreas, small intestine, and middle back. Continue to breathe yellow energy into these organs and areas several times.

11. Move your awareness down to your Second Chakra, called the Social Center, located two inches below the navel. Slowly breathe the light in and out of your Second Center, watching it turn into a beautiful shade of orange. Breathe the color orange into your large intestine, reproductive organs, bladder, kidneys, spleen, and lower back. Allow the color to circulate and strengthen the energy from that center. Continue to breathe the color orange in and out of that Chakra.

12. As you continue to breathe, slowly bring your awareness to your First Chakra, called the Survival Center, located at the base of your spine. Take a deep breath in and watch it turn into a beautiful shade of red. Breathe the red color in and out of the base of your spine, filling it with grounding red energy. As you breathe this color in and out, slowly let it circulate in and around your genitals, filling up your legs, moving past your knees and ankles, through your feet, and out your toes.

13. After you have finished breathing in the color red to your First Chakra, slowly watch the color red in your legs and Survival Center turn back to a beautiful, glowing white light. See the white light filling up your legs, moving up through your Social Center, filling up your intestines and your lower back, continuing to move upward toward your solar plexus, filling up your stomach, all your major organs, and the middle of your back. Continue to breathe this beautiful white light up into your Heart Chakra, filling up your chest, upper back, arms, and hands. Allow your breath to continue to bring the white light up into your throat and to the back of your neck, circulating it in and through your mouth. With your next breath, move the white light up into your Third Eye, breathing it into your eyes, nose, and ears. Continue to breathe the white light

up into your head and circulate it around in the Crown Chakra. Finally breathe the white light up and out the top of your head, returning it to its safe, natural resting place, in your Eighth Chakra six inches above the top of your head, where it will always illuminate your path.

14. Take a deep breath in, and slowly bring your attention back to your body. Take another deep breath in and bring your attention back into the room, and when you are ready you can open your eyes.

15. Make some notes. Take notice if any color seemed scarce, abundant, or difficult to visualize. If so, go to your list of the Chakras and read what things each Chakra oversees and is responsible for. Try to connect how those things are working or not working in your life. Decide whether you need more or less of that color, then try to bring those colors into your energy field through the foods you eat, the colors you wear that day, and additional color breathing.

TWO WAYS TO APPLY THE COLOR BREATHING MEDITATION

I. Color-Breathing Meditation as a Daily Chakra Tune-Up

Some people choose fifteen minutes every morning before they start their day to practice this meditation, while others choose the time just before they go to bed. There is no correct way, so don't worry about doing it wrong. With practice it will become easier, especially if you try to create a routine that will keep you consistent and structured. If you have difficulty remembering all the Chakras at first, it may help to have a friend guide you through the meditation; or you can purchase my recorded version on CD,★ so that you can have me guiding you through all the colors without having to remember the sequencing or order.

★Color Meditation CDs can be purchased through my NSP&A website, www.fengshui-santopietro.com

This meditation should take you a minimum of fifteen minutes. Gradually extend the time as you add more breathing time to each color in the meditation.

II. Color Breathing as a Health/Chakra Diagnostic Tool

Part A. ESPs of Illness (Writing Exercise)

Take out your health biography (the one I urged you to do back in chapter 2), and look at some of the current issues you are addressing regarding your health. Choose one particular health or health-related issue that you want to work on. Now take a separate piece of paper and specifically write that health issue down. Include all your feelings about it (fears, resistance), then write down all the ESPs of that particular illness that you can list. Claim the area where you are going to do your meditation for 20 minutes as a "sacred space" where you can minimize interruptions, and place the list on your lap, inside a red envelope. Perform the Three Secrets Reinforcement Blessing and remember to visualize in nine segments the health situation being resolved. (See chapter 9.)

Part B. Locating the Main Chakra in Which Your Health Concern Is Lodged

Get comfortable, for the next part of this exercise begins the Color Breathing Meditation, outlined above, but this time with a specific goal: to help you locate the Chakra(s) where the core of the illness is vibrationally lodged. Follow the same meditation guidelines as above, but instead of using your color breathing as a general color-breathing meditation, you will now be looking specifically for a Chakra in your system that feels to you to be the most blocked and in need of your attention.

Part C. Specific Color Breathing

Take notice of which Chakras you had the most difficulty with, either because you couldn't see the color, because you fell asleep during the color breathing or just before you arrived at that color, or because something felt blocked, wrong, or otherwise problematic. Once you've identified the

Chakra that is of concern, bring yourself properly out of the meditation (follow the steps listed in the closing chapter exercise, Color Breathing Meditations, on pages 246–50)—otherwise you might feel spacey and a little disoriented—and for the next nine consecutive days spend time doing your daily color-breathing exercise, allowing yourself to spend a little extra time each day on the Chakra in question and breathing more breaths of that color into the Chakra. Then add another step (below) to help breathe the Chakra that needs healing in and through the healing energy of the heart. This serves to help you energetically break the internal matrix grid in your Chakra energy system that might be contributing to holding your illness in place.

While in the above meditiation and once you have identified the Chakra and color that you will be working on, close your eyes and, on your next inhalation, breathe into this Chakra and visualize your inhalation as the same color as the Chakra. Then pull your breath up (or down) to your Heart Chakra and watch your breath turn to a beautiful shade of the color green as you release your exhalation of green out of an imaginary opening in the center of your Heart Chakra. Do nine complete inhalations and exhalations to help stimulate and energize the Chakra that is holding the core energy of your illness. By pulling that color through the use of your breath and moving it up and out of the Heart Chakra, what you are actually doing is raising the vibration of your particular health issue by processing the very powerful healing vibration of the heart energy. This helps break down and transmute the illness through the use of color as a vibrational medicine. Practice this breathing exercise for 27 days, with nine full inhales and exhales each day.

Part D. Place Your Red Envelope in the Health Gua (Center) Under Your Mattress

Take your red envelope and put inside it the list containing health concerns and your intentions. Place it under your mattress, in the Health/middle gua position, and sleep on it for the same 27 nights that you are doing your specific color-breathing meditation. Each morning, perform the Three Secrets Reinforcement Blessing on the red envelope, and visualize the health issue being transmuted and resolved.

NINE HALLMARKS OF THE EMOTIONAL AND SPIRITUAL REVOLUTION AND THEIR IMPACT ON YOUR HEALTH

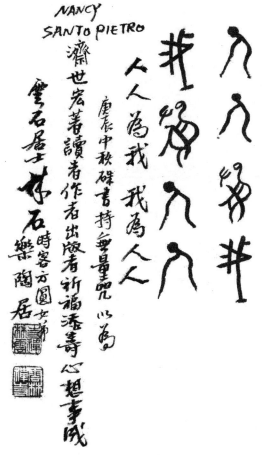

"Everyone for me; I for everyone."

CALLIGRAPHY BY H. H. PROFESSOR THOMAS LIN YUN RINPOCHE

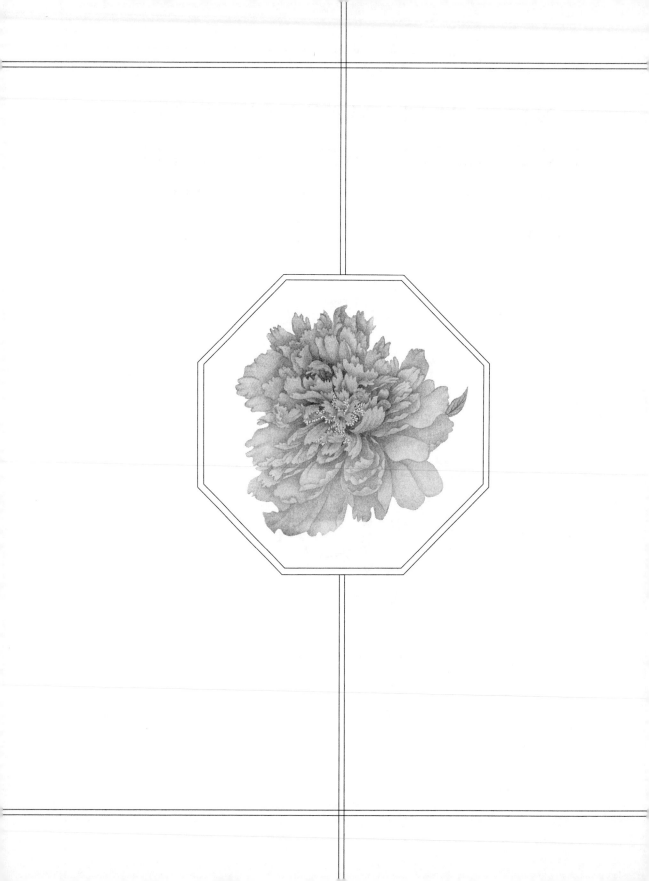

ALTHOUGH TALKING ABOUT the underpinnings of illness is a wonderful start, the actual changes that need to be made are sometimes very hard because we have to face, uncover, and deal with things that are painful about others and ourselves. Most of us were taught to suppress our emotions and to be logical. But in spite of that conditioning process, life unfolded and we began to experience all the things we had been taught to suppress. As a result, many of us developed an inner conflict, and our souls and hearts became very confused about how to act and which way to be.

Most of us have grown up trying to apply many of the new teachings as well as to incorporate the primary rules we learned from our parents and during childhood, only to experience disastrous results as we tried to mix two different belief systems. The "new world" thinkings see the mind as a vehicle and not as the driver; they encourage a heart that acts first and a mind that thinks later. Subsequently, every act of love and personal growth becomes "higher powered" and raises the vibration of the whole planet, whether or not that was its original intention.

So, as we become more evolved, it can actually be very scary, because the rules change drastically. Although the rewards are greater, so are the risks. This is the gift that comes with enlightenment and also its horror, because we are constantly faced with different rules and a different grid.

As the changes begin to occur in your life, in spite of all your efforts to stop them or slow them down, you'll realize that your emotions and responses are different from how you were accustomed to responding in the past. Randomness and uncertainty can be very overwhelming at times, and you can feel very much out of control. Many of us shut down out of fear and confusion, in an effort to control the changes, while others get depressed or ill. This is probably the most confusing hallmark of the shift, because at times it even becomes hard to recognize yourself, much less your responses to the changes.

Author Gregg Braden, in his groundbreaking book *Awakening to Zero Point: The Collective Initiation,* writes, "You may be happy to discover, as I was, that you are not imagining these changes and shifts—they are real and coming into full dominance." Braden, a former scientist, explains that many measurable changes are currently happening on Earth, and are contributing to what is happening to us on an emotional and physiological level. These changes are a direct result of changes in Earth's geomagnetic field. In his book he explains that Earth's geomagnetic field is currently at 1.5. Although known to fluctuate (based on the Kelvin scale of 1 through 10, with 5 being the midpoint), we are now at 1.5, significantly on the lower end, and heading toward "Zero Point." When Zero Point happens, it will cause a major change in the Earth's vibrational frequency and, in turn, a change in the matrix of our own personal frequency. The changes that will occur will alter the biochemistry of our bodies, influencing the chemical voltage and frequency to which different molecules such as DNA respond.[9] **This change is what the New Age refers to as the Paradigm Shift.** Although it will take place over several years, it will pick up speed at the end of 2001—and into the year 2002. Life-changing events can surface during these times, as the whole paradigm attempts to rebalance itself while our familiar matrix begins to break.

Braden states that the decrease of Earth's magnetic field, and the simultaneous slowing of the planet's rotation, have created the energetic opportunity to change the vibrational patterns that determine how we *feel, love, fear, judge, need, and hurt.* The denser the magnetic field on the planet, the more we are locked in to the emotional and energetic patterns that are passed on and calcified from generation to generation. Because of this energetic lock-in, emotional, spiritual, and physical healing and growth take longer.

As we move through this energetic shift, we are discovering that the decreased magnetic fields are allowing our body frequency to shift to one that will resonate to a new, higher vibrational level. The higher frequency allows our personal vibrational frequency to be less dense. Less density in our vibration will accelerate our ability to change more quickly through the use of our emotions. These changes can at first feel drastic or even overwhelming but they nonetheless need to, and will, happen, if our lives, world, and illnesses are going to heal and transmute.

OUR GREATEST CHALLENGE: ACCEPTING THAT SOME THINGS JUST WON'T MAKE ANY RATIONAL SENSE

As the internal changes start happening in your life, you will soon realize, if only by default, that it's imperative to start looking at your life and your illness through another set of lenses. You will slowly begin to surrender to the reality that what you can't see will influence you more than what you can see. The invisible lines of energy and vibrational patterns that pass through and around you create your life and contribute to your illness. We used to think that illness was something that "just happened" to us, but we understand now that every illness has a consciousness, and that we have to treat all its parts in order for a complete healing to take place. It doesn't matter if you exercise every day, eat brown rice, and chant for hours on end. If your personal energy field and your environment are laden with old patterns, negative thoughts, and unbalanced vibrations, disease will manifest. I'm not discouraging you from living a healthy lifestyle, but the truth is, if you deal with your life, feel your feelings, and show up to face the hard stuff, you might have a better chance at having a longer, healthier life, even if you don't always eat right or exercise.

We know now that the old structure has to go in order for the healing process to come in. We must allow ourselves to fall apart to the degree needed, in order for something new to develop. Not until we are ready to be broken can we completely break through and change. Some of us will go willingly, while others need to be pushed, but either way the healing process for our illness demands that we let go.

We have worked so hard to try to keep it together and not to fall apart, as we were taught, but what we truly need to do is the exact opposite! Getting out of our own way and loosening our grip on our old life is what we need to do so the new health we are creating can flow in. This is precisely what will help us get through the changes and the shifts sooner.

Don't hesitate to ask yourself the hard questions. Be honest and dare to find out what you are made of! Don't be afraid to talk about your illness, death, and dying. Find friends, counselors, and support groups who are not threatened or scared by what's happening in your life. It's part of the new way to use our emotions to cut through fear and shame and enhance the healing process. Remember that the amount of distance you keep from your illness emotionally, spiritually, and physically is the same exact distance you hold yourself from healing or resolving it. Say what you mean and mean what you say, and you will see life's great mystery unfolding right before your very eyes. *The challenges of your illness will test your spiritual and emotional strength; although you will be emotionally weakened, please know that if you hang in there long enough you will be spiritually strengthened in return.* Your spiritual connection with a higher power will be enhanced, because the universe promises to walk with you through the fires, to send you all the helpful people that it can muster up, as you face and embrace your healing work.

As the tenets of the new consciousness for health and healing go into effect, you will be faced with the many new challenges that expanded awareness can bring. Sometimes change means moving, other times it may mean switching careers. Probably the most difficult change to face is the ending of a relationship that worked well for you when you and your partner were both on a similar level of consciousness. Sometimes this is the price we have to pay for introspection and spiritual growth. All these changes and upheavals on the surface, and beneath it, can conjure up a lot of feelings, fears, and growing pains. These issues, if left unresolved, underprocessed, and/or suppressed, can lead to a host of problems and health-related conditions because often the individual who is going through the expansion and illness doesn't even realize what's happening. Without understanding the energy shifts that are occurring in your life and around your illness, you are left totally clueless and fearful, and you may blame yourself for lack of stability, constant changes, relationships that end, and your illness.

Without a frame of reference, an illness can look like random chaos. For many individuals, this causes a knee-jerk response to resist the changes and shut down. This will only lead to more chaos and subsequent depression, anxiety, and illness.

As we learn to manage these changes and times more elegantly and with a better understanding of what is actually going on, the smoother the transition will be for everyone. The transitions listed below are ones that I have encountered throughout my work as a Feng Shui consultant, psychotherapist, and healer. In working with individuals over the past 18 years, I have found that being stuck in some of these transitions was a major underpinning to many of their illnesses, diseases, and sufferings. By learning how these transitions manifest through your Chakra Energy System and the Feng Shui Design of your home, you will be able to identify where your blocks and issues are, and where they are located in your body and home. This formula will give you yet another approach to help you disarm your illness. Each level of the Paradigm Shift is associated with a corresponding Chakra and Feng Shui gua, as well as several different types of illnesses that can manifest because of the avoidance or challanges these issues or concepts can bring.

If you aren't sick or facing a disease, this information can help prevent illness, allowing you to bring to the surface some of your challenges and work toward shifting them to their highest vibration and resolution.

The Nine Hallmarks of the Emotional and Spiritual Revolution (also known as the twenty-first century Paradigm Shift),[10] listed below, depict the many changes that we, as a people and as a planet, are going through in consciousness and thought-forms. Energy always follows thought. This list highlights some of the great thought transitions of our time, and shows how these bigger-picture issues are manifesting through individual lives and influencing their emotional, spiritual, and physical health. I believe that with all these shifts and new ways to look at our lives, this time period will be remembered as the one in which the world woke up, both spiritually and emotionally.

NINE HALLMARKS OF THE EMOTIONAL AND SPIRITUAL REVOLUTION

1. From *Scarcity to Abundance* (Survival Chakra and Wealth Gua)

This shift is probably one of the most eagerly awaited on the planet. At one time or another most of us have faced the fear that comes along with feeling like there is not enough. Not enough love, money, health, or time to do the things we want or need to do. Socially we have seen an escalation in poverty that has affected not only Third World countries but big, prosperous countries as well. This level of scarcity was created by a premise in our old belief system that there wasn't enough, and that only the deserving and the lucky would have access to what was available. These fears became engraved in our thought patterns and then calcified in our genetic programming. The energetic response to scarcity is fear. When people are functioning from a base of fear, their only recourse is to entrench and protect themselves. When a society is fear-based, it creates rigid rules to ensure some security, although it is usually a very false sense of security.

On a Chakra level, the challenge of survival issues is addressed in our first energy center, located at the base of the spine, our survival center. Fear throws everything and everyone it touches into a primary mode of survival because First Chakra consciousness doesn't yet understand and trust the other levels of consciousness, whose rules state that abundance is a birthright for all, not just for a chosen few. The way this truth is "owned" by the individual is through the changing of his or her level of consciousness. Without a major shift in understanding our right to prosperity, an intellectual knowledge of this information is not enough.

As we enter into the twenty-first century and what is now being referred to as the "paradigm shift," everything has begun to change. During this current period, scientists have documented that the rotation of the earth has slowed down somewhat, in addition to discovering an anomaly in our compass direction of true north. This shift is almost 15 percent away from prior accurate readings.[11] As these planetary changes occur, many individuals will be able to access a new game plan that will change the way they see their self-worth. As we move more into the vibration of abundance, we will see a revamping in government, more unity among nations, and a political climate that will restore our faith in humanity. These are opportunities that will bring us new jobs and relationships and open us to a more expansive level of receiving. The challenge of this level is that sometimes when we outgrow a job, a salary, or a relationship that is supporting us financially, we are forced to make the change before the new source of abundance has manifested. This in-between period can be very stressful and sometimes create feelings of distrust of our own intuition and decision-making abilities. As we address and face this conflict directly, we also face all the fears and uncertainties that go with our ability to provide for ourselves and care for our needs. The transition period from scarcity to abundance will bring with it a newfound sense of prosperity and trust in the higher plan.

Scarcity to Abundance:
Its Impact on Your Chakras, Feng Shui, and Health

This shift triggers all unresolved issues associated with the First or Base Chakra, the Survival Center, which oversees all issues of wealth and abundance. When it is constricted, resisted, or blocked, it can manifest in health-related problems such as leg, knee, and foot disorders, sciatica, phlebitis, broken ankles, water retention, lower-body weight gain, colon and prostate cancer, and impotence.

Chakra Color-Breathing Remedies. Color-breathe nine consecutive breaths of the color *red* into your Base Chakra each morning for nine mornings. For the next nine mornings, do an "alternating color-breathing" exercise in which you inhale the red energy into your Base Chakra, and exhale the same breath out the Heart Chakra in the color *green*. For the next nine mornings repeat the first color-breathing sequence above, for a total of 27 days. If any of the emotional, spiritual, or physical issues are still present, stop color breathing for nine days, then repeat the above 27-day sequence again.

Feng Shui Adjustment Remedies. Adjust *all* the Wealth areas in your home, and make all needed repairs to your Wealth guas. Augment the areas with brass wind chimes, fish tanks, a water fountain, a 40- or 50-mm clear or AB Feng Shui crystal on a red string in multiples of nine, and a bright red object, or paint the space in hues of purple or lavender. Perform the Three Secrets Reinforcement Blessing (see chapter 9), with all adjustments.

2. From *Procreation* to *Co-Creation* (Social Chakra and Family Gua)

This is a very crucial stage in the transition to higher levels of consciousness and healing. This shift is one of the first red flags that we are moving out of our survival issues as a planet, where we always considered the self first, and into a broader understanding that we are part of a greater whole. The new concept of co-creation also allows us to open up to the different levels, outside of human life, and acknowledge that other forms of life exist and that we have a responsibility to include them in all our creation endeavors. This shift is reflected in the interest in spirit guides, angels, devas, nature spirits, and the like, and it coincides with the Second Chakra, the Social Center.

The act of procreation, in our former thinking, was mainly to expand the family unit as extensions of self. It was also about expanding the Earth's population, bringing more souls into the world to serve the planet, to manifest their destiny, and to complete their soul's work here. Although the primary motivation for having children should be an expression of love, often it happens as an outcome of societal expectations, family values, and religious conditioning. Many people from the last generation, when asked why they got married and had children, will say, "Well, that's what you did in those days." They're not being crude or insensitive about having children, just honest about not having really thought it through. As times begin to change, many women and men find themselves caught between two worlds. Some may choose not to marry and/or have children. They may feel a pull toward developing their careers instead, and make their chosen work, projects, students, clients, and contributions to the planet as important to them as having children is to others. They may choose to focus their life's work on the things that they are creating and giving birth to, and see humankind as their extended family. As the concept of the family changes, so do traditional family structures. Reconstituted families, gay and lesbian relationships and families, single parents, parents who are separated or divorced, children who are adopted or are conceived through in vitro fertilization are all part of this very stressful shift that identifies socially who we are and how we fit in. This shift in consciousness and social expectations can initially bring the individual and the new type of family a lot of challenges and pressure from outside sources.

In the new shift in consciousness toward a co-creative process, we begin to understand that we are all part of the larger family of humankind and also part of all other life force on the planet. As we begin to recognize that we live in a world that includes all of God's creatures, human, animal, and mineral alike, we start to recognize that the way we go about our decision-making processes and judgments needs to change. It is during this shift that we begin to open up to other ways of seeing what a valuable life is, and that there is a variety of possible family structures. Other helpful extensions of our bigger-picture families, from a spiritual perspective, now include spirit guides, nature spirits, vegetable and flower devas, angel guides, deities, and the like. We begin to see the significance in that all life must be included in the decisions that we make on a daily basis. This all-encompassing concept allows us to step fully into understanding the importance of living life as part of a co-creative group and process.

This means that we can no longer blithely cut trees down and not consider the impact on the planet and other life-forms that depend on those trees for shelter and sustenance. We can no longer pollute our air and waters and not suffer greatly for it. As this shift occurs, we will begin to honor and cherish all that God has created and treat it as we would our own child, acting as if the air is our brother and the Earth our mother. This new perspective helps us plan renovations, construction, and other expansive technologies with all of the elements in the animal and mineral kingdom acknowledged and considered. We begin to understand the deeper meaning of life and more of the spiritual reasons why we incarnate. We understand that each soul has a purpose and a personal mission that accompanies its journey. With this shift children are conceived as an act of love *and* as a gift to the universe, so that the child can live out the karma he or she has come here to experience. We also begin to realize that the energy force that joins us in bringing children into the world is the same one that helps us birth all creative projects, writings, books, artwork, theories, discoveries, new ideas, and brilliant concepts.

As we begin to co-create with God and all living things on the planet, we open ourselves to greater guidance and providence, understanding that our contribution to the planet always takes into consideration the higher good of all. We are less concerned about what *we* want for our children; instead our support is motivated by what *they* want for themselves and the work they are here to contribute. We birth our projects and then release them to the world in whatever way they need to unfold, because other principles and energies are now involved that are helping us with the project, theory, or child, and walking with it through its next stage on its evolutionary path. It is in this shift that we learn to release the inner programming that tells us we have to do certain things alone, without help, and that individual accomplishments are the goal.

Procreation to Co-Creation:
Its Impact on Your Chakras, Feng Shui, and Health

This shift triggers all unresolved issues associated with the Second Chakra, the Social Center, which oversees family, pregnancies, childhood and co-dependency issues; addictions to food, drugs, alcohol, and sex; and childhood traumas and abuses. Health-related issues that may evolve here because of a resistance or a block to this shift are difficult pregnancies, reproductive-organ problems, depression, addictions, lower-back problems, and bladder, kidney, uterus, and urinary tract infections.

Chakra Color-Breathing Remedies. Color-breathe nine consecutive breaths of the color *orange* into your Second Chakra every morning for nine days. For the next nine mornings, do an "alternating color-breathing" exercise in which you inhale the color orange into your Social Chakra and exhale the same breath out the Throat Chakra in the color *light blue.* Then, for the next nine mornings, repeat the first color sequence above for a total of 27 days. If any of the emotional, spiritual, or physical issues are still present, stop color breathing for nine days, then repeat the 27-day sequence above.

Feng Shui Adjustment Remedies. Adjust *all* the Family areas in your home, and then make all needed repairs to the Family guas. Augment the areas with mirrors, a 40- or 50-mm Feng Shui clear or green crystal on a red string in multiples of nine, live plants, or an orange object, or paint the area green. Remember to perform the Three Secrets Reinforcement Blessing with all adjustments (see chapter 9).

3. From *Fear to Trust*
(Will Chakra and Career Gua)

As we grow and shift to higher levels of consciousness, one of the wonderful gifts that come as by-products of this transition is the ability to disconnect and be released from many of your fears. *The more you expand your level of consciousness, the less fear you will have, because the less fear you will need.* As we understand more of the bigger picture of why we are here, we also gain an understanding of how to transcend and transmute energy. This shift teaches us that fear is just a temporary illusion designed by our intellect to hold us back from moving forward. Why would the mind want to do this? Because, as expansive as the mind is, it is also very limiting. The main purpose of the mind is to provide us with an organ that allows us to think, store information, *and* rationalize our world and some of our actions. The innate ability to rationalize is what separates and makes us different from any other species. This incredible organ backfired when we overpowered it by giving it vetoing rights over the consciousness of our heart, feelings, and intuition. When the mind comes across something it doesn't understand or hasn't experienced yet, it recoils and constricts. The emotion that it produces when it's in a constriction mode is *fear.* Fear is always the by-product of rational constriction, and constriction is the opposite of expansion. But when our parents teach us, through eliciting fear, not to run into the streets or play with fire, we believe it to be a true and necessary component of the learning process.

Because it appeals to our sense of rationale, we buy into the notion that when fear appears, it means we must unequivocally avoid the fear-evoking situation. We are also taught that certain aspects of life, pain, and desire are to be feared. Unfortunately, we bought this teaching, hook, line, and sinker, because we were never given any alternatives to ponder. We have all been taught that fear is a necessary part of life that teaches us the all-important lesson of discernment. *But actually the only thing that fear teaches us is to be afraid.* Discernment can be taught through *awareness,* and through awareness we learn trust. Trust in your ability to care for yourself, trust in your relationship with God, and trust that you will be okay, *especially during times of change, illness, and chaos.* Although on a day-to-day basis you might be facing very real problems or personal illness, try to hold the thought that on a spiritual level, all is well in your life. The very scary things that you might be facing have been orchestrated perfectly to bring the exact set of experiences needed to help you process the issue at its core.

As we switch consciousness levels, we earn the right to trust in all the intangibles that are here to assist us and reduce our fears. When we begin to believe that we are connected with the universe and the higher powers that be, we realize on an even deeper level that whatever is happening to us, even illness, is not just a random occurrence. Our old thinking and level of con-

sciousness, in attempting to provide us with a sense of safety, unintention-
ally misused the emotion of fear. Fear of not having enough money, fear of
not being loved, fear of dying and living are all manifestations of limited
thinking, not awareness. The world around us further reinforces our fears
with horror stories in newspapers, dramas, murder mysteries, and violent
television shows. *Fear moves you farther and farther away from your birthright of
inner peace, abundance, and greatness as it cleverly whispers in your ear that you are
not safe.* Emmanuel says, "Fear tells you, 'I want to make you safe.' Love says,
'You are safe.'"[12] As an emotion, fear was created to slow down expansion;
trust, on the other hand, was created to accelerate our expansion. With each
shift in consciousness, we move closer to the main objective of our incarnation: to seek and manifest love in our lives and in the lives of others.

In the past, many of our beliefs were based on the fear principle; it actually helped many of us to feel safe. We knew what the rules were, and what
was expected of us. Although it provided a false sense of safety, it also gave us
a sense of boundaries, of where things began and ended. It defined our sense
of limits, but what contributed to it becoming a problem was that many of
these rules were based in fear. This level of consciousness approached everything from the "I" position: How is this going to affect *me*? It is a dimension
of consciousness that is very rooted in our inner desire to stay in control. As
we move away from this kind of thinking, we also grow out of the pervasive
feeling of impending doom that shadows our sense of safety. As we move into
more expansive levels of thinking, we trust that our lives are guided and begin
to understand our life's purpose; we develop a spiritual frame of reference on
which to base all our experiences. It takes trust to the level of knowing without second-guessing all that is happening in your life.

Fear to Trust:
Its Impact on Your Chakras, Feng Shui, and Health

This shift triggers unresolved issues associated with the Third Chakra, the
Will Center, which oversees our physical energy, adrenals, gut, stomach,
pancreas, gallbladder, upper intestine, liver, energy drive, intelligence, and
career issues. It is here that we store all our fears, angers, and guilts. The types
of illnesses that can emerge, if you are having a difficult time with this particular shift, are stomach ulcers, diabetes, gastrointestinal problems, middle-

back pain, exhaustion, depression, anxiety, chronic fatigue syndrome, viruses, insomnia, certain cancers, and almost any other illness that has its roots in faulty digestion, lack of nutrient absorption, or fear.

Chakra Color-Breathing Remedies. Color-breathe nine consecutive breaths of the color *yellow* into your solar plexus, every morning for nine consecutive days. For the next nine mornings, do an "alternating color-breathing" exercise in which you inhale the color yellow into your solar plexus and exhale the same breath through your "third eye"/Sixth Chakra in the color *indigo.* Then, for the next nine mornings, repeat the first sequence. If any of the emotional, spiritual, or physical issues are still present, stop color breathing for nine days, then repeat the 27-day sequence above.

Feng Shui Adjustment Remedies. Adjust *all* the Career areas in your home, and make all needed repairs to your Career guas. Augment the areas with brass wind chimes, indoor fountains, mirrors, artworks, water scenes, or paint something in the area black. Remember to perform the Three Secrets Reinforcement Blessing with all adjustments (see chapter 9).

4. From *Conditional Love* to *Unconditional Love* (Heart Chakra and Relationship Gua)

As we move through the different layers of expanded consciousness, it is very important that we look at how we were taught to understand, expect, and experience love. Love, although easy for us to express and acknowledge as children, is a very difficult emotion for adults. Most of us were taught from a very young age that love was something that you would feel only for that "special someone," and that when we realized we had those feelings, we should not act impulsively in sharing them, but give them great thought and consideration. We were encouraged to be shy about love and to protect ourselves from having our hearts broken or hurt in the process. A lot of rules and conditions came with our programming on love, which indirectly caused us to be calculating and controlling about feeling love and sharing in its joy spontaneously. This took the beauty away from the gift love was meant to be. Many of us were taught to fear love, as wanting and needing it may eventually hurt us. Often we were raised with parents who were struggling with their own limitations, having acquired similar beliefs from their parents.

In turn, many of us grew up and sought out partners who re-created our original love wounds, thus reinforcing our pain and confusion about love. The love issue is the emotional dynamic most in need of healing because without a healthy love relationship (be it with a partner, friend, or self), it's impossible to grow, heal, and do our work on the planet.

As we work toward expanding our consciousness, we automatically find ourselves resonating to a higher level and vibration of love energy. But even with this new level of consciousness, quite often we still attract people, places, and things that open old love-related wounds. In addition, as our vibration level increases, so does the level at which we feel things. Many people might actually find themselves growing and evolving to a higher frequency, only to find that certain situations feel even more painful and confusing than they did in the past. You might even be surprised to find that you have actually pulled in situations that seem old, with patterns that sometimes seem even worse than past situations. The reason for this interesting conundrum is that, from an energetic perspective, *love tends to bring up everything that's unlike itself.* This means that unresolved issues will be pulled in, brought to the surface, and magnified in order to be addressed and healed.

As we enter this new level of consciousness, love takes on a whole new expansion, because we come to understand that everyone and everything that enters our life is part of the divine plan. This doesn't mean we have to like it all, or that we deserve a bad relationship or an illness, but understanding the purpose behind these events helps us put the seeming randomness of the event into another perspective. It helps to empower us by putting more of the responsibility in our own hands, where we can truly do something about it. It is at this consciousness shift that we begin to have a heart expansion and become able to hold more love, unconditionally, for ourselves, for others, and for the co-creative kingdom of which we are a part. This is where our relationships and relationship patterns start to shift, as we find ourselves reevaluating our values, attractions, partners, and desires, and sometimes that means having to make radical changes in our current relationships.

These shifts are a natural part of the energy changes, but can be quite upsetting to partnerships and long-term plans. If a deep love is involved, or children, money, or possessions, the conflicts are even more intense and stressful. Often, clients who are requesting a Feng Shui consultation or private Therapeutic Chakra Feng Shui sessions with me are facing these issues head-on, and they can be very painful at first, as one realizes that one needs to move on from a loved one or a relationship. The long-term effects of resisting this part of the expansion and shift leave many people depressed, frustrated, and in unhappy relationships that they have outgrown and that no longer serve them. But many individuals, myself included, have opted at different times to stay in situations that aren't completely working because the familiarity of the relationship outweighs the enormous fear of what a change might or might not bring. As we expand our level of consciousness, everything that is left unprocessed is then repeated, but at a higher frequency with a bit more emotion, bringing with it more purging. This clearing and expansion into unconditional love moves many individuals energetically toward working with larger communities or overseeing programs that serve the higher good of society at large.

Conditional Love to Unconditional Love:
Its Impact on Your Chakras, Feng Shui, and Health

This consciousness shift triggers all unresolved issues associated with the Fourth Chakra, the Heart Center, which oversees all issues of connecting with self, others, nature, spirit, God, and our ability and capacity to love and be loved. When this principle is challenged in any way, it can reduce the amount of ch'i flow to the Heart Chakra, manifesting in illnesses such as heart disease, high blood pressure, respiratory infections, lung disease, carpal tunnel syndrome, arthritis of the hands or spine, shoulder, arms, and upper-back injuries.

Chakra Color-Breathing Remedies. Color-breathe nine consecutive breaths of the color *green* into your Heart Chakra, every morning for nine consecutive days. For the next nine mornings, do an "alternating color-breathing" exercise in which you inhale the color green into your Heart Chakra and exhale the same breath in *purple* energy out of your Crown Chakra, located at the top of your head. Repeat the first sequence again for nine days, for a total of 27 days. If any of the emotional, spiritual, or physical issues are still present, stop color breathing for nine days, then repeat the above 27-day sequence again.

Feng Shui Adjustment Remedies. Adjust *all* the Relationship areas in your home and make all needed repairs to your Relationship guas. Augment those areas with live plants, mirrors, brighter lighting, or a 40- or 50-mm clear or pink Feng Shui crystal on a red string in multiples of nine. You can also augment these areas with green objects or paint the room pink. Remember to perform the Three Secrets Reinforcement Blessing with all adjustments (see chapter 9).

5. From *False Self to Authentic Self* (Throat Chakra and Children-Creativity Gua)

In our old level of consciousness, many of us were taught to be who we are based on how others wanted or perceived us to be. We became mirrored extensions of what our parents wanted for us, what society thought we should do, and what limitations our gender roles carved out for us. We lived in a world where getting approval was important, and putting others' needs before our own was something that elicited approval and rewards. Being a good person, doing what we were told, and being liked were often the goals that motivated us. As we twisted ourselves into soft, nicely shaped pretzels just to get by without someone discovering our little secrets, we moved farther and farther away from who we really were. In an effort to please others, we willingly became our false selves. Often we didn't even know that we were turning into someone we were not, until our life, for various reasons, started changing and we found ourselves with no idea who we really were, or what we truly wanted.

Because of the false messages that we fed our inner compass, we had to develop ways of coping and living with this false self that we created. This inner wound is at the core of our addictions to alcohol, drugs, sex, food, debt, codependency, avoidance, and denial. The farther we move away from our true self, the farther away we also move from our own divinity. Our divine self is our spiritually attuned self who is directly connected to our higher power. The more we move away from our higher power (whomever we worship), the more we feel lost, and the more our pain increases. This process of being disconnected from the self puts us on a false path that subsequently follows a different soul route.

On the other hand, as our levels of consciousness expand, in a very accelerated fashion many of us are thrown very quickly into our authentic self. This is the more evolved part of the self that is more honest, real, and willing to show up for life. This consciousness shift also means that this person has to step up to the plate and take an honest look at who they are and who they are not. They must also be willing to address those less desirable "shadow parts" of themselves, and then take on the challenging task of bringing those pieces into the light, to be exposed and transformed. This is a very hard piece of work, especially if one has lived most of one's life with a false self. The universe is always willing to lend a hand as it lovingly places people, places, and things on your path to help put a crack in the façade, so to speak, helping the true self emerge.

This step is extremely challenging. Often when individuals are faced with the task of having to be painfully honest with themselves, they shut down, go into denial, or attempt to re-create their old life. Very quickly they discover that they cannot go back for very long, and the only direction that the universe will fully support is forward, and on to the new level of expansion.

False Self to Authentic Self: Its Impact on Your Chakras, Feng Shui, and Health

This shift triggers all unresolved issues associated with the Fifth Chakra, the Throat Center, which oversees all issues of identity. It's the center that oversees all of the creative works that we bring to the world, our sense of healthy versus unhealthy authority, our ability to speak up for ourselves, and all unresolved adolescent issues, and processes we go through that make it okay to be in the world as our true selves. If there is resistance to this necessary transition, it can manifest through various illnesses such as thyroid or endocrine imbalances, sore throats, chronic neck pain, and tooth and gum disease.

Chakra Color-Breathing Remedies. Color-breathe nine consecutive breaths of the color *sky blue* into the center of your Throat Chakra, for nine consecutive mornings. For the next nine mornings, do an "alternating color-breathing" exercise in which you inhale the color sky blue into your Throat Chakra and exhale with the same breath out of your Social Chakra, located two inches below your navel, in the color *orange.* Then, for the next nine mornings, repeat the first sequence to complete a total of 27 days. If any of the emotional, spiritual, or physical issues are still present, stop color breathing for nine days, then repeat the above 27-day sequence.

Feng Shui Adjustment Remedies. Adjust *all* the Children/Creativity areas of your home and make all the needed repairs to your Children/Creativity guas. Augment those areas by adding brass wind chimes, a 40-mm clear Feng Shui crystal, plants, mirrors, or any light-blue object, or paint the areas white. Remember to perform the Three Secrets Reinforcement Blessing with all adjustments (see chapter 9).

6. From *Analytical Thinking to Intuitive Knowing* (Third Eye Chakra and Knowledge Gua)

One of the most obvious signs that we are moving out of our old ways of thinking is that the way we assess and process things begins to change radically. Most of us were taught to rely mainly on analytical thinking as a way to understand our world and the way we should function in it. Analytical thinking has created many wonderful technologies that have advanced our culture, society, and world. These technological breakthroughs have allowed us to enjoy modern conveniences such as television, laser surgery, the Internet, and, of course, home computers (like the one I used to write this book). We owe a great debt to analytical thinking, for in many ways it has enhanced our lives and our stay here on the planet.

The thinking tool of logic is very important, for it allows us to advance toward, and then beyond, our wildest imagination. Analytical thinking has taught us to base our decisions on what we can logically deduce. If we are not able to figure something out or intellectually understand it, we can always fall back on our linear skills of reasoning to assess a situation and come up with a solution. It is through this process that the mind is given a lot of power. We were taught that we should allow the function of the mind to decide our actions for us, and reach decisions based on what we can see, feel, touch, taste, hear, or measure. Truth, in this way of thinking, is based on what the five senses can verify. It is how we arrived at our judgments, rationale, and conclusions for most of our business and personal decisions.

Because this thinking is so ensconced in logic, anything that cannot be proved or validated by the five senses is often disregarded. The flaws in this type of thinking start to emerge as we begin to grow into the next level of consciousness, because it is at this level that we start to take notice that our system of logic is not working the same way anymore. We begin to notice that some of our internal decisions are based on how we *feel,* and not necessarily on what we *know.* Our gut feelings start to get our attention, as we begin to give credence to the inner voices that guide us toward an alternative decision. Our intuition is now not something that we just dismiss as a "hunch," but a real resource that we need to learn to listen to for guidance. This shift slowly starts moving us into a place where we begin to work with our intuition and draw on it to validate what we intuitively know, as opposed to what we intellectually know. We can then expand on the use of our five senses and integrate them with our intuition as we begin to experience how we can use them in tandem.

On our new, more expanded level of consciousness, we not only hear external things, but thoughts and voices inside us as well (not, it must be noted, the kinds of voices that can send you off to "Shady Pines" for a lengthy stay). In our old way of thinking, you might be considered crazy if you shared such experiences, but in an expanded level of consciousness, you are slowed down, so that you can hear this very loud thinking, clearly.

As time goes on, you will welcome this guidance, for this shift in thinking will encourage you to reach for tools such as meditation and yoga to bring you closer to deciphering your life's path and direction. If you try to explain this experience to a person who is still locked in to analytic thinking, it will not necessarily be well received.

If, while trying to engage with your friends and lovers, you feel as though you have lost the ability to communicate comfortably with them, use this as a marker. It is usually a sign that you have moved out of your old ways of thinking. This is especially hard when you begin to realize that friends and family members with whom you were once close are now starting to feel distant. This aspect of the shift and expansion can bring feelings of sadness, pain, loss, abandonment, fears, and the like. This is a very difficult part of the transition, because as we grow and our consciousness expands, the people around us do not grow or shift at the same time. If we are not able to find common ground, the relationship then has to change, or possibly end.

Another fallout from this shift is the impact on your work and your ability to stay in your job or with your usual group of friends, because when you begin to acknowledge this inner knowing and use your intuition, it automatically moves you into a place of truth. It may be the truth of a situation, of a relationship, or of a particular person. Once we move into a place of inner knowing, it becomes harder to deny what we know. Sometimes that knowing means taking an honest look at the different people, places, and things in one's life. The truth then forces us to take action, which can cause a lot of change and upheaval.

As we move into higher levels of consciousness, we begin to recognize that we have been given additional abilities to intuit our lives, as we make more and more of our decisions from an internal place of knowing as opposed to an exclusively intellectual one. As we expand, more ways of accessing information are made available to us.

Analytical Thinking to Intuitive Knowing: Its Impact on Your Chakras, Feng Shui, and Health

This shift triggers unresolved issues associated with the Sixth Chakra, the Third Eye, which oversees our ability to see the truth, access intuition, and remember past lives. When this shift is blocked or energetically obstructed, it can manifest through various ailments, including those of the physical eyes, vision problems, cataracts, as well as allergies, sinus problems, hearing losses, ear infections, headaches, congestion, spaciness, aneurysms, systemic illnesses, and the inability to see things clearly.

Chakra Color-Breathing Remedies. Color-breathe nine consecutive breaths of the color *indigo* into your Third Eye each morning for nine days. For the next nine mornings, do an "alternative color-breathing" exercise, inhaling the color indigo into your Third Eye and exhaling the color *yellow* out of your solar plexus. Then, for the next nine mornings, repeat the first sequence, for a total of 27 days. If any of the emotional, spiritual, or physical challenges are still present, stop color breathing for nine days, then repeat the above 27-day sequence.

Feng Shui Adjustment Remedies. Adjust *all* the Knowledge areas in your home and make all needed repairs to your Knowledge guas. Augment the Knowledge guas with a 40- or 50-mm blue (or clear) Feng Shui crystal on a red string in multiples of nine, an indoor water fountain, brass wind chimes, mirrors, or any indigo-colored object, or paint the area in shades of blue. Remember to perform the Three Secrets Reinforcement Blessing with all adjustments (see chapter 9).

7. From *Cruise Control to Accelerated Speed* (Crown Chakra and Fame Gua)

As we approach this new shift, the speed at which our lives unfold rapidly accelerates. At first you may not recognize what is happening because what you are personally experiencing will occur in what seems like a vacuum. First, one change will occur, and then another. Not until we view our lives in retrospect will we see the amount of change that has transpired. Often the changes happen so quickly that they are internal and can only be felt by you. As you change levels of consciousness, you also go through personality and perceptual changes as well. You may feel the urge to leave a relationship or change jobs or careers, or consider moving to a different location. These changes may be prompted by a "gut feeling" rather than by a concrete and secure opportunity, for when leaving our old ways of being, the ways we make decisions also change. This can be scary at first; you may feel as though your life has become unglued. You will actually seem more scattered and unfocused at first. This can be quite disconcerting, especially while others appear to be calm, and their lives stable. Changes will happen more abruptly than they may have in the past, and often without notice. This is also because in our old levels of consciousness we diligently lived by a set of time references that created the daily structure in which our lives functioned. We knew how long an hour or a day was, and that twelve months made a year. With that information in place, we set out to live our lives and make our goals and changes fit into time frames that included the traditional nine-to-five workday, twelve-o'clock lunches, and downtime weekends consisting of Saturdays and Sundays.

Time can become a stress factor, and a form of limitation, when we shift to new levels of understanding and consciousness. As the speed of our life accelerates, the way we have measured time, by the old calendar, loses its meaning. Without realizing this, at first we may try to apply our old frame of reference to our current life schedule at the new level, which can result in a feeling that our timing mechanism is a bit off. Knowing about this specific time change gives you the right to use my favorite excuse, whenever

I'm running behind (borrowed from my friend Dr. Heather Anne Harder): *"Sorry, I don't do Earth time very well!"*

After you acclimate to your new time frame, you will discover that things that would normally have taken even two to five years to process or accomplish may take only a few months. Because things are moving so quickly, certain things will transpire in a very accelerated way. This may sound like lots of fun, for things that you want may come to pass more quickly, but in order for those new things to be brought into your life, other things may need to change and be cleared out first. These shifts mean *changes,* and change, no matter how well intended, can be disruptive and sometimes not so much fun. Your life will change, and sometimes that means the people, places, and things in your life will change also.

Most of us are experiencing this time shift, in one way or another. If your life is not going through some major reevaluations, changes, or spurts of growth, you are probably resisting the transition on some level; this is common, and is something we all do at different times throughout the shift.

Whatever you do, don't try to force it, and don't feel bad or left out. In the right time, in divine order, it will find you. Just when your soul is ready to make those changes, it will gently place you right into the fast lane, and there you will go.

During this shift in acceleration, you will have the desire to create and manifest more things. But until you fully understand how to manage the energy and time shifts, you may, without realizing it, overextend yourself. This time transition often shows itself behaviorally in individuals who take on more and more responsibilities. This dynamic is different from that of the overachiever or the workaholic of our previous consciousness, because what distinguishes the two behaviors from each other is motivation. In our new, expanded level of consciousness, our motivational force is to become more involved and part of the bigger picture by contributing the gifts that we are here to share. Understanding our life's work more clearly, we understand what is needed from us during these times of profound changes.

In addition, any decisions that are related to time factors—such as having a baby before you get too old, staying in your company till you get the pension, or waiting till the kids are grown to go back to school—can get challenged in a very accelerated way. Sometimes if we find ourselves retooling our life plans based around other people's needs, this can create a delayed response. The types of illnesses listed below can occur when you delay life-plan changes based on other people's neds. Not focusing on what you are being called to do will throw off the soul's internal time clock, which keeps you on track with your own life's schedule. Remember, as these shifts unfold, it's important to keep your life as balanced as you can, whatever your level of consciousness. Honor your own time needs first, and make sure that you are doing all the things you require and desire, in order to take the best care of yourself that you can.

Cruise Control to Accelerated Speed: Its Impact on Your Chakras, Feng Shui, and Health

This shift triggers all unresolved issues associated with the Seventh Chakra, the Crown Center, which oversees our path, destiny, and the work that we are here to do. Illnesses that may occur, if this point of transition is blocked or constricted, include those that have to do with the blood or blood disorders, various cancers, brain injuries, tumors, Alzheimer's, multiple sclerosis, systemic and atypical diseases, and strange or rare illnesses.

Chakra Color-Breathing Remedies. Color-breathe nine consecutive breaths of the color *violet* (or purple) into the Crown Chakra, located at the top of your head, for nine mornings. For the next nine mornings, do an "alternating color-breathing" exercise, inhaling the color violet into the Crown Chakra and exhaling the color *green* from the Heart Chakra, nine breaths for nine consecutive mornings. Then, for the next nine mornings, repeat the first sequence, for a total of 27 consecutive days. If any of the emotional, spiritual, or physical challenges still exist, stop color breathing for nine days, then repeat the 27-day sequence above.

Feng Shui Adjustment Remedies. Adjust *all* of the Fame areas in your home, and make all necessary repairs to your Fame guas. Augment those areas with a 40- or 50-mm clear (or red) Feng Shui crystal on a red string in multiples of nine, any pictures or artwork with depth and color, nine red ribbons, or any green object, plants, bright lights, or paint the area in vibrant shades of red. Remember to perform the Three Secrets Reinforcement Blessing with all adjustments (see chapter 9).

8. From *Blame to Responsibility* (Transpersonal Chakra and Helpful People Gua)

In our very early years we were all taught the very wonderful social skill of blame. We all know what blame is, right? It is the process by which we shift the responsibility from one person, place, or thing onto another so we don't have to claim our part in a particular situation. It was originally intended to hold others accountable for their actions, but it quickly became misused. We've all done it at one time or another. It's an integral component of human behavior, a knee-jerk reaction. The process of shifting blame to others has contributed to keeping people unaccountable for their actions, and therefore absolving them of responsibility.

The freedom that higher levels of consciousness affords us does not come without a price: *Along with that freedom comes responsibility for all that we do and don't do in our lives and with the people who are placed in our lives.* This very significant shift will profoundly affect our actions and the very core of our moral structure. Over the years, the abdication of responsibility has contributed to everything from parents justifying child abuse to governments not meeting the needs of the people they serve. The "blame game" has given us permission to ignore our social, political, and spiritual responsibilities.

As a psychotherapist I often saw the therapeutic value in blaming, for it initially helped hold others accountable for some horrendous behaviors, in addition to helping a lot of clients understand what had happened to them in their childhoods or in their unhappy relationships. Previously, many of those clients, especially those with histories of abuse, had spent their whole lives erroneously blaming themselves for the pain and disappointments they had endured. Often I found that blaming others was the exact emotional precursor needed to help many of these people over the hump of self-blame (which is at the opposite end of the spectrum). This dynamic has kept many individuals trapped forever in a victim role. The problem with the blame response is that many people get stuck there and never get around to taking responsibility for their own lives and recognizing that for some reason their soul has summoned this particular challenge to somehow heal or transmute something.

Blame should not be confused with ascribing responsibility where responsibility is due. Sometimes people do horrible things that one deems unforgivable, and that's a choice individuals have to make. But even if we choose not to forgive, we still need to move on.

As we begin to shift consciousness and start to take more responsibility for our lives, we begin our ascension out of victimhood and into true healing, and we open up to other types of knowledge and ways of perceiving things. One of the signals that you are shifting gears is your understanding of why certain things happen to you in your life. It is at this level that you start to consider other factors that have created your life's experiences besides your family of origin, your childhood, and a few lucky breaks. You start to consider your purpose in life, along with karmic factors and the possibilities of past-life influences. You take more responsibility for what is or isn't happening in your life. This thinking spills over into how we view and treat one another; into how governments create their policies; and into the way we treat all the creatures that reside on the planet. We start to see ourselves as powerful beings who can use our own personal divine power to walk our path with dignity and help make the changes, in our life and in the world, that we came to make. We understand that we are all here with a purpose, and that *everything* we have experienced in our lives can be transmuted into something higher, as we come to understand that there are no junk experiences.

Blame to Responsibility:
Its Impact on Your Chakras, Feng Shui, and Health

This shift can trigger all unresolved issues associated with the Eighth Chakra, the Transpersonal Center, located six inches above your head. This area is where the body splits off and is half in spirit and half in body. It is the center that oversees the soul's path, as opposed to the Seventh Chakra, which mainly oversees one's life path during one's incarnation on Earth. This center does not carry physical illness per se, because illness as we understand it manifests in the physical body and not technically in the same way in an etheric body. What this center does do is hold the nonphysical vibrational counterparts, or miasms, of all the illnesses that can occur in the Seventh Chakra and in other Chakras as well. Miasms are not a predisposition to any illness, just an "energetic possibility" that certain illnesses can occur for that individual. When we are not connected to our spirit or to accessing help on a spiritual level, and we are cut off from seeing all the signposts that keep us on our path, we can get sick—not as a form of punishment, but as a means of helping us find our way back, *or back home.* This energetic separation from our higher self can act as the catalyst to developing almost any illness.

Chakra Color-Breathing Remedies. Color-breathe nine consecutive breaths of *white* light in and out of your Transpersonal Chakra, located six inches above the top of your head and also throughout your whole body, every morning for nine days. Then do an "alternating color-breathing" exercise and inhale a breath of white light into your Transpersonal Center, six inches above your head, and exhale *green* energy out of the Heart Chakra. Do nine breaths for nine mornings. Repeat the first sequence for nine more mornings, for a total of 27 days. Then stop color breathing for nine days. If the emotional, spiritual, or physical challenges still exist, repeat the complete color-breathing sequence for an additional 27 days.

Feng Shui Adjustment Remedies. Adjust *all* the Helpful People areas in your home, and make all necessary repairs to your Helpful People guas. Augment those areas with brass wind chimes, water fountains, and bright lighting; photos of deities, mentors, and supportive people; create altars and hang mirrors. Add gray-colored objects and paint the space white or gray. Remember to perform the Three Secrets Reinforcement Blessing with all adjustments (see chapter 9).

9. From *Traditional Medicine to Vibrational Medicine* (Overall Vibration/Health and Center Gua)

As we move into the world of invisible energy, we begin to draw to ourselves many new ways to problem-solve, and many of those ways are different from what our old ways of thinking offered us. Most of us were taught that our problems should first be analyzed, and the solutions based on what's practical, rational, tried and true. Most such solutions were safe, predictable, and conformed to the status quo. They were the ones that made the most intellectual sense, for they were based on intellectual reasoning. In Black Hat Feng Shui we refer to such solutions as "mundane solutions" (see chapter 9).

For instance, if you're having a difficult time finding work, a good piece of advice might be to go back to school and get another degree in a different field, or, if you would like to buy your own home, to go to a local bank and apply for a loan. These are all approaches that make sense from a traditional point of view. They are based in logic, with an understanding that is germane to the way things were approached within that level of consciousness. But going back to school doesn't assure us a well-paid job, any more than applying for a loan guarantees us a house. Unknown factors including general circumstances, energy patterns, access to opportunities and karmic baggage also have a significant impact on what happens or doesn't happen in our lives. The Chinese believe that five things strongly influence our fate: education, karma, good deeds, good luck, and Feng Shui.

Most of us approach our health care and choices of medical treatment from a similar point of view. The majority of traditional treatment plans are based on after-the-fact interventions based on test results, followed by prescriptions of synthetic chemicals that we manufacture in laboratories.

The problem with traditional medicine doesn't lie solely in the type of treatment, but in the way that it omits other very important information. Although traditional medicine has brought us some wonderful breakthroughs in the areas of diagnostics, transplants, and surgery, it often fails by neglecting to treat and address the whole being.

As we expand our state of awareness, we become much more receptive to alternative ways of healing and problem-solving. It is in this new place of awareness that we embrace our intuition and our ability to see, know, feel, and sense things to which we may not have been open before; it is from this level of consciousness that we seek out new ways to understand and transcend the everyday problems and the health challenges we are facing.

Many cures for illness that are based on a Feng Shui or Chakra perspective are not derived from logic, as we were taught it. Transcendental in nature, these treatments often don't make much rational sense. Keep in mind, as you read in the next chapter, that they do make a lot of sense, just on a different level. Within their own realm of invisible energy and vibrational patterns, however, they have a rigor and a very clear purpose unique to their own level of consciousness.

That's why, for example, it may be pointless to try to persuade your mother to change her diet to help alleviate arthritis discomfort (I know this one personally). Although the connection between food and arthritis pain might be obvious to you, if the sufferer is not open to new and sometimes revolutionary treatments, the well-intended suggestions might fall on deaf ears.

As mentioned earlier, you will find that as your consciousness grows, your life begins to accelerate, and your physical body scrambles to maintain homeostasis. It is because of this new level of consciousness and understanding about life, energy, sickness, and disease that we are in need of new medicines that will align with our newfound perspective on health. We have developed a need for new tools to help us manage and treat our life and our health from a vibrational perspective. These vibrational medicines are often rejected by people with different levels of consciousness, because it just isn't within their present capacity to see how these alternative solutions can work.

As we increase our understanding of the invisible realms of knowledge and how they work, we begin to attract information on those tools that are available now to assist us. This phenomenon is part of why you found this book—or *why it found you.*

We are now beginning to understand that we are more than just a body and mind, and that we possess a soul, a spirit, and are connected to a consciousness far greater than ourselves. It is at this consciousness level that we become open to using tools of divination—pendulums, tarot cards, angel cards, crop-circle cards, and medicine cards, to name a few. At other levels we may also find ourselves consulting the *I Ching,* meditating, going to psychics and medical intuitives for guidance. It is here where we begin to explore numerology, consult astrologers, or explore past lives, and, of course, utilize Feng Shui and the Chakras as complementary medicines for our healing process.

Traditional Medicine to Vibrational Medicines:
Its Impact on Your Chakras, Feng Shui, and Health

Many of us are most familiar with traditional medicines as treatments for acute and chronic illnesses. As new ways of seeing and treating illnesses are presented to us, many of us find ourselves with one foot in each camp, trying to find the balance between modalities. Actually, most of those reading this book will fall into this category. When faced with an illness, overwhelming fear often clouds our inner clarity and treatment choices. To help you bridge the gap and choose what's right for you from the best of both medicine worlds, use the color-breathing exercises below to help you become very focused and clear on arriving at the right decision for you and your healing process.

Chakra Color-Breathing Remedies. This health-related transition corresponds to the overall vibration of your body and the collective energy system of all the Chakras. Color-breathe nine complete breaths of either *golden* or *white* light into your whole vibration, and into every organ, cell, muscle, tissue, and bone, all sick or diseased areas, and your total body. Do this for a minimum of 27 mornings, nine complete breaths each morning. To further strengthen the above cure, try alternating your color-breathing meditation with nine inhalations of *white* light, and nine exhalations of *yellow golden* light for an additional 27 consecutive days.

Feng Shui Adjustment Remedies. Adjust *all* the center Health areas and make all the needed repairs to your Health guas. Augment those areas with a 40- or 50-mm clear Feng Shui crystal, thriving plants, increased lighting, brass wind chimes, and any multicolored rainbow objects, or paint the area in shades of yellow. Remember to perform the Three Secrets Reinforcement Blessing with all Feng Shui adjustments, choices, and cures. Keep in mind that if you want to raise the effectiveness of the color cures bless them, too, with the Three Secrets Reinforcement Blessing (see chapter 9).

WHAT IS NEEDED FOR A SMOOTH AND SUCCESSFUL TRANSITION?

As these nine shifts start to unfold (and they have been doing so ever since the 1960s and the "free love" movement), it's important that you understand the psychological concepts that will be of help to you in making your transitions smooth and successful. The three principles that follow will give you a frame of reference that you can use to help you put the fallout from the transition period into perspective. These concepts will help you manage your life, and eventually your health, in ways that will allay your fears and reassure you that although you are going through difficult times, you are on the right track.

Three Principles for Easing the Transitions

1. ***Minimize resistance.*** When we are in a time of change, it is a common reaction to consciously (or, more often, unconsciously) resist the change. Even if you are the one who initiated the change, or it is a change that is obviously for the better, from an energetic standpoint we all go through a phase of resistance. This isn't a bad thing or even a negative reflection on you, but basic human nature. This is a very common occurrence because any situation in your life, even your particular illness, has an energy field around it, and whatever has an energy field around it also has a life force. Whenever a life force is present, and it feels as though it is in danger of annihilation, it will react to the situation by fighting for its life. So you will have to learn how to work with resistance when it surfaces. As you move forward into your healing process, you may become uncomfortable, and you may be very tempted to let resistance get its way. Stay strong and see through the resistance, and don't allow yourself to be manipulated by it.

2. ***Do not be seduced by the fear.*** As you start delving more and more into the underpinnings of your illness or health concern, it is easy and common to become afraid. Sometimes the roots of fear are quite old, but as they resurface during the purging process, often they feel as real as they did as when you first experienced them. At other times the fears are unfounded, just the ghost of our frightened inner child that still resides in our consciousness. In Native American teachings, fear is referred to as the Great Coyote, a master of trickery and illusions. It will disguise itself as truth, in as many variations and disguises as it can concoct, just to fool you into believing that you shouldn't be doing what you're doing, or that you're making the wrong choices.

   As the world starts changing around you—sometimes initially not for the better—life will become scary. If your long-term marriage is ending or if you have been diagnosed with a serious illness, there is no way around it; the unknown will be frightening. Feel the fear, have your doubts, but move forward anyway. Do not let the fear convince you otherwise that you are doomed and without a benevolent higher power or personal path. Your guides are right by your side, surrounding you, waiting for you to call on them, to acknowledge their presence and your need for assistance.

3. *Acknowledge chaos as change.* As the shifts begin to happen, chaos is inevitable to a certain degree. As we break down old patterns, belief systems, and ways of being, people, places, and things will begin to shift and move toward reordering themselves. The time between the way things were and the way they will be can seem very chaotic. The old is torn down, and before it can be rebuilt, the time period in between can look like it is in demolition. If we fixate on just that middle segment of the process, we will feel hopeless and devastated, without a vision of the new, more expansive change in times ahead. We then lock in to this phase and build our reality around it, as if it were a permanent state of affairs. Often we act as if the chaos itself were the final destination and not just a stepping-stone along the way to something greater. Sometimes it's hard for the universe to reorder things for your higher good, without dismantling the exact things that contributed to the problem or health crisis to begin with. But it is during that time that true change occurs. As the universe helps rebuild things for you on a more personal level, it is also simultaneously changing bigger vibrational patterns and planetary thought-forms that held the energetic space in the world for your problem or illness to exist.

TWELVE ISSUES TO ADDRESS AND PROCESS AS THE OLD MATRIX BEGINS TO CRACK

The twelve issues to address and process, which I outline below, are designed to give you further guidance on the various things you should do as your old thinking and consciousness begin to shift. These suggestions will assist you in addressing and processing many more aspects of the ESPs of your illness and, in turn, further accelerate your healing and transformation.

1. *Make amends/bring closure* to as many old situations and past relationships as you possibly can. Make this pilgrimage every few months until you are dealing with things and situations as they happen, with no backlash or stagnant energy accrual.

2. *Address your relationship patterns* and take responsibility for the part you had in creating toxic dynamics and causing unintentional harm. Work on changing your patterns by being honest and emotionally "showing up" for every day and every thing that needs to be addressed. Release with love and compassion all significant relationships that no longer serve either partner's growth or life path.

3. *Face the reality of impermanence* as things start technically to move away from you, change, or possibly leave your life. Know that everything is borrowed, and that all of your partners and relationships are basically on loan from the universe. Try to return them in the same shape or better than when they first arrived.

4. *Release all attachments* to things of the mundane world that no longer serve you. Let go of clutter, unwanted gifts, old self-images, and locked-in ways of being in the world. Nothing is worth holding on to that doesn't serve your highest good. Keep in mind that in the end we leave even our bodies behind. If we can do that with our bodies, we can surely let go of other things.

5. *Discover your genius.* Before incarnating, we were given special gifts and talents to share with the world, and we agreed to use them for the higher good. Find those latent or subtle talents, and put all your energy into developing them and sharing them with the world. This is what you agreed to do, so let the rest fall by the wayside for someone else to address.

6. *Expose your shadow.* Unearth the parts of yourself of which you are embarrassed, and that hold your deepest, darkest secrets. These are the

exact things that lurk in our shadow and manifest unresolved through our illnesses. By exposing these secrets to God, other people, and ourselves, we are fulfilling our promise to the personal work we said we would do, and supporting our healing process.

7. ***Confront your inner saboteur,*** the part of you that creeps up and pulls the rug out from under you just as you have made some progress, worked through some major issue, or taken a big risk. It's the part of yourself that wants to keep things the way they were when they were on a prior, more familiar level, because quite often, change, although wanted, can be scary.

8. ***Frustrations are grist for the mill.*** Setbacks are created to help you hone your focus and get to what's really important. Delays are the "divine buffer of time," purposely placed to create the correct timing for the event or situation to unfold or manifest.

9. ***Take good care of yourself.*** You too are on loan from the universe. Most of us take better care of the books we borrow from the library than we do ourselves. The physical body that the universe lent you during your stay here needs to be cared for, loved, pampered, exercised, fed good food, nurtured, and emotionally and energetically kept in good shape. When you are sick, take it as a sign that you are in need of some more of everything on the list above. This is not a choice or an option, but an agreed obligation that you have to your life and body, especially when you are sick.

10. ***Redefine illness and death.*** As you start to experience the shift in your life, it's important that you move away from seeing sickness as a punishment, and death as a random tragedy. Instead, reconsider the idea that life is something we've chosen, incarnation is a privilege, and all the issues, illnesses, and even deaths have a higher and deeper meaning than just the pain and suffering they bring. Empowerment through the crisis, illness, or loss comes from owning the experience from the soul's perspective, and not from the personality's limited view.

11. ***Embrace your insanity.*** As things start changing and falling apart, our worst insanity, expressed in the ways we react and try to control things will surface. And in turn we will try to blame or discredit others, or project our madness onto them, especially on the ones we love and often are closest to. Try to own your own brand of insanity, and be as honest as you can about what is being triggered and coming up for you. Look long and hard at where you are the most insane, and then make your amends and try to take the right actions.

12. ***Celebrate Your SQ!*** We are all born with an IQ (intelligence quotient), but what we haven't been told is that we are also born with an SQ, or Stupidity Quotient. Personally, this is my favorite part of being in my life. Why? Because we spend so much unnecessary time covering up our inadequacies, while trying to pretend that we are good at everything, we know how to do it all, and we aren't in need of any help. When you acknowledge and embrace all the things that you don't know or don't understand, you automatically free yourself from the debilitating façade of the cover-up. This ownership allows you to hire professionals to do the things that you are totally ignorant about, ask for help from others when you need it, and lean on a benevolent higher power to bring in the helpful people we all desperately need. When we can smile and own our insufficiencies, life gets so much easier. Just try being who you are and where you are in your life, and let that suffice. *There is so much more integrity in being disliked for who you truly are, than in being someone who is liked for something he or she is not.*

As Emmanuel says, "Who you are is a necessary step to becoming who you will be."[13]

Closing Chapter Exercise

Review the "Nine Hallmarks of the Spiritual Revolution" and pick three that you feel you are currently being challenged by. List how they are manifesting in your life, what aspects of your life they are affecting, and three possible solutions for each one that will help you move through the transition more smoothly. Please note that many of these shifts and hallmarks overlap. Try to connect with the one that fits your issues most closely. Check the health-related manifestations and your likes and dislikes of certain colors, then check the corresponding areas of your home that may be in disrepair. All these pieces, when analyzed, will help you decide which pieces of the transition you are being affected by and may be contributing to your current illness. Make sure you list your fears, reasons for resistance, and ways that you can approach the changes differently. Review any illnesses you have currently, or had in the past. Try to connect your illness with the emotional and spiritual transition that is taking place. Do your color-breathing exercise (see the end of chapter 7 for more details), and make your Feng Shui adjustments accordingly. Keep in mind that even if you are not currently ill, you can still review the Nine Hallmarks and see which issues apply to you. Follow the same procedures listed as a preventive means for shoring up your Chakras and various guas of your home to head off any potential illnesses.

CHAPTER NINE

TRANSCENDENTAL CURES

Spiritual Prescriptions for What Ails You

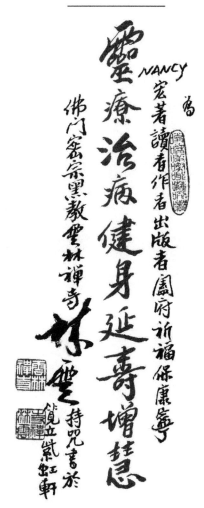

*"Spiritual Healing Cures Illnesses, Strengthens the Body,
Prolongs Longevity, and Increases Wisdom."*

CALLIGRAPHY BY H. H. PROFESSOR THOMAS LIN YUN RINPOCHE

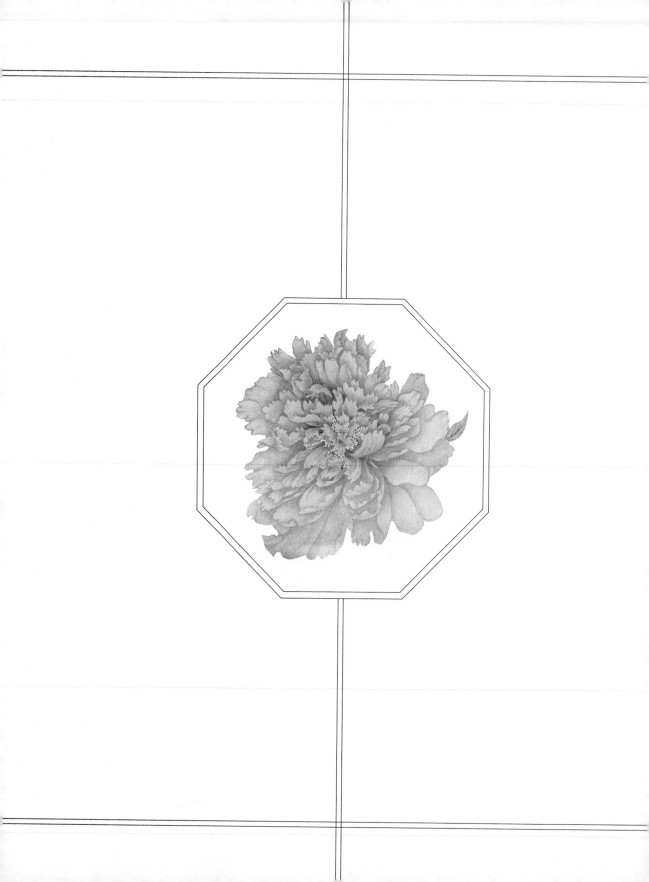

MANY ROADS, MANY SCHOOLS

ALTHOUGH FENG SHUI has been around for over 4,000 years, we in the West are just now beginning to receive its benefits. In 1989, when I first began to study Feng Shui, it was hard enough to find a class on the subject, let alone an article or a book. Information on the subject was mostly written in Chinese and was almost nonexistent in English. My colleague Sarah Rossbach almost single-handedly changed all this when she wrote the first book on Feng Shui from the Black Hat School perspective in English. Sarah has indirectly touched each of you who are reading this book, because without those teachings I would not be writing on these principles today. I am deeply indebted to her for her ingenuity and her contribution to my life and work, and to the spiritual growth of the world.

When my first book, *Feng Shui: Harmony by Design* (Perigee), was published in 1996, there were only two other books written in English on the subject of Black Hat Sect Feng Shui, both by Sarah Rossbach. I was only the second author to be published in English on its principles! That was a real honor for me to be part of such a great spiritual movement and distinguished lineage. But now there are so many more books available that the sheer volume of information can very often be confusing. The main reason for this is that as Feng Shui teachings become more available, what the books and articles fail to tell you is that there are many different schools of thought and approaches to the Feng Shui process. But the specifics on the different schools of Feng Shui are not as important as being aware that the differences exist, so that you're not overwhelmed when one article tells you to put your bed on one wall, only to find that another, equally well intended article suggests to place the same bed in another location.

As you come to know the various schools and principles, you will be able to make a decision on what school of thought resonates to your liking, and which principles you would most like to follow and implement. All schools of Feng Shui thought are equally good and share the same objective: to create environments that assist people and help transform their lives for the better. No one school is intrinsically better than another, but you will develop preferences based on the energetic compatibility between you and the teachings. All schools of thought should be honored, respected, and explored before you make a decision based on what feels right to you.

THE THREE MAIN FENG SHUI SCHOOLS OF THOUGHT

Although there are as many schools of thought in Feng Shui as there are regions in China, it's easiest for us to narrow them down to three main areas for our purposes here. The oldest and one of the most basic schools is the "form school," started by average commoners and farmers who basically wanted to plant their rice where it would have the best chance of growing and flourishing. They would call in the "Feng Shui priest," as such persons were called at the time, and he (even today, not many women practice Feng Shui professionally in Asia) would look around at the surrounding environment and try to assess the impact of the various shapes on the crop and on the owners of the crop. The main environmental objects and shapes considered at that time were mountains and mountain ranges. The priest would assess the shape of a mountain to see if it was auspicious or inauspicious, and then ascribe an element to it, based on its shape and form. For example, if the mountain was pointed and came to a high peak, that range would be considered a Fire element. Then the priest would assess whether the element of Fire would be compatible with the site and with the farmer's personal elements.

Placement was also known to be important to good Feng Shui Design. By placing the rice crop with water in front of it and mountains behind, you would be utilizing the natural elements of nature to support the goals and objectives of the individual. The water would nourish the crop and the mountains would protect it from the harsh winds. With those supports in place, the chances for that crop to thrive were increased. A healthy crop would mean a well-fed family; a well-fed family would mean a healthy family. An abundant crop would also create a surplus of rice that could be sold and would thus bring prosperity. By aligning the crop with the forces of nature, nature would innately support the farmer and all his endeavors; thus Feng Shui was born; its name in fact means "wind and water."

A second group of schools are referred to as the "traditional schools," or better known as the "compass schools." Many schools fall into this category: San-yuan, San-he, Jyiou-shing, Ling-nan, Tao, Dza, Yin-Yang, Flying Stars, Five Pillars, etc. Their main common characteristic is that they follow a traditional approach and employ a "compass" (also known as a *lo p'an*) as their primary measuring tool. They emphasize the importance of tangible, objective factors and things that can be seen or measured. In addition, they utilize "absolute direction" (east, west, north, and south) and astrological information. When you are reading a book or article that makes reference to placing a piece of furniture in a specific direction you will know, even if it is not clearly stated, that the point of reference is that of one of the traditional, or "compass," schools.

The third school, and probably the most popular here in the United States, is the one that is the basis for this book, the Black Hat Sect Tibetan Tantric Buddhism School (or BTB). This school was brought to the States by my mentor and teacher, His Holiness Grandmaster Thomas Lin Yun Rinpoche. Professor Lin is the Head Master and Spiritual Leader of the Third and Fourth Stages of the Black Hat Sect Tibetan Tantric School of Feng Shui. The First Stage originated in India before Buddhism existed. The Second Stage occurred when Indian Buddhism spread to Tibet, where it converged with the native religion, called Bon. In Tibet, the Buddhists split into five different sects, each one named after the distinctive color of the clothes/hats they wore. The Five Sects became known as the Red, Yellow, Green, Multicolored, and Black. Four of the sects remained in Tibet, with their monks leading a monastic life. The Black Hat Sect, however, broke tradition and migrated to China to spread its teachings and directly be with the people.

BTB spent most of its time in its Third Stage in China, where it developed many of its Feng Shui principles, theories, and cures. Professor Lin Rinpoche, leader of the Third and Fourth Stage BTB, brought these teachings to the United States in the mid-1980s. Throughout his 35 years of practice, he has incorporated other disciplines into Black Hat Feng Shui, to enhance its effectiveness and reflect the needs and issues of modern society. Black Hat Feng Shui incorporates various studies such as modern medicine, psychology, architecture, art, urban planning, holistic healing, aromatherapy, meditation, ch'i cultivation, and spirituality.

The additional ways that BTB incorporates traditional teachings differs from other schools in terms of approach and application. The main features that distinguish BTB are that instead of using the *lo p'an* compass or absolute directions to determine where the different gua locations are, we superimpose the Bagua; we emphasize *yi* factors, which are intangible or invisible elements, to determine placement and cures; our emphasis is on the "mouths of the ch'i," or entranceways for determining the proper placement of the Bagua and the location of its guas. BTB is rooted in spirituality and its emphasis is on cultivating one's own energy; we use both mundane and transcendental solutions and for our Feng Shui assessments we analyze both the visible and invisible factors equally. We conduct Blessings Ceremonies, use the Three Secrets Reinforcement Blessing, and, whenever appropriate, employ the use of the "Red Envelope Ritual."

MUNDANE VERSUS TRANSCENDENTAL SOLUTIONS

The two ways that we attempt to adjust the Feng Shui in our lives are through *mundane* and *transcendental* cures. Mundane cures are solutions that are practical, reasonable, and deemed logical by most of the population. Transcendental cures are solutions that are considered more mystical and spiritual in nature, and don't necessarily follow any rules accessible to logic or intellect. Both sets of solutions—and I cannot emphasize this enough— are equally important because they need to work in tandem to maximize their effectiveness.

To give a concrete example, let's say that you are tired a lot and are having a difficult time breathing. You believe that your symptoms are stress-related due to unhealthy activity, so you call in a Feng Shui consultant to assist you with the work-related issues. After a thorough assessment of your home, several different solutions including mundane and transcendental cures might be suggested. For example, the consultant may recommend that you see a holistic doctor, get a checkup, talk with a career counselor, or consider taking a vacation. All these types of suggestions can be considered common responses and in Feng Shui are referred to as "mundane solutions." In addition, the Feng Shui consultant might also suggest placing wind chimes in all your entranceways (entranceways oversee the respiratory system), hanging a crystal on a nine-inch red string in the center of every room (the center of the room oversees the Health Gua), and placing a mirror in the Relationship gua of your bedroom (the Relationship gua connects with the Heart Chakra, which oversees the lungs). These examples of "transcendental solutions" make no sense, but Professor Lin believes that many of them can be up to 120 percent effective, as opposed to the 20- or 30-percent effectiveness of mundane solutions. Transcendental solutions are those that are borrowed from more advanced levels of consciousness, because, in the expansion of or understanding of energy and how the invisible factors work, we begin to incorporate sound, color, vibration, and other means of healing that don't require speech or tangible proof. Hanging a crystal ball on a nine-inch red string in an area where there is no light makes no rational sense, so we call it transcendental. What we are actually doing is reaching out into a more advanced level of "spiritual technology" for solutions that will solve the problems of the prior level of consciousness.

Transcendental solutions have three basic premises that need to be considered in order for you to decide whether you agree with them. *The first premise* is believing there are valid systems and realms of knowledge that we cannot intellectually understand. *The second premise* is that these systems are valid and function on a higher order, enlisting the help and expertise of other spiritual forces. *The third premise* is that you accept and understand that the process is part of a co-creative effort to work with all the invisible forces of nature collectively, to rebalance energy and to shift and heal the whole planet. Although working with energy is an invisible and, at times, intangible process, energy exists everywhere and has a profound effect on all our lives. And just because we are creating change through an invisible energy system doesn't make it any less valid or real.

The Chinese have been using energy in their medical practices for centuries. Acupuncture, Chinese herbal medicine, and shiatsu massage are just a few examples of the many healing modalities that have made their way West and have become not only popular but also accepted as respectable alternatives to Western medicine. When a doctor or acupuncturist inserts a needle in a certain part of your body to stimulate blocked ch'i, what he or she is really doing is placing the needle (or the fingertips, in shiatsu) on an energy pathway in the body that is referred to as a meridian. These meridians, which are invisible, connect to different organs and regulate the flow of ch'i in a person's body. Blocked meridians mean blocked energy, which creates a reduced flow of the life force. The meridians correspond to the organs and their related systems in the body, affecting their health and well-being.

The same invisible system of energy or ch'i that governs these healing modalities also oversees the Feng Shui process. *Feng Shui is like acupuncture for your home.* The same life force of ch'i that lives invisibly in the body also lives invisibly outside the body in your home, office, and outdoor environments. So, when you place a crystal ball in your Wealth corner to stimulate ch'i flow, you are actually using that particular adjustment item the same way acupuncturists use their needles and shiatsu practitioners use their fingertips to move and unblock ch'i.

If the idea of transcendental cures seems foolish to you, remember that research and science have always had a way of making the unexplainable acceptable. Imagine yourself two hundred years ago, trying to explain the Concorde, or even a basic airplane! The idea would have been inconceivable to most people, and looked upon as wild fantasy. What about sending a man to the moon? *Today's modern technologies were yesterday's impossibilities.* Having television and music coming from a box in your own home? We are the generation that has been chosen to explore many previously unexplainable things and, when we are done, to make them as matter-of-fact to the next millennium as booking a flight to Florida is to us now.

Transcendental cures, although mystical by nature, come from the same realm of knowledge as all new ideas. At our core, we are spiritual beings living in human form during this incarnation, and the information we receive, be it to develop the wheel or discover penicillin, all comes from the same spiritual realm. When we fully grasp this concept, we will no longer need to separate certain types of knowledge from one another. We will understand that many new ideas and ways to solve problems in our lives are considered new, odd, or impossible only because at one time they did not exist as part of our consciousness. Ironically, these solutions have actually always existed; they were just waiting for us to arrive at a particular need *and* time where we could grasp their concepts, usage, and value as means to further support and enrich our lives.

As discussed in chapter 7, we are basically units of white light that emit and receive energy through the seven energy centers in our bodies called Chakras. When our "receiving line of energy" connects with an "emitting line of energy" from another source or person, we are then able to draw on an idea or a solution to a particular problem. That is how, from an energetic standpoint, all ideas, inventions, scientific theories, medical breakthroughs, and spiritual guidance occur.

Most of the time these ideas are energetically picked up by many people simultaneously, only to be publicly shared by the few individuals who, as part of their life's mission, bring that particular idea to the people. For example, how many times have you had an idea for an invention, only to find that someone else has already developed it? What about the scientists who fight over who discovered a particular cure first, or the musicians litigating over who wrote a tune? That is why we had to develop systems for copyrighting and patenting our ideas. The significant point here is that when the time is right and the idea is ready to manifest itself in our world, many people, often at the same time, receive the same notion. Timing is the key, and personal karma will dictate who will bring it into the world.

You may not be the only one to receive an inspiration from the universe, but it may be your calling to take the actions to make it real. That's why it is so important to stay open and clear throughout your life, especially during times of difficulty and transition, so the universe's guidance and your life's work can come through. The more open you are, the more help and direction you will be able to receive. That is another reason why it is important for you to stay focused and relaxed, meditate, take a walk on the beach, listen to your favorite music, feed the birds, pet the dog, and take some quiet time to think. These are all the ways we connect with the guidance that is available to us.

It has been said that prayer is the format that gives us the opportunity to talk to our higher power (whatever name we give it), and meditation is the format that allows that power to speak back to us. I believe that transcendental solutions are one of the ways that we gain access to the divine interventions from the other side that we so often pray for and call upon. Black Hat Sect Feng Shui, through its Buddhist teachings, draws on these solutions and makes them available to *all* people, to help them improve the quality of their lives.

BLACK HAT SECT TRANSCENDENTAL CURES

Hundreds of Transcendental Cures are available through the teachings of Black Hat Sect Feng Shui, for healing everything from pregnancy problems to career difficulties. These cures are seen as sacred information: highly respected, honored, and taken very seriously. They should not be shared indiscriminately, even if your intention is good and the cure is intended for your spouse, best friend, or closest relative. Share them only with those who are willing and ready to receive them. Many times these cures will fall on deaf ears, if the individual you are trying to assist has a different level of consciousness. Try to honor where they are also, without judgment.

The best litmus test to determine whether an individual is ready to receive a cure, and whether you are ready to dispense it, is if both parties are willing to participate in the Red Envelope Ritual. ***Whenever you share these cures with others, no matter who they are, you must receive at least one red envelope with every cure given*** (see page 313). This ritual honors the exchange of ancient sacred information, protects you spiritually, and gives the person receiving the cure the opportunity to participate in the healing process.

In addition, to really activate the cures, you must perform the Three Secrets Reinforcement Blessing, explained on the next page. Utilizing these two very important methods is the proper protocol for working in the transcendental realm. **Do not cut corners here,** because this is where we do the big stretch and reach up and out to borrow some assistance. *The Red Envelope Ritual keeps you spiritually and energetically protected during the exchange of information.* The force that truly activates the power behind the cure is the act of transmitting the information orally to the person who is sincerely asking for the help. This is how these cures were honored and passed down from teacher to student for the past 4,000 years. Please acknowledge your good karma in finding these transcendental solutions, for when used correctly, with the right intentions, they can change lives. In return, honor your fortunate findings by respectfully following the proper protocol of the Red Envelope Ritual.

The Three Secrets Reinforcement Blessing

One of the most important transcendental principles in Black Hat Feng Shui is the very special and powerful blessing known as the Three Secrets Reinforcement. It combines three very important concepts: the Body Secret, the Speech Secret, and the Mind Secret. When performed together, these three can raise the effectiveness of any transcendental blessing or cure. After you have completed making your Feng Shui adjustments, moving your furniture around, and hanging your plants, crystals, and wind chimes, go back and bless all the changes by using the Three Secrets Reinforcement Blessing. You will also use the Three Secrets Reinforcement Blessing to bless all the red envelopes that you receive from clients, friends, and family members for shared cures, Feng Shui adjustment suggestions, and remedies.

1. The Body Secret

This secret comes in the form of a *mudra,* which is a hand or body gesture that conveys an unspoken message. In our everyday life, we are not strangers to the use of hand mudras; we use them all the time, to convey a variety of messages. The most common ones are our greeting handshake, placing a finger to our lips to convey silence, or shaking a clenched fist to convey anger. Throughout the ages we have used these gestures over and over again. In the Black Hat Sect, we use a variety of these mudras to convey a specific spiritual objective. Each mudra is used to emphasize a different intention.

The Mind-Calming Mudra (Fig. 35) is usually accompanied by the Speech Secret Mantra "The Heart Sutra," and is used to calm the mind and the heart, bringing serenity and balance back to a situation fast. Cup your left hand over your right and place your thumbs together.

Fig. 35. Mind-Calming Mudra

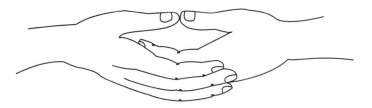

The Ousting Mudra (Fig. 36) is usually accompanied by the Speech Secret Mantra "The Six True Words," and is used to rid oneself or one's home of unwanted issues, bad luck, or obstacles. Extend pointer and pinky fingers, and use the thumb to "flick out" the two middle fingers. Women should use their right hand, men their left hand.

Fig. 36. Ousting Mudra

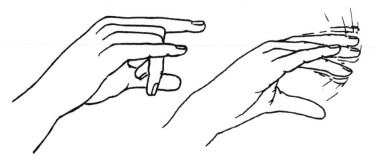

2. The Speech Secret

The second element of the Three Secrets Reinforcement is the Speech Secret, which is the reciting of a group of words that convey a certain intention or request. These phrases, when said repeatedly through the power of the Speech Secret, are called *mantras*. Just like the Body Secret, the secret of speech is something that we are also very familiar with in our daily lives. For example, using provoking curse words can easily get you into a fight, and shouting "Fire!" is usually a signal for someone needing help. Words are very powerful, for they evoke feelings, convey messages, and resonate to various tones that imply a certain attitude. Each mantra used in Black Hat Feng Shui emphasizes a different intention or objective. Many different mantras are used in Feng Shui, but the two most common are listed below. These mantras are used in conjunction with the mudras listed above. All are usually repeated nine times each, or in multiples of nine such as 18, 27, 36, up to 108 times.

The Mind-Calming Mantra (Heart Sutra)
(in Two Different Dialects)

Tibetan:

Gatè Gatè Boro Gatè Boro Sun Gatè Bodhi So Po He

(*Gatè* is pronounced *Gatay*.)

Chinese/Mandarin:

Getè Getè Para Getè Para Sum Getè Bodhi Swaha

(*Gete* is pronounced *Jetti*.)

This mantra is usually accompanied by the Mind-Calming Mudra. Loosely translated, it means: Go or run (Getè Getè) to the other side of the shore or nirvana (Para Getè), many, or numerous, times (Para Sum Getè)—being aware of all truths, knowing all things and having wisdom and omniscience—and do so quickly (Swaha).

The Six True Words Mantra

Om Ma Ni Pad Me Hum

This mantra is the most commonly recited, and can be used with the Ousting Mudra. Loosely translated, it means, "I bow to the jewel in the lotus blossom," or "I see the God within you and I acknowledge and bow to that light."

3. The Mind Secret

This secret is in the form of how we think and use the power of conscious intentions. It is the part of the Three Secrets Reinforcement Blessing where you visualize the outcome of your prayers, requests, and wishes. As you position your hands in a mudra position and recite a mantra nine times, you should also *visualize, in nine steps,* the positive results you desire to achieve. If you wanted to improve your health, for instance, you could do it this way:

1. Think about when you first became sick.
2. Visualize the organ or body area that is ill.
3. Your ch'i begins to feel stronger.
4. You receive the name of a new doctor.
5. That doctor gives you the correct medication to help you heal.
6. Your energy starts to improve even more.
7. You see yourself doing things that you weren't able to do before, like exercising again.
8. You see yourself on vacation, swimming and healthy.
9. You see yourself fully recovered, enjoying life.

There is really no "right" way to do this part of the visualization. Just trust your instincts and visually create nine segments of what you want to establish. You may find that at the beginning it is very hard to do all Three Secrets at once, so feel free to take your time. Do the mudra (Body Secret) and mantra (Speech Secret) together nine times, and then, while your hands are still in the mudra, do the nine-part creative visualization (Mind Secret). After a while, with experience and practice, you will be able to do them all at once. Either way, both methods will work. The more often you do the mudras and mantras, the stronger your ch'i will become and the more spiritual power you will have to help others and yourself make changes. Professor Lin always says, "What is most important is your sincerity." I also believe that if you combine your sincerity along with your willingness to do what's necessary to change, things will manifest themselves quickly and appropriately.

The remedies that have been suggested in this book, particularly the Transcendental Cures in this chapter, were carefully selected by me, and I received approval to share them with you from Professor Lin, who is their original source. The cures that follow can be used for several purposes, but they all can be used for supporting health, clearing stagnant energy from the body or one's space, and transmuting disease and illness.

The Golden Cicada Shedding Its Shell

Perform this Transcendental Cure between 11:00 A.M. and 1:00 P.M. or between 11:00 P.M. and 1:00 A.M. on Chinese New Year's Eve, the Western New Year's Eve, your birthday, during a run of bad luck, to remove bad luck from past years, to attain good luck in the coming year, during difficult times of change or transformation, and when you are sick or have an illness.

Various items that you will need:

- one fresh new egg bought specifically for this cure
- a new, unopened bottle of high-proof liquor
- 0.9 grams or a pinch of cinnabar powder (approximately ¼ teaspoon)
- an eye dropper (for measuring)
- a paper or plastic bag
- a location higher than your dining room table

The following steps should be carried out without interference between the hours listed above:

1. Purchase a new egg. While purchasing the egg, do not talk with anybody or show anyone the egg.
2. Hard-boil the egg. Make sure the egg is at room temperature before placing it in the hot boiling water; this will reduce the likelihood of its cracking. (The eggshell needs to be in perfect condition, with no cracks, after cooking. If it cracks, you'll need to begin the cure again.)
3. Set the boiled egg aside. Put the cinnabar powder in your palm (women use left palm; men use right). Squeeze drops of liquor into the cinnabar power. The number of drops should be equivalent to your Chinese age (your real age plus 1). Do not be concerned if the liquor overflows and drips down the side of your palm. Mix the cinnabar powder and the liquor together with the middle finger of your right hand if you are a woman, your left hand if you are a man.
4. Roll the egg into the mixture on your palm, dyeing it red (like an Easter egg). Put the dyed egg aside. Rub your hands together, visualizing that bad luck and negative ch'i are being sealed off. You may wash your hands (very thoroughly) only when they are dry. Recite the mantra *Om Ma Ni Pad Me Hum* nine times.
5. Take the dyed egg and a paper sack and go outdoors to a place where the elevation is higher than your dining table. Once there, peel off the eggshell. Reinforce your act with the Three Secrets

Reinforcement Blessing, using the Six True Words Mantra and the Ousting Mudra, visualizing that all bad luck, problems, poor health, and negative ch'i are being completely removed. See yourself as that egg, with your outer vibration and sickness being peeled away, and the new healthy self hatched. Place *every piece* of the removed eggshell inside the paper sack. Do not leave any pieces of the eggshell behind; check the ground for any dropped pieces.

6. Continue with the reinforcement of the Three Secrets as you consume *the parts of the egg that have no cinnabar powder on them,* or you can just take a bite of the egg and be sure to include a piece each of the white and yellow sections, and specifically make sure there is no red cinnabar powder on it. **(Cinnabar is mercury sulfide and is poisonous, so handle with care and take necessary precautions if small children or pets are around.)** Take the remainder of the egg and scatter it in the four compass directions, making an offering to all the energy and spirits that need to be fed. Toss the remaining egg upward with an open palm feeding all the "hungry ghosts."

7. Then, while holding the paper sack containing the eggshells, take at least one hundred steps in the direction that points you *away* from your house.

8. Recite the Six True Words Mantra, *Om Ma Ni Pad Me Hum,* do the Three Secrets Reinforcement Blessing nine times, and throw away the sack along with the eggshell pieces. Visualize that you have thrown away all your bad luck and sickness—old and new. Do not look back in the direction that you have discarded the shells. When finished, return home with your newly birthed self.

The Great Sunshine Buddha Meditation

This is a very powerful cure to use for all health-related problems and depression. Repeat the following three phases nine times each morning for 27 consecutive days. If you cannot be exposed to sunlight for all 27 days, you can make the gesture and motions as you point up to the sky or place yourself near a window. What is most important is that you practice this for 27 days in a row, and that you clearly visualize the light consuming all the stagnant, sick ch'i in your body. If you are seriously ill, to make this meditation more powerful practice it nine times a day (81 times in total) for 27 consecutive days. If you happen to skip a day, you will need to start over again from day one.

Phase 1

1. Stand with your feet shoulders' width apart, hands above your head, with head and palms turned up to the sky.
2. Visualize sunlight entering your body through the center of each palm and the middle of your forehead (your Third Eye Chakra), moving through your body, and then exiting from the bottoms of your feet.
3. Lower your hands to your side.

Phase 2

1. Start from the same standing posture as in Phase 1.
2. Visualize sunlight entering your body again through the above-mentioned points. It races to the bottoms of your feet, then bounces upward and speedily travels out of your body through the three entering points.
3. Lower your hands to your side.

Phase 3

1. Take the same standing posture as in Phase 1.
2. Visualize sunlight entering your body again the same way, except that when it reaches the bottoms of your feet, it rises upward slowly and moves in a spiraling motion throughout your body, removing all the pains and sick cells from the unhealthy parts of your body.
3. Lower your hands and relax.
4. Perform the Three Secrets Reinforcement Blessing.

Cinnabar (Jusha) Cures

A. **Sealing the Doors.** This very powerful cure can be used in your home or office to clear away negative ch'i that has accumulated during times of misfortune, illness, robberies, or a recent death.

Ingredients needed:

- 1 teaspoon of Jusha (cinnabar/mercury sulfide) powder
- 1 teaspoon of Syong Huang (realgar/arsenic sulfide) powder
- new, unopened bottle of a high-proof liquor
- eye dropper
- small sacred bowl for mixing (not one that will be used for foods as Jusha can be poisonous)

Take the liquor and add the number of drops that equal each individual's Chinese age (real age plus one year) to the Jusha and realgar. If you are doing a whole large family's home or an office space, you can use 99 drops to represent the whole group. Between 11:00 A.M. and 1:00 P.M., close all the doors and windows, combine the mixture, and walk through the house *dotting the inside of every closed door,* energetically sealing it shut and locking out all the harmful and unbalanced ch'i. Do this with the windows, too. Each door gets three dots (with your middle finger) of the mixture up the side and on the top where the door closes to the frame (see Fig. 37). Double doors can get an extra dot at the top where the two doors close and meet the frame. Also add three dots to all the beds, stove, desks, and any other important items that you want to clear. While dotting these various objects and areas, use the Three Secrets Reinforcement with the Ousting Mudra and Six True Words Mantra, and visualize that all the sick or negative ch'i is leaving your home and the space is being filled up with good, positive, and harmonious ch'i. Add water to the remaining mixture and pour a little bit down each drain and toilet in the house, visualizing that all the bad ch'i is stopped from rising up and going back up into the house. **Wash your hands thoroughly** and visualize that all the sick ch'i is being washed away from your hands, body, and your house.

Fig. 37. Sealing the Doors

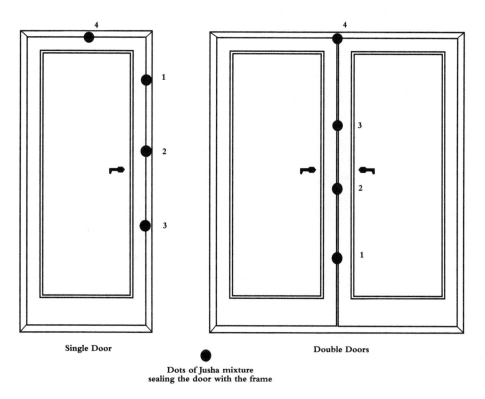

Single Door

Double Doors

**Dots of Jusha mixture
sealing the door with the frame**

B. *Interior/Exterior Transcendental House Clearing with Blessed Rice.* This cure can be used for clearing the exterior space around your home as well as the interior space for negative and imbalanced energy. Prepare the Jusha as you did in the "Sealing the Doors" cure above, with two minor changes. You add the Jusha (without the realgar) and the alcohol to approximately half a bowl of uncooked rice. You then use your middle finger to mix the rice with the alcohol and Jusha while chanting the *Om Ma Ni Pad Me Hum* mantra 108 times. Afterward, walk around the perimeter of the inside or outside of the house, tossing the rice with an open hand in an upward motion, while visualizing all the negative or sick ch'i scattering away. Perform the Three Secrets Reinforcement Blessing. You can also use this cure for remedying the Feng Shui of a home that has a bed sharing a bathroom or kitchen wall (see chapters 5 and 6). In addition, throw a handful of the rice and Jusha mixture down the toilet, close the lid, and flush. Visualize that the toilet or the kitchen appliance that is of concern will have no effect on the individual's health. This cure can also be used to remedy a bathroom that is located over an entranceway. These are various layouts that can make you very ill. Please keep in mind that Jusha is poisonous and care should be taken, especially when you're using it where small children and pets reside.

Bamboo Flute Cures (for Health)

A. ***Backaches and Spine Problems.*** Place one bamboo flute, with red tassels on both ends, between your mattress and box spring, running parallel to the length of your body. The mouthpiece of the flute should be toward your head. (See Fig. 38a.) Bless the cure with the Three Secrets Reinforcement Blessing, visualizing the health problem and any pain lifting away, and good health restored. Leave the flute under the mattress until your back is healed or as a preventive measure, indefinitely. For serious back or spine problems, use method B, under Fig. 38a.

B. ***Unfocused Energy, Low Physical Stamina, Insomnia, Depression, Anxiety, and Low Energy, or to Increase Emotional Strength and Improve Overall Constitution.*** Place two bamboo flutes with red tassels in an *upside-down* V (Λ) position, with the point of the Λ facing toward the head. The third flute should be sitting directly on that point. Place this three-flute configuration in the bed where you sleep, between your mattress and box spring. (See Fig. 38b.) This shape represents the Chinese character for "human." Make sure that you place all three mouthpieces at the top end of the flutes, with all three flutes facing the same direction.

Figs. 38a and 38b. Proper Bamboo Flute Cure Positions

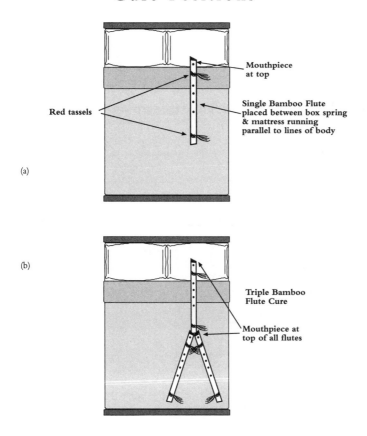

(a)

Mouthpiece
at top

Red tassels

Single Bamboo Flute
placed between box spring
& mattress running
parallel to lines of body

(b)

Triple Bamboo
Flute Cure

Mouthpiece at
top of all flutes

Mirror Cures (for Health)

A. ***Insomnia, Migraines, Eye Problems, or Heart Ailments (Single Mirror Cure).*** Place a three-inch round mirror between the mattress and box spring (mirrored side facing up toward the body) under the body area with which you are having a health problem, and perform the Three Secrets Reinforcement Blessing. For example, to cure insomnia, place the mirror under your head area between the box spring and mattress with the mirror side toward the body. For heart problems, place the mirror under the heart area between the mattress and box spring with the mirror side toward the body (see Fig. 39a). Keep the mirror in that location for a minimum of 27 days or until you heal.

B. *Respiratory, Asthma, Breathing, or Lung Problems (Double Mirror Cure).* Place a two-inch-round mirror at the bottom of a bamboo pen holder, with the mirror inside, facing upward. Place the bamboo pen holder, with the mirror inside, under the bed, directly in alignment with the area or organ that you wish to heal. To make the cure stronger, add the same size round mirror on the ceiling directly above the area that you are trying to heal, with the mirrored side facing down toward the body (see Fig. 39b). Make sure you use an authentic bamboo pen holder (see the NSP&A website). Reinforce with the Three Secrets Reinforcement Blessing.

Figs. 39a and 39b. Mirror Cures for Health

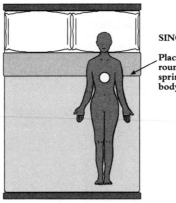

SINGLE MIRROR CURE

Place a two-inch- or three-inch-round mirror in between box spring and mattress under the body area you are trying to heal.

(a)

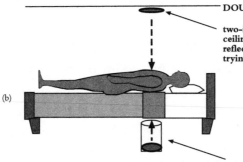

DOULE MIRROR CURE

two-inch-round mirror secured to ceiling, mirror side facing down reflecting body area you are trying to heal.

(b)

Place a large mouth bamboo cup/pen holder with a two-inch-round mirror at the bottom (with mirror side directly facing up) under the body area that you are trying to heal. Place the cup and mirror in direct alignment with the two-inch mirror on the ceiling facing down over the same body area.

THE RITUAL OF THE RED ENVELOPE: A BLACK HAT TRADITION

When Transcendental Cures are offered, the giver needs to request of the receiver at least one, three, or nine new red envelopes, depending on how many cures were dispensed. Nine envelopes are usually given to the person with the cures when the receiver wants to express his or her greatest respect and thanks to the giver, but one or three are acceptable if only one or two cures are prescribed. These envelopes can be traditional Chinese red "money envelopes" *(hong pao)* or any red envelopes made of construction paper or bought at a local card shop. The important thing is that they were *never* used before and that after you complete the exchange ritual they will be discarded and *never used again.* Inside *each* red envelope is a token monetary gift. The offering in each can be as little as 45 cents or a dollar bill when it is being offered to a nonprofessional. When the envelopes are being presented to a Black Hat Sect Feng Shui expert or consultant, then the practitioner's fee goes inside one of the nine red envelopes with a dollar bill in each of the other eight. After the envelopes are received, before spending the money or even opening the envelope, the consultant or cure giver must sleep with it under his or her pillow or mattress for one night after blessing the envelopes with the Three Secrets Reinforcement Blessing. **It is important to remember that *everyone,* layperson and practitioner alike, needs to follow the Red Envelope Ritual, whether you share the cures with friends, family, or clients.** If you find that you are uncomfortable asking for the red envelopes, or if the person you are sharing the cures with doesn't want to follow through on providing them, accept those signs as an indication that you are not yet ready to share the information or the other person, for whatever reason, is not ready to receive it. Knowing when to help and when not to help is a very valuable and important skill to have. It is very important that you take this part of the Feng Shui process seriously, then try to be patient with yourself and the process; trust that you will know when it's the right time to share the information with others.

CREATING A SACRED HEALING SPACE

From a Feng Shui perspective, our homes are always significant in terms of our life events, but when we are sick they become even more priceless, because nine out of ten times our homes are where we return to heal. It is the all-encompassing place where we make decisions, make love, and make life unfold. In reading through this book, you can see how important the environment and its elements are, even if the factors aren't immediately tangible. *But that invisible exterior environment acts like a mirror for our invisible inner home, the sacred place deep inside of us.* When we become sick, it's our inner home that is off, hurting, and carrying some old, unreleased wound. So, by giving attention to our environment through Feng Shui adjustments, what we are really doing is indirectly making the changes that can eventually help shift the interior wounds and act as a catalyst for the true healing we need.

We owe it to ourselves to be in a place of constant contact and awareness with our environment, for it is there that we can begin our healing process in a concrete way. But the idea and concept of a "healing space" is different for every one of us. Color, location, and the amount of space that we would ideally need all become variables that factor into our concept of what that ideal space would look like. All those variables are based on our different personal frequencies, our vibration's specific needs and requirements, our personal tastes, and the dimensional level of consciousness on which we are living.

To list what makes one environment more healing than another would almost be impossible, but what we do know now is that beyond the particulars, there are certain elements that help create and sustain a healing space. These elements are important to helping a space hold its vibrational pattern in a stable, consistent way, which in turn supports the environmental energies that are needed during a time of illness or in a healing crisis. There are seven elements that are, in my opinion, unequivocally essential for any healing environment, no matter how big or small your space is. Those things are sacred objects, spiritual/inspirational guidance materials, life force, color, altars, space-clearing rituals, and blessing ceremonies.

Simple Elements of a Healing Environment

1. **Sacred Power Objects.** These are our "spiritual transition objects" that carry healing energy and intentions, and act as a conduit to connect us to the higher realms and our guides. Make sure you add to the list any personal objects that are special to you and impart a peaceful, loving, and healing feeling. The object may remind you of a special time, place, or person. It could represent to you a mentor, a spiritual leader, or a deity to whom you pray, or is helping you to heal. The only requirement is that it feels either powerful or sacred to you. Such objects may include bells or cymbals, statues or representations of deities, rocks, seashells, driftwood, feathers, photographs, and incense.

2. **Spiritual/Inspirational Guidance Materials.** I recommend that you have a collection of your favorite spiritual books on life concepts or healing in or near your Sacred Healing Space. In addition, make sure you have a few different oracles for helping you make decisions and gain clarity through everyday uncertainties and dilemmas around your illness or treatment plan. When you are grounded and thinking clearly, it is easy to make decisions and take action, but when you are sick, stressed, or in fear, those are the times when the oracles can guide you and connect you to other etheric sources for guidance. Some of the oracles I use and recommend are Sphericals, Crop Circle Cards, Angel Cards, Runes, the *I Ching,* Medicine Cards, and Affirmation Cards. Find the ones that speak to you, have a healing message, and resonate to your personal truth. Also, keep a beautiful journal and a pen near you at all times to help you purge and document any thoughts or inspirations.

3. **Life Force.** It is very hard to heal in an environment that is void of life force. When we are ill, it is our internal life force that is compromised and low, so it is precisely at that time that we are in need of additional life force to support us. When we are surrounded with various life forces, our auras absorb their energies and in turn help us heal. If other life-force elements aren't able to live and/or thrive in your home, it's only logical that

you won't be able to, either. Trying to get well in an energetically depressing environment is very difficult. Life force reminds the innate intelligence of the body to resonate toward life, and subsequently healing. Life force is present in everything from beautiful lush plants and nine live bamboo stalks to water fountains and fish tanks. Other wonderful life-force supports are playful dogs, purring cats, and singing birds. Music can also be a life-force adjustment, especially music that contains chanting or mesmerizing mantras. All music carries life force, because sound and tones activate the Chakras. Music makes you feel good, and want to move, sing, and dance. When you're able to tap your feet and feel the beat, that's always a good sign that a healing of some sort is on the way.

4. ***Color.*** As all the information throughout this book has pointed out, color is an integral part of who we are intrinsically. It is the "healing medicine of the gods." Our souls are a beam of white light that breaks down into the various Chakras in the body, with each having a corresponding color and vibration. When white, gray, or monochromatic walls and upholstery surround us, our innate energy bodies do not get fed or fueled.

Our Chakras interact with the Feng Shui of our environment, and together they energetically create our lives. Color is an important component in how completely and quickly we heal. Color is another form of life force that stimulates, activates, and encourages us to emote. When we are trying to heal our illnesses through working on the ESP underpinnings, color will help us feel our feelings. An absence of color will keep us locked in and checked out. All-white walls can contribute to bouts of anxiety and depression, because ch'i has a very hard time adhering to white, which creates a ricocheting effect and throws all the energy patterns into chaos. This doesn't mean that you can't use white in your home at all; one room with other accent colors or white on the trim or ceiling is fine. But try to be mindful of what your color quotient is throughout your home and your life, and then act accordingly. The transcendental use of color can and will help you heal.

5. ***Creating an Altar.*** Within your sacred space, it is always very important to create an altar of some kind. An altar doesn't have to be all spir-

itual in nature, just an area that you put aside to place things that are important to you and have special meaning. It could be on a windowsill, a shelf, a mantel, the floor, or the edge of your bathtub. Wherever you have been drawn to create it is probably the exact place it needs to be. Once you have "claimed your space," you'll know within that space where the altar should be. Keep in mind what your conscious intentions are; if one of them is to meditate, if you want to use it for relaxing and thinking, then make sure you have enough space around the altar so you can sit by it. All your efforts to make this a consciously planned place will activate the ch'i around the altar and throughout your home. Once you determine where your altar is going to be (you can have several), the next step is making offerings and placing the objects on that altar. A partial list of items you can use to create an altar includes candles, feathers, crystals, and all of the sacred objects listed above. Feel free to add anything else that will help you personalize your altar and have it reflect you and your intentions. Remember that wherever you place your altar, you will enhance that area's Feng Shui. Your altar, in addition, will become a powerful adjustment for that gua.

6. *Space-Clearing Rituals.* Crisis, trauma, and sickness, in our lives and in our homes, often give off an electrical or emotional charge that, even long after the event or situation has come to pass, still remains in the space, in the walls, and even absorbed in the furniture. When you are creating a healing space, it's important that you regularly keep that space (and your whole home) clear of emotional and physical debris. Leftover stagnant energy that remains in the environment can easily be reabsorbed into your energy field and into the Feng Shui of the surrounding environment, keeping you energetically and physically ill with the old grief, crisis, sickness situation, or despair. The following are two methods of space clearing that I use and always recommend.

    Burning white sage. Purchase either loose leaves or a tied bundle of white sage called a "smudge stick," light one end, then blow out the flame and "walk the smoke" around the whole perimeter of each room and each door frame, and outlining every window. Visualize that the burning sage is smoking out all the unwanted and stagnant energy in the space. Make sure you keep a fireproof tray under the burning sage, as it will shed some ashes as it burns down. Walk through your home from the farthest end, backing up and out toward the front door, leading the unwanted energy out. Do this as often as needed (weekly, monthly).

Purification by Fire. For this method you'll need an old coffee cup, Epsom salts, rubbing alcohol, and a Pyrex dish or kitchen pot. Place an inch of Epsom salts in the cup and cover it with the rubbing alcohol. The level of the alcohol should be just slightly above the Epsom salts approximately ¼ of an inch over, no more. Then place the cup in the fireproof pan (in case the cup breaks) and take the cup and pan into the room you want to clear. Place it on a stable, secure platform or the floor and make sure there are no flammable materials in close proximity. Tilt the cup and light the alcohol and salt mixture with a long wooden kitchen match. Sit by the fire (but not dangerously close), and as you watch the flame moving up and down, eating up all the sick or negative energy in the room, state out loud all the things, issues, or people that you want to let go of. The fire will burn for approximately 10 to 20 minutes. Use a different cup and mixture for each room you want to clear, and when you are finished, let each cup cool down first, then *throw it away, as soon as it is safe to do so, with the dried-up salts inside.* Do not reuse the cups. Do this method once every two weeks or monthly.

7. *Blessing Ceremonies: Purifying a Home During Difficult Times.* Sometimes we run into a stretch of bad luck, and it seems as if whatever we do turns out other than the way we planned. The loss of a job, the end of a relationship, or the passing on of someone dear to us can take its toll on our energy and the energy in our homes. During difficult times or after a specific event, it is very helpful to realign the energy of your home. "Tracing the Nine Stars" is a Transcendental Cure from Professor Lin Yun, used by the Black Hat Sect School of Feng Shui. Its objective is to transform a negative energy trend in a home into a flow of positive energy. Take out your overall floor plan and trace the nine Bagua points as illustrated, starting with (1) the Family section, continuing to (2) the Wealth section, (3) the Center section, (4) Helpful People, (5) Children, (6) Knowledge, (7) Fame, (8) Career, and (9) Marriage. (See Fig. 40.)

Fig. 40. Tracing the Nine Stars

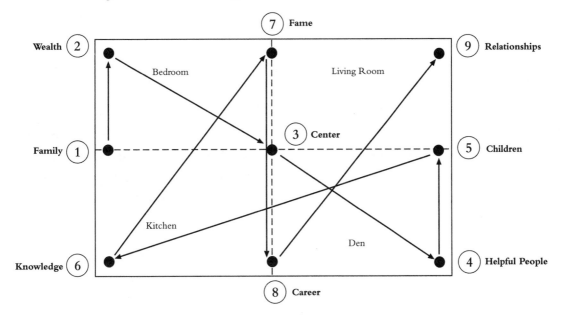

Then walk over to the first point, the Family section of your house, and call on the light of Buddha (or whomever you worship) and ask for his/her energy to be added to yours in purifying your home, regarding your family and the possible underpinnings to your illness, health concern, or other challenges. Then recite the Mind-Calming Mantra while positioning your hands in a Mind-Calming Mudra and recite nine times: *Gatè Gatè, Boro Gatè, Boro Sun Gatè, Bodhi So Po He* (*Gatè* is pronounced *Gatay* in Tibetan, or feel free to chant it in Chinese as listed earlier in this chapter). Starting with the Family section (see Fig. 40), walk to each Bagua point and send your energy to each gua by either touching the point or discussing the area that it is connected to and sending your ch'i out to it. Follow this format to the ninth point, the Marriage section. Send your energy, along with Buddha's (or whoever's) blessing, to each point, clearing the space and raising its vibration with your light.

INTERIOR SPACE CLEARING

When you begin to create a sacred space within your home, what you are actually doing is creating that same sacred space within yourself. One of Feng Shui's main points is that nothing exists outside you that does not already exist inside you. *So the next important and crucial step in your healing and recovery process is to do your internal space clearing, for that is the precious space in which your soul resides while you are here on the planet.* The way that you came to understand the importance of your outer environment and its influence on your life applies even more to your internal sacred space within. There are a few specific emotional, spiritual, and psychological issues that must be addressed if we are to do our inner space clearing, get to our truth, and explore and process the ESPs of your illness.

Practical Spirituality

Where are you spiritually? How are you making sense of your illness, your struggles, and your daily life? When we begin to think about God, religion, and developing a spiritual practice, it's important not to see spirituality as something that exists outside of yourself, as we have learned from more structured religions. Spirituality is something that you co-create with God, and in turn, that partnership creates a frame of reference that will help structure your life. It will provide you with a set of beliefs and principles to live by. Without some frame of spiritual reference, life becomes very random and scary, with no constructive place to put your illness. *Randomness happens when you are not in alignment with a benevolent higher power, so part of your healing process will be to sort out your feelings about God and create a perspective that will anchor your life and fuel your recovery.*

There are more people on the planet that are spiritually bankrupt than financially broke! How much savings do you have in your spiritual bank account? How often do you make your deposits? Are you saving for a rainy day? Your spirituality is something that you must learn to invest in every day, so that when you need it in a crisis, you will have a wealth of credit to draw on.

A while ago a report appeared on my local news channel that stated scientists have now determined that the frontal lobe of the brain, which they knew oversaw our immune system functioning, is the same part of the brain that also oversees our relationship and experience with prayer, faith, and religion. Scientists are now starting to make the link between praying, meditation, having a strong spiritual belief system, and the recovery process. This reinforces the idea that when we trust in a higher power that we can pray to, cry to, or tug on for guidance and assistance, we heal, transcend, and move through our healing crisis more quickly and with a lot less chaos.

Figuring out how to incorporate your beliefs into an everyday practice in a very real way will make your faith stronger. As you design your own unique brand of spirituality, you create a set of beliefs and principles that are practical and reflect who you are and your everyday life. You decide when and how to pray, meditate, and commune with nature and God. That way you will find hundreds of ways to experience and live what spirit means to you, and not have to follow a set of man-made rules.

Revise what you have learned about what a spiritual person is or does, and know that the everyday practice of spirituality has more to do with walking the dog, feeding the kids, being honest and authentic, and showing up for your life in the face of all crisis and duress. Even with a full-fledged change in one's spiritual beliefs, under siege we still tend to go back to some of our primary conditioning and dogma.

Even though my spiritual beliefs are so much more eclectic now and are a synthesis of many religions, when something terrible happens, my knee-jerk reaction is to try to figure out what I did to deserve this. Fortunately, it never lasts very long, but occasionally those old Catholic beliefs do still come up, even for me.

You Have the Spiritual Power to Heal Your Life

The most powerful connection that you will ever have in your lifetime is a spiritual connection with a higher being. I say that not from a religious point of view, but from an energetic perspective. For when we connect spiritually, we make that connection from our Heart Chakra. It is from that energy center that our physical being connects vertically and receives its energy and color fuel from the universe.

When we draw our energy from the universal source, we are absorbing energy that is always plentiful and specially designed for us; when we try to access our sense of power through means outside of ourselves, such as other people and things, we usually wind up feeling frustrated, limited, and codependent on that external energy force. So, the more we strengthen our spiritual connection and own our power, the more energy we will have to access the things we desire and illuminate the path that we chose to walk. The more you comfortably own your personal power, the more you are able to believe that you can transmute your illness.

Boxing with God

Once you come to accept a benevolent higher power into your life and your healing process, the next step is to take notice of how you are relating to that power. Often the same old religious/higher authority tapes that are programmed in our minds since childhood will seep through to our newfound belief system. Religion contains a lot of structure and dogma. Spirituality differs from this mainly in that it "cuts out the middleman" and acknowledges that you can have direct access to God, *because a piece of God exists within you.*

Many orthodox religions teach us to fear God. Spirituality instead encourages you to take full responsibility for your own actions and not to blame God for what's gone wrong in your life. These two very different spiritual principles have actually created a somewhat similar response in you, because both, in their own ways, have prevented you from having all your *feelings* regarding God. On the one hand, if your life is all your own doing, then how can you get mad at God about being sick, losing a loved one, or getting fired from your job? On the other hand, if you believe in a God that exists outside of you, and you get angry at Him because you're sick or lonely, then you really might make him even more mad at you, and the chances are slim to none that you will ever get better; even worse, you might be punished some more.

If we are going to have an enriching, wonderful, and healing relationship with God, we have to be willing and feel safe enough to have all our feelings regarding Him. That means we allow ourselves to love him, depend on him, and *get angry with him, if needed.* Anger is part of our human set of emotions that God created. He knew that we would need to experience all of them, including anger, in order to have a full human experience. So if, in your life and in your healing process, you find yourself feeling angry at God because you're sick or have been hurt or abandoned, *go ahead and let Him have it*. He won't flip out and run away, or run out and buy a box of bonbons and eat them to soothe His feelings. He won't do any of these things, because he understands human emotions and limitations and loves us unconditionally. Remember, He created these feelings himself, with a purpose for their use.

Sometimes, in order to get better and heal, we need to get mad at God first and then many others. As with any human relationship, we have to feel safe enough to have *all* our feelings, particularly the "ugly" ones, to know that we are still loved and won't be abandoned. The problem that arises with being angry is not with having those very real feelings, but staying stuck in them and in a continual place of blaming others for what is happening or not happening in your life. Challenge your perceptions of God; and revise them to include a benevolent higher power.

IF NOT NOW, *WHEN?* IT ISN'T THAT LONG A STAY

Often we do not seriously think about death and dying until we are faced with a sickness, an accident, losing someone we love, or our own mortality. But the truth is that in many ways life is only a part-time job, and no one gets to stay longer here than they need to. Living forever was never the intended purpose of being born. We are here to work out certain issues and make certain significant contributions to the world. When our job is done and our work is completed, we return home.

Although you may find that thought depressing or scary, for many people it can feel like a relief or, even better, a reprieve. When you realize that *it really isn't that long a stay,* the "small stuff," normal life frustrations, and everyday contradictions become less significant. Make the best use of your time here, and attempt to do all the things you said you would do.

IF YOU'RE LIVING LIFE TO THE FULLEST, PLEASE RAISE YOUR RIGHT FOOT!

Most of us spend our time driving through life with our foot on the brake. A lot of energy is spent on controlling the speed at which we live, with much effort focused on trying to avoid some of the inevitable pieces of life that, in spite of all we do, will happen anyway. Take your foot off the brake today, because the truth is, *you are not really driving anyway.*

When you decide to relinquish personal control and opt to co-create your life with all living things and also partner with a higher power, you find yourself and your life on an "Accelerated Path" (which is also the title of my Feng Shui and Chakra Consultant Training Program). This path will guide you toward enhancing the quality of your emotional, spiritual, and physical health. The journey of life improves as you include spirit more, because then even the hard times and setbacks are seen as part of the divine plan. This perspective makes life a bit more manageable, especially during difficult times.

The Earth is a very difficult schoolroom, and those of us who have chosen to incarnate during this very tumultuous time on the planet knew in advance what was coming and what would be needed. I also believe we were aware that what eventually would matter the most was *how* we lived and how we dealt with the challenges and tasks that were presented to us, not *how long* we lived.

We were aware that living in human form would require us to face reality, be authentic, and live through the emotional carnage that came with loving and losing, experiencing deep feelings, and having some sad memories.

We knew that the future would be somewhat veiled, and that often we would be confused by life, by our loved ones, and by the causes of hardships and illness. But we also knew, deep inside, that the gift of life was a privilege, an opportunity to do service and heal more aspects of ourselves.

Now we are so immersed in our day-to-day struggles, faced with so many conflicts, disappointments, and illnesses, it is very easy to lose sight of the incredible beauty and freedom that came with the gift of living.

We all agreed to leave the world in much better shape than when we entered it, and to love and cherish all of God's creations, no matter what our differences were. So, as testament to that original promise, healthy or sick, enlightened or not, we still have to check in with ourselves periodically and make sure we are on track and living the life we were committed to live.

The stay here is quite short, not just for people who are sick, but for everyone. ***In my opinion, worse than having to die is having to live with the sad reality of leaving behind a graveyard of dreams.*** At the end, the things we never did, said, or experienced are the things that are the most regretted and unresolved by the soul. It's been observed that no one on their deathbed ever said, "Boy, I wish I'd spent more time at the office!"

Can you live every day of your life as if it were your last? Embracing our own immortality shouldn't serve to depress us, but instead to motivate us to be present, to bring closure, to right wrongs, to make amends, and to have an enjoyable life.

If your illness is not terminal, can you live your life as if it were? Think for a minute. If you just found out that you were going to die today, what would you feel the most unresolved about? What calls would you make, or what letters would you write? Check your home and office; if you died tomorrow, would everything be in order? Can papers or important documents be found? Would your friends or children have to clean up any messes, emotional or physical, that you left behind? Can you die with integrity, knowing that you did more than the best you could, but *everything* you could to take care of your own business and life? Can you embrace your illness and see it as an opportunity to resolve other issues that might have gone unattended?

Keep in mind that the chaos illness creates was perfectly orchestrated for you, but it was not created for you or by you so that you could avoid it. It was created so that your soul could learn how to navigate through it, to strengthen your coping abilities and help you hone and keep focus on your center and the importance of your life.

DON'T JUDGE YOUR SICKNESS OR DEATH AS A SIGN OF FAILURE

Although talking about death and dying might be uncomfortable for some, ultimately we are all better off for addressing it openly before it happens.

Many individuals finish their work here and leave the planet in what seems like a very short time or sudden way. These exits are some of the hardest losses for the loved ones who remain behind to make sense of or process.

As we start to understand the bigger picture of life, we begin to see that we co-create life with God, and that death, very often, is the soul's choice (not always the personality's choice) and not just a horrible human tragedy that happens randomly to people. In understanding this concept, we become freer to let the person that we lost and loved go on to the next level of their life and soul's growth. This is genuinely the greatest gift we can give someone who has passed on to the Yin life or afterlife, the blessing and support they need to move forward with their spirit's evolutionary work.

The soul is in constant contact with the higher realms, checking in often on what to do, and even when to go. Often we program in many exits and probabilities for times that we can leave and go home. Try not to jump to conclusions; see things for what they really are, and not from the limited perspective of your personality, but from the expanded view of your soul.

Closing Chapter Story

Back in 1998, I had to fly to Texas with one of my associates, to speak at a conference where I was being given the "Lightworker of the Year" award. Until the last few days before I left, I was really ambivalent about going because there were so many things I was working on for my nonprofit program, Feng Shui Across America. On my third night in Houston, I woke up in a cold sweat from a very vivid dream. In the dream I was looking over my body, which was lying on the kitchen floor of my home, and I appeared to be dead. In the dream I kept thinking, What did I die from? I didn't look sick or injured in any way, but I was definitely dead. Although I have had many different kinds of dreams or nightmares, there was something about this dream that I just couldn't shake.

The following day, while still in Texas, I got a call from a friend who was checking on my apartment while I was gone. She told me that when she'd come to water the plants the prior evening, there was an overwhelming smell of gas in the house. She'd had to call in an emergency crew, who tested the house and found an extremely serious gas leak! The dream I had the day before suddenly made sense, and affected me even more after hearing about the gas leak. I realized that in my dream I was overcome by the gas leak!

Two weeks after I got home from my Texas trip, I picked up a call at my office, only to hear the voice of a former employee sounding so relieved to hear my voice. When I asked her what was wrong, she hesitantly told me that she'd sent something in the mail to me at my home address a few weeks ago, only to have it returned to her by the post office with the word "Deceased" stamped over my name! It was very humbling. I remember thinking, "Oops, that was a close call!"

As if that weren't enough, almost a year later the saga continued. I applied for an additional credit card machine for my office, only to be turned down because when they did a credit check, they found me listed as deceased! I was then cut off from all my banking and credit accounts; several institutions somehow had been notified to put a freeze on all my accounts because they thought I was using Nancy's identity to perpetrate fraud! I traced the source back to the Department of Social Security, which had somehow been notified that I was deceased and by law had to notify all the affected financial and credit institutions. They even had a specific date of death for me! It was unbelievable!

Just for the record, if you are ever erroneously listed as dead, it's very hard to prove you're not. A dear friend and colleague told me that it was a probability that I'd programmed in, just in case I'd needed to leave and go home at that juncture. In retrospect, who I was at that time in many ways has died. It was the part of me that was still engaging in some of my old behaviors and ways of thinking that stemmed from the period of my life when I was still sick. But, in truth, even for me, the whole thing was very freaky!

I guess I decided to stay, otherwise this book would never have been written. When I thought about it, what happened to me made perfect sense because sometimes I'll do just about anything to get out of writing!

We forget that there are so many things out there that we are spared from. Try not to forget that what we don't get is often a blessing in disguise. So when you take a few moments out of your hectic life to pray, remember to thank God for all you have . . . but also don't forget to thank God for all the things that you don't have!

CHAPTER TEN

A MULTILEVEL APPROACH TO DISARMING 15 CHALLENGING ILLNESSES

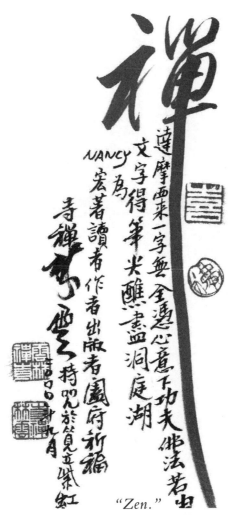

"Zen."

CALLIGRAPHY BY H. H. PROFESSOR THOMAS LIN YUN RINPOCHE

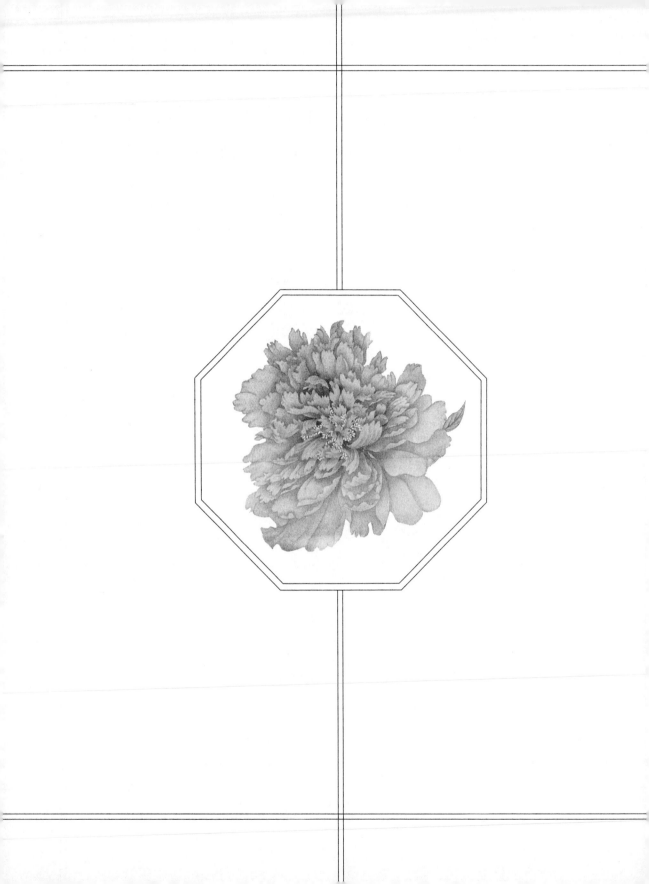

VIBRATIONAL MEDICINE, VIBRATIONAL HEALING

EVERY ORGAN, tissue, bone, and system in our bodies is in a constant state of vibration. That vibration is unique to a single soul, with no two on the planet (or elsewhere) exactly alike. When things in our life become stressful, or when an unexpected illness erupts, it can easily throw our very delicate personal resonance out of balance and alignment. When we are not in sync with our innate rhythm, everything from our biochemistry to our heart rate can be thrown off, and over time, if not corrected, this can lead to various mental, emotional, and physical diseases. Vibrational healing consists of methods that we can use to help the body return to its original nature and the pattern of its true vibration and homeostasis.

By applying an outside stimulus or "vibrational medicine" such as homeopathy, acupuncture, flower essences, color, sound, crystals, and aroma, we can very gently persuade the body to change its existing energy pattern and move back toward a more conducive and balanced one. These powerful modalities have the ability to change our energetic and molecular structure through mirroring back a healthy resonance and stimulating our innate flow of ch'i. These various medicines vibrate to a similar energy frequency as our bodies, Chakras, and souls. As we apply these various modalities, our bodies, through the scientific phenomenon known as "sympathetic resonance," are reminded of their true vibrational nature, and respond by returning back to a state of health.

Healing through sound, scent, crystals, and color has been utilized for thousands of years as "transformational tools" for discovering ourselves emotionally, spiritually, and physically. Although we have discovered that there are certain oils, sounds, and crystals that resonate to specific Chakras and areas of the body, none of this information is written in stone. Every day we are discovering more and more information, and working diligently to uncover hidden meanings and vibrational cures.

So, by all means follow these lists and use their wisdom to guide you in your healing journey, but it is of great importance to remember to honor your own intuition and judgment as well. If something doesn't feel right to you, or if there is a cure or remedy that you would rather not explore, trust that inner voice and proceed accordingly. Also keep in mind that because some of this information is new and unfamiliar to you, you may be using its unfamiliarity as an excuse not to stretch past your "comfort zone," so you might need to rethink your response: Are you being intuitive or resistant?

When new information is revealed to you, you need to trust that the information offered is of a karmic nature, in perfect divine order, and that, yes, your prayers have been heard. Quite often the help we need, deserve, and pray for comes to us disguised. We often inadvertently turn it away because most of us are more limited in our ability to receive what we need than to actually ask for what we need. Our openness to absorbing these "vibrational gifts" is just as important as the courage it takes to find them.

INCORPORATING THE HEALING POWER OF SOUND, CRYSTALS, AND ESSENTIAL OILS

Sound and Tone Healing

Robin Spiegel, massage therapist and sound, color, and aromatherapy healer of Rye, New York, states that the dictionary defines the verb *heal* as "to make whole or sound." Our nervous system and our energy field are profoundly affected by vibration, sound, tone, and frequency. Before the ears hear sound, it is first received by our auric field, which then sends ch'i impulses to the nervous system via our various vibrational fields. Our physical bodies, minds, spirits, and emotions are vibratory fields that are affected by these impulses. On a conscious level, sound elicits emotional and thought-provoking responses, but on a subconscious level, it affects all of the cells in our bodies. If healing and balance is created in your energy (auric) field before it reaches your nervous system, it can help prevent illness or disease from manifesting.

In sound healing, whether we use tuning forks, quartz "singing bowls," musical instruments, tones from our voices, or chanting to music, we are working with the vibrational field around our bodies, in an effort to return it to a harmonious balance. The use of your conscious intention is as important as the tools you are using for the healing.

The sound that our nervous system makes is a low hum that changes constantly throughout the day as situations and the surrounding variables change. Different frequencies of tuning forks are available for us to use, measured in cycles per second (cps), which is the speed of the wave of the sound energy. Humans hear approximately 16 to 16,000 cps, whereas dolphins, for instance, can project and receive information at approximately 180,000 cps!

Lightly hold the stem of the tuning fork, and gently tap the body of the fork with your knee and bring it to your ears. The fork will ring for approximately 20 to 25 seconds, while your body eagerly adjusts its vibration to the frequency of the sound it hears. This positive impact that sound has on the overall body can work in reverse, also; noise pollution, loud music, or disruptive sounds can throw off the body's equilibrium, creating ill health.

Now available are several tuning-fork sets for you to purchase and work with. A full-octave set of eight forks is called the harmonic spectrum, and each fork vibrates to and makes the sound of a different note of the major scale: C, D, E, F, G, A, B, and high C. Each of these notes corresponds to a different Chakra in the body and a different gua in Feng Shui. C corresponds to the First Chakra, the Survival Center, D to the second Chakra, the Social Center, and so forth. These forks resonate from 256 cps to 512 cps. If there is a specific Chakra or gua out of balance, the sound of a particular note can help return the Chakra or Feng Shui gua to a state of health and equilibrium.

There is also a set of forks called Ottos, which create low sounds and are wonderful for grounding and focusing purposes. The set also includes an additional Otto tuning fork, which resonates to the vibration of *Om* at 32 cps to 136 cps. *Om* is the universal tone that incorporates all sounds, because it resonates to the sound of God; that is why it is used universally as a common chant for meditation.

Angel tuners, sometimes referred to as crystal tuners, are very powerful tuning forks that you can use with quartz crystals and semiprecious stones. These tuning forks can be used to help clear away any stagnant or energetic debris in your home and office. They are also very powerful space-clearing tools that can be activated by gently tapping a quartz crystal with the tuning fork and pressing the stem of the fork to the base of the crystal, and then holding that crystal with the fork attached in a certain gua in your home or office. The crystal's healing abilities will become vibrationally magnified by the tuning fork—and in turn resonate to the gua that is out of sync, to help restore it to balance. A second way you can use the tuning forks in a gua is by striking them on your hand or against another tuning fork, allowing them to use their innate vibration to readjust the gua you want to strengthen. In addition, both methods, with and without crystals, can be used on and over the body to adjust the vibrational pattern of the Chakras.

Sound has the ability to rearrange molecular structure and create change on an extremely profound level. The healing possibilities, in conjunction with other vibrational medicines such as crystals, sounds, color, and oils, are limitless. For more information on what notes resonate with what guas and Chakras, see the multilevel charts at the end of this chapter.[14]

The Six Ch'i Healing Sounds Meditation

This is a very powerful active meditation to strengthen your health or to dismantle the matrix of certain illnesses. Each organ in the body, just like everything else, resonates to a certain vibration, frequency, color, and sound. By learning the different sounds to which each of the organs listed below resonates, you can help adjust the vibration of your internal body ch'i and support your health and healing process. In addition, this meditation introduces you to the most powerful and most often prayed-to Buddha of Healing, called

Medicine Buddha. If you are healthy and want to use this meditation as a preventive, health-strengthening practice, then perform this meditation every day for 27 days. *Please note: If you are healthy and using this meditation, make sure you place emphasis on the exhalation of each sound you make.* If you are sick and are using this meditation to assist you in getting better, perform this meditation nine times a day for 27 days. *If you are sick, make sure you do not place any emphasis at the end of your exhale.* These small but important nuances will help you strengthen the power and focus of this meditation. Remember to bless each meditation with the Three Secrets Reinforcement (see chapter 9).

The Six Healing Sounds Meditation

1. *Hsi* ("**shee**"): the three body cavities (Respiratory, Digestive, and Excretory systems; see Figs. 11a and 11b)
2. *Chwei* ("**chew-way**"): Kidneys
3. *Sz* ("**sss-u**" or "**sue**"): Lungs
4. *He* ("**huh**"—this sound should come from the back of the throat, with your tongue touching the roof of the mouth): Heart
5. *Hu* ("**whoo**"—like the sound of the wind): Spleen and Pancreas
6. *Hsyu* (ssh-u): Liver and Gallbladder

How to Practice the Meditation

1. Put your hands in a Mind-Calming Mudra position (see chapter 9, pages 301–2), placing your left hand cupped over your right, with thumbs touching each other. Rest this hand gesture at the level of your heart. Visualize that everything is calm, quiet, and dissolved into a peaceful void.

2. Recite the Mind-Calming Mantra nine times: *Getè, Getè, Para Getè, Para Sum Getè, Bodhi Swaha* (Mandarin) or *Gatè Gatè, Boro Gatè, Boro Sun Gatè, Bodhi So Po He* (Tibetan).

3. Visualize that the Blue Medicine Buddha is sitting before you on a lotus-shaped throne, holding a medicine bowl in his left hand and a *ling-chih*

(a hard fungus believed to have supernatural powers) in his right hand. Also visualize that all your family members, relatives, and close friends are with you, meditating in front of the Blue Medicine Buddha. (Also include any others whom you want to bless, and see them sitting next to you, side by side.)

4. Concentrate on your breathing. Visualize all the organs in the body, and the body itself, becoming crystalline, sparkling, radiating light. See this light filling up your body and traveling to all your blood cells, organs, tissues, muscles, and bones, healing them and clearing away any stagnant energy, blocking illness or disease. Spend extra time and focus on the areas that are ill or diseased.

5. Take a deep breath, and as part of your exhalation, pronounce each of the Six Healing Sounds, explained below, three or nine times:

Hsi (**"shee"**): Visualize the three visceral cavities of your body (the respiratory, digestive, and excretory systems) and see that they are strong and functioning at their best. Imagine that a bright, luminescent light is passing through them, healing all imbalances and releasing all stagnant energies and emotional memories that have contributed to your illness. See the Medicine Buddha coming toward you with his *ling-chih* and medicine bowl, healing all diseases of your circulatory, digestive, and excretory systems. Visualize the same thing for all your friends and family members who have joined you for this meditation.

Chwei (**"chew-way"**): Visualize that your kidneys are radiating beautiful healing light, and that they are strong and functioning well. Healthy light is flowing through them and clearing away any of the unhealthy ch'i from every one of its cells, tissues, and emotional memory bank. See the Medicine Buddha coming toward you with his *ling-chih* and medicine bowl, healing all the imbalances or sicknesses of your kidneys. Visualize this for all your friends and relatives who have joined you in this meditation.

Sz (**"sss–u" or "sue"**): Visualize that your lungs are radiating light, and that they are clear and operating well. Each breath is bringing in healthy ch'i for your body and exhaling all negative and illness ch'i, and all stagnant energy that is stored in the lungs' emotional memory. See the Medicine Buddha coming toward you with his *ling-chih* and medicine bowl, dispensing healing for your lungs. Visualize this for all your friends and family who have joined you in this meditation.

He ("huh"): Visualize your heart radiating a pure, strong, healing light, all its muscles, chambers, veins, and arteries flowing with healing ch'i and light, releasing any blocks, scars, or sickness of any kind, including ill ch'i from the heart's emotional memory. See the Medicine Buddha coming toward you with his *ling-chih* and medicine bowl, healing any imbalances or diseases of your heart. Visualize this for your friends and family members as well.

Hu ("whoo," a sound like the wind): Visualize that your spleen is filled with and radiating beautiful, healing light, and that it is strong and functioning well. Healthy light is flowing in and around it, clearing away any sick, imbalanced, or emotionally taxing ch'i. See the Medicine Buddha coming toward you with his *ling-chih* and his medicine bowl, healing any sickness or past issues associated with your spleen. Visualize this for all your friends and family members who have joined you in this meditation.

Hsyu ("ssh-u"): Visualize your liver and gallbladder radiating pure light and that all ill ch'i is being released from their cells, tissues, and emotional memory. See the Medicine Buddha coming toward you with his *ling-chih* and medicine bowl, treating any illness or imbalance of your gallbladder or liver. Send this light and visualization process to any friends and relatives who are also with you in this meditation.

Visualize all the organs in the body becoming crystallized and radiating light. A slowly blooming lotus flower appears with eight petals in the center of your heart. Sitting on top of the lotus is a Buddha. As he slowly expands, he fills up your whole body. The Buddha is you, and you are the Buddha, possessing his perfect wisdom, compassion, prosperity, and healing abilities.

Visualize that you are sending out this internal Buddha light for all kinds of healing to yourself, your friends, family, the six realms of existence, all those who are suffering and sick, all the Buddhas and deities that support you, all your teachers, mentors, Professor Lin Yun, and the person who gave you this healing meditation. Recite the Mind-Calming Mantra nine times, take a deep breath in, and open your eyes.

Don't worry too much about the actual pronunciation of the Chinese words; make your best effort but reciting them from your heart, and knowing that they are powerful, are what make them work. The more spiritually connected you are, and the more you work on cultivating your ch'i, the more powerful this mantra will be for you. Professor Lin believes that we all have a Buddha that lives inside of us, and if your heart is calm and clear, that Buddha in you is able to come out. Meditating, praying, and working toward being your authentic self will create an opening for your Buddha inside to appear. Draw on that divine and expansive part of yourself, for it will help give you strength and direction during fragile times and in periods of confusion.

Quartz Crystals and Semiprecious Stones

When used in combination with conscious intentions, crystals and gemstones can amplify your thoughts, raise the vibrational levels of your ch'i, and enhance the Feng Shui of your home. All crystals and gemstones have special properties and vibrate at certain frequencies, that in turn can resonate to the different areas of your life, the different Chakras in your body, and various health conditions. When used on an altar, in a car, in different parts of your home, or carried on your person, they will work toward healing imbalances and shoring up weaker areas of energy. Natural crystals also bring in the element of Earth wherever they are placed, because they are thousands of years old and mined from the earth.

Make sure to clear the energy fields of any crystal before you activate it for your personal use. (Instructions for clearing stones follow the table of crystals below.) You will notice on the charts that follow that many crystals listed are primarily for the Heart Chakra/Relationship gua, and that many of the descriptions do not list a specific health problem. This is because to prescribe a crystal for a particular illness would limit all the various psychological and emotional underpinnings (ESPs) that significantly contributed to the physical manifestation of that illness to begin with. The way I have listed the descriptions and properties gives you a range to pick for yourself the issues that you feel are germane to you and your illness.

If you take a quick look at the Transcendental Cure called Tracing the Nine Stars, page 319, you will see that the star trace begins in the Family gua and exits out of the Relationship gua. This is because everything, including our lives, starts out with the family, only to come full circle to where we have to deal with those unresolved issues one more time before we can actually release them, through our adult life and relationships. Many of the underlying issues of your illness will have some root cause in one of those guas and corresponding Chakras. In addition, the Heart Chakra is the energetic balancing beam in the body because it has three body Chakras above it and three below it. Keeping that Chakra clear and balanced should be a priority. Equilibrium is essential, especially as you are going through a health crisis or your healing process.

If you are incorporating crystals into your overall vibrational medicine treatment plan, or as an adjunct to your current treatment plan, feel free to carry, wear, meditate on, and bathe with the stone that resonates to the particular Chakra, gua, or illness that you are addressing. Use any crystal that feels vibrationally correct and toward which you innately gravitate. Always feel free to bypass my charts and suggestions, if you feel drawn to certain crystals or aromatherapy oils that might not align perfectly with the information provided. We are learning together how to decipher the correct and various vibrations that each crystal carries. If something doesn't feel right or align with you completely, acquiesce to your inner authority and follow your own intuitive knowing.

When using the stones, make sure you clear them first and then frequently, for they will absorb all your discharged energy and emotions (see clearing instructions following the chart below). This will stagnate their energy fields and render them useless, as they start spewing back to you and the environment all the muck and aspects of the illness that they have absorbed.

CRYSTAL AND GEMSTONE PROPERTIES[15]

Crystal/ Gemstone		Chakra Centers Feng Shui Guas
Agate	Encourages acceptance, grounding, emotional and physical balance. Raises consciousness, helps digestion.	First Chakra Survival Center/ Wealth Gua

continued

Moss agate	Encourages acceptance, self-confidence, and security. Relieves hypoglycemia and depression.	First Chakra, Survival Center; Wealth Gua
Botswana agate (from Africa)	Relieves depression, helps in quitting smoking. Relieves breathing/lung-related problems.	Fourth Chakra, Heart Center; Relationship Gua
Amethyst	Assists opening to path and spirituality in a grounded way. Encourages creativity, sobriety, courage, intuition, self-esteem. Assists in restful sleeping.	Seventh Chakra, Crown Center; Fame Gua
Aquamarine	Calming, improves mental clarity, enhances self-expression, clears adolescent issues, helps one come into one's own and mature.	Fifth Chakra, Throat Center; Children Gua
Aventurine (green quartz)	Encourages joy, lightens the heart, improves mental clarity. Promotes calming, positive attitude.	Fourth Chakra, Heart Center; Relationship Gua
Carnelian	Strengthens body and mind, promotes creativity. Relieves lower-back problems, strengthens reproductive organs, helps address and release incest, addictions, early childhood issues, and sexuality-related issues.	Second Chakra, Social Center; Family Gua
Citrine	Breaks up energy blocks in the body, strengthens will, vision, balance, self-confidence. Helps in letting go of addictions.	Second Chakra, Social Center; Family Gua
Clear quartz	Powerful transmitter. Amplifies and directs thought-form. Healing energy balancer, promotes clarity, attunes one to higher self.	Overall Vibration, All Chakras; All Guas
Emerald	Improves relationships, meditation. Relaxant, heart balancer. Strengthens clairvoyance and psychic abilities, aids in relieving mental illness.	Fourth Chakra, Heart Center; Relationship Gua
Fluorite	Relieves arthritis. Strengthens ability to perceive higher levels of reality. Clears air of psychic clutter. Connects you to your higher path, while grounding you in Earth reality.	First and Seventh Chakras together, Survival and the Crown Centers; Wealth and Fame Guas
Garnet	Improves blood and oxygen circulation, especially in lungs, skin, legs, feet, and intestines. Promotes heat, energy, and vitality. Stimulates imagination, self-esteem, and healthy willpower. Calms anger.	First Chakra, Survival Center; Wealth Gua

Hematite	Improves blood disorders. Increases self-esteem, aids in astral projection. Protection.	Third Chakra, Solar plexus/Will Center; Career Gua
Jade	Blood cleanser. Strengthens immune system and kidneys. Generates Divine Love. Encourages altruistic nature and expression of feelings. Protects from injuries and accidents.	Fourth Chakra, Heart Center; Relationship Gua
Lapis lazuli	Increases psychic abilities, opens Third Eye. Throat—increases expression. Cleansing. Aligns etheric, mental, spiritual bodies. Thought amplifier.	Sixth Chakra, Third Eye Center; Career Gua
Malachite	Balances right/left brain. Strengthens body and mind during mental illness and over-toxification. Protects against radiation. Promotes tissue regeneration. Inspires giving of self, self-expression. Assists vision on all levels. Absorbs anger. Soothes stomach problems.	Third Chakra, Solar Plexus/Will Center; Knowledge Gua
Pyrite	Digestive aid, good for red corpuscles. Eases anxiety, frustration, depression. Good for circulation. Money magnet.	Third Chakra, Solar plexus/Will Center; Career Gua
Rhodochrosite	Cleanses subconscious. Strengthens self-identity. Combines the healing properties of the Heart Chakra with the strengthening power of white light.	Fourth Chakra, Heart Center; Relationship Gua
Rose quartz	Increases confidence, personal expression, and creativity. Emotional balance—self-love. For "heartbreak"—opening to universal love. Comfort.	Fourth Chakra, Heart Center; Relationship Gua
Rutilated quartz	Breaks old patterns, childhood blockages. Tissue regeneration, builds immune system. Eases depression. Releases father issues.	Second Chakra, Social Center; Family Gua
Smoky quartz	Increases fertility, creativity, joy. Balances emotional energy, grounding. Strengthens adrenals, aids protein assimilation.	Second Chakra, Social Center; Family Gua
Sodalite	Encourages harmony, balance, courage, communication. Strengthens lymphatic system, alleviates subconscious fear and guilt.	Sixth Chakra-Third Eye Center; Third Chakra-Solar Plexus Center; Knowledge/Career Gua

A MULTILEVEL APPROACH TO DISARMING IS CHALLENGING ILLNESSES

continued

Tourmaline	Dispels fear, negativity, grief. Promotes healthy environment, tranquil sleep, balance in relationships, self-expression. Eases compulsiveness.	Various Chakras, depending on the color of the tourmaline Various Guas
Black tourmaline	Eases arthritis, strengthens adrenals. Protects against negativity. Grounding.	First Chakra Survival Center; Wealth Gua
Green tourmaline	Strengthens immune system, balances heart energy. Helps release emotional under-pinning to physical heart problems.	Fourth Chakra, Heart Center; Relationship Gua
Blue tourmaline	Encourages communication and self-expression. Enhances speaking out and creativity. Strengthens lungs.	Fifth Chakra, Throat Center; Children's Gua
Watermelon tourmaline	Stimulates other tourmalines, strengthens their effect. Balancer, strengthens heart and endocrine glands.	Fourth Chakra, Heart Center; Relationship Gua
Pink (rubellite) tourmaline	Heart balancer. Increases depth of insight and perception. Creativity, fertility. Balances passivity/aggression.	Fourth and Sixth Chakras, Heart/Third Eye Centers; Relationship and Knowledge Guas
Tourmaline in quartz	Attunement to higher self, increases spiritual understanding, promotes peace.	Seventh Chakra, Crown Center; Fame Gua

Crystals and gemstones have sensitive energy fields, which can easily pick up energy from humans and other sources. Assume that other admirers have handled all these stones before they found their way to you. To remove any imprinted energy, clearing the object immediately after purchase is recommended, in addition to clearing the stones every few months thereafter. One of the following two methods may be used:

1. Dissolve one heaping teaspoon of sea salt per quart of water (springwater is prefer-able, though not essential). Immerse your crystal or gemstone in the solution for three to seven days. Afterward, place them in the sunlight to recharge.

2. Pass the crystal or gemstone through the rising smoke of a piece of burning white sage or smudge stick 27 times. This method is recommended for any "power object," including a crystal or gemstone, that has been soldered, glued, or drilled in any way. Also, certain crystals that have a metal as part of their composition, such as hematite or pyrite, which are metal ores—or amber, which is a resin—should not be cleansed in a saltwater solution, as this will harm their finish.

Therapeutic Grade Essential Oils

For thousands of years in ancient Egypt, Greece, China, India, and the Middle East, the art and science of using essential oils for healing was a highly developed and well-respected sacred process. The plant kingdom has made an incredible amount of healing information available to us, and the scent aspect of the oils is only a part of the offering that we receive from the plants and trees from which they come. Each of the essential oils, just like the tones, colors, and Chakras, vibrates to a different frequency and contains various healing properties that help restore the body to balance.

Essential oils are highly concentrated extracts distilled from flowers, trees, leaves, roots, and seeds. Only 5 percent of the essential oils being produced in the world today are being used for therapeutic purposes. The majority are used primarily in the perfume, food-flavoring, and pharmaceutical industries. Not all oils are the same. It is important to note that there are five major grades of oils, all having different degrees of quality: (1) industrial; (2) food-grade; (3) fragrance-grade; (4) perfume grade; and (5) therapeutic grade.

Pure *therapeutic grade essential oils* are the only grade I recommend for healing ourselves and our environments. They take anywhere from three to 28 times longer to distill because they are distilled at a slower speed and at a lower temperature, maintaining the molecular structure of the plant, which keeps their ch'i alive and their life force active. All the other grades of oil have had their molecules fractured during the very rapid distillation process. The pure extracted oils carry the essence, life force, and distinctive "fingerprint" of that particular oil without any major damage to its core vibration.

The oils enter our body in two very important ways: they travel on and through the olfactory nerves, which lead from the nose to the brain, and they are absorbed through our pores and hair follicles. It takes approximately 15 minutes to 12 hours for these oils to be fully absorbed, but the body and the environment can start reacting to them in as little as three seconds from the time they make contact. The oils can be experienced in many ways: through massage or steam inhalation, or when used in a diffuser, bath, compress, base oil, or lotion.

Please note that there is much controversy regarding the internal use of essential oils. French medical practitioners often use them internally, but they are well trained in the exact preparation for this method. Here in the United States, this is not common practice. In general, using oils internally is not the best method of absorption, for there is a strong possibility of irritating the stomach lining and ingesting toxic amounts.

We Have Borrowed the Language from Music to Describe the Oils

Notes: Base, Middle, and Top

As you first begin to start working with the oils, feel free to experiment; blend and mix them together. You can also use your intuition to guide you, or you can follow the guidelines below and in the chart at the end of this chapter, to form a well-balanced blend. We've borrowed musical terminology to describe the oils. *Base note oils* (such as sandalwood) strengthen and ground the blend, draw the oil into our skin, and are connected to the Survival, Social, and Solar Plexus Chakras, our lower three. *Middle note oils* smooth the sharp edges and provide softness (geranium, lavender), offering healing to the Solar Plexus and Heart Chakras. *Top note oils* are generally uplifting and penetrating, and will give you the first scent and impression of the blend (bergamot, lemon). Top notes assist the Throat, Crown, and Transpersonal Centers, our higher three Chakras.

As we are now discovering, many oils are available to help treat illnesses and vibrational imbalances. It is important to learn the different properties each oil possesses, because this will help you in your choice. Just as each person on the planet has a different personality and gift to offer us, so does each oil. To choose an oil, look at all its properties and see which one suits you best, or smell them and see which ones your sense of smell responds to most favorably. Sometimes the smells that we actually don't like are the ones we need the most. Literally hundreds of oils are available to you for their healing purposes. For the purposes of this book, I have briefly described 22 of the most commonly used essential oils. The oils are powerful and usually just a few drops are needed to add to a bath or to a base oil in a diffuser for positive results. For more in-depth information on aromatherapy, *Aromatherapy A–Z,* by Patricia Davis, and *Colour Scents: Healing with Colour and Aroma,* by Suzy Chiazzari, are two excellent books on the subject (see the list of suggested reading at the end of this book).

ESSENTIAL OILS AND THEIR HEALING PROPERTIES[16]

ESSENTIAL OIL	PROPERTIES	USED FOR	STIMULATES AND HEALS CHAKRA(s)	ATTRIBUTES
Lavender	calming; balancing, soothing; sedating; cleansing	anti-inflammatory; influenza; anxiety; depression	1st, 4th, 7th	Acts as a "nurturing mom"; will detoxify and release anything that is not unconditional love; support for financial management; connects with Higher Self and beyond.
Lemon	refreshing; uplifting; purifies; stimulates; enlivens; circulates congested ch'i	mental clarity; helps to release anger; resentment, judgment; detoxifying, helps fight infections; liver congestion or deficiency (hot compress w/ rosemary oil, 20 minutes); osteoporosis	3rd, 5th	Purifies self and environment; helps you find another way to see things clearly; brings energy of being here and now; opens you to new beginnings; good for studying and concentration.
Peppermint	uplifting; master balancer; calming; clarifying; awakening; penetrating; inspiring; energizing	digestive aid, stomach pains, nausea, flatulence, vomiting, diarrhea; impotence; mental alertness; helps with feelings of helplessness—stops negative flow of thoughts	1st, 7th	Do not use more than a week—weakens nervous system; no more than three drops in a bath; use peppermint *early* in the day, so as not to disturb sleep; works on supporting your self-acceptance; stimulates all immune functioning.
Blood orange	warming; cheering; soothing; calming; creativity; balancing; energizing; lighthearted; courageous	anxiety, worry, addiction; antidepressant; diarrhea, constipation	2nd	"Spontaneous joy"; *only* up to three drops in a bath (can cause irritation and burning); good for healing sexual abuse; good for pregnant women, elderly, babies; untouched innocence restored.
Eucalyptus	powerful cleanser of negativity; grounding; strengthening; stimulating; centering; expanding; supports growth and success	anti-inflammatory; colds, coughs; asthma; heated emotions, irrational thoughts, temper tantrums, mood swings, congestion	4th	Helps with facing challenges, transitions, and success; opens up respiratory tract and improves breathing; opens up heart and throat.
Rosemary	stimulating; uplifting; strengthens; sharpens; piercing; centers; brings clarity; stabilizing	arthritis; headaches and migraines; heart tonic; muscular aches and pains	1st, 4th, 5th, 7th	*Do not use* if you are pregnant or have epilepsy or high blood pressure; strengthens circulatory, respiratory, and nervous systems; reduces swelling from fibroids.

continued

Oil	Properties	Uses	Chakras	Description
Sandalwood	calming; relaxing; openness; harmonizing; balancing; alleviates confusion; sense of well-being; meditative; enlightenment	antidepressant; reduces nervous tension; diarrhea; urinary tract, bladder infections	1st, 5th, 6th, 7th	Brings us in union with the divine; used in rituals, meditation, and ceremonies; helps us to cut ties with the past; helps overall being stay focused and grounded.
Jasmine	warming; sensual; relaxing; reassuring; aware; uplifting; intuitive; inspirational; joyful; euphoric	aphrodisiac; increases self-confidence and optimism; reduces menstrual cramps and pain; aids spiritual development	1st, 2nd, 4th	Jasmine is the "king of oils", "oil of the angels"—helps draw angelic beings to you; helps with assertion; fun, positive energy for creativity.
Geranium	balancing; expansive; creative; stabilizing; uplifting	anti-cancer; stabilizes emotions; hormone balancer; stimulates lymphatic system	4th, 5th	Aids the creative process and our ability to perform and function; helps us to move beyond our comfort zone; helps us to stay positive and hopeful.
Ylang-ylang	calming; sedative; focusing; joyous; assertiveness	aphrodisiac; impotence, frigidity (fear, nervousness); anger; self-esteem	2nd, 4th	"Divine sexuality" oil; can place oil in Relationship area, bedroom, and Marriage gua to enhance sexuality; balances Yin/Yang energies and masculine/feminine aspects of self; use small amounts for short periods of time, otherwise can be irritating, causing headaches and nausea.
Rose	purifying; sedative; cleansing; regulating	heart disease; uterus tonic; grief; tonic effect on circulatory, digestive, and nervous systems	4th, 7th	"The queen of the flowers"; heals by opening the heart; helps all systems of the body balance and regulate.
Neroli	calming; relaxing; stabilizing; clearing; sedative; joy; peacefulness; contentment	antidepressant; sedative for children; anxiety; enhances the creative process	2nd, 3rd, 4th	Holds the essence of Quan Yin, the Buddhist Goddess of Compassion; Leonardo da Vinci used it when he was creating artwork.
Fennel	assertiveness; confidence; focusing; clearing; motivating; courageous; clarifying	eating disorders, alcoholism; digestive aid	2nd, 3rd, 4th	Psychic protector (1 drop on solar plexus—rub in counterclockwise motion); renews our interest in life; releases creative blocks; opens us to our own inner wisdom; avoid during pregnancy or if you have epilepsy.
Marjoram	penetrating; increased confidence; comforting; strengthening	arthritis and rheumatism; high blood pressure and heart conditions; calms nervous system tension; lower backaches	2nd, 4th, 5th	Warming and comforting to heart—lifts sadness, grief, and loneliness; use only in small doses, as it can block emotions; "Joy of the Mountain" and "herb of happiness"; avoid when pregnant.

Cinnamon	invigorating; energizing; aggressive	flu, colds, coughs; antiviral and antifungal; bladder infections; stimulant	1st, 2nd	Use very small amounts, as it is toxic for many people and can cause painful skin reactions; used to bring in financial prosperity.
Chamomile	soothing; sedative; relaxing; encourages patience	PMS, menstrual pain, and menopause; reduces insomnia; releases emotions linked to past; dispels anger and fear	5th	Use over throat to help express true feelings; Mild enough to use on children and elderly.
Bergamot	joyous; refreshing; uplifting; motivating	urinary tract infections; supports quitting smoking; reduces hopelessness; restores self-confidence	2nd, 3rd, 4th	Expands the heart energy; helps to see both sides of a situation.
Vetiver	grounding; centering; calming; protecting	strengthening circulation; reducing emotional burnout; helps mind focus; supports taking action; helps mind focus	1st, 3rd	Brings energies of all major Chakras into harmony and alignment with one another; psychic protector—apply 1 drop to solar plexus and rub in counterclockwise direction; helps us to find purpose in life.
Tea tree	centers; calms; purifies; heals	immune stimulant; antiviral and antifungal; respiratory—asthma, bronchitis, congestion, coughs; disinfects wounds; protects the psyche	6th, 7th	Opens Sixth Chakra; helps us to release our fears and anxieties and to trust in higher guidance; dissolves negativity before reaching subtle bodies.
Frankincense	comforting; stabilizing; centering; purifying; restorative; protection; meditative; enlightening	chronic bronchitis and asthma; strengthens immune system; reduces swollen lymph glands in neck; calms emotions and mind	7th, 5th	Used to drive out stagnant/negative ch'i; helps break links with the past; connects us with our higher self; one of the most valuable for respiratory/lungs.
Cedarwood	grounding; strengthening; powerful; focusing; stabilizing; improves concentration	arthritis/rheumatism; urinary tract infections; strengthens circulatory system; helps diffuse anger, aggression, and fear	1st, 2nd, 3rd, 7th	Provides an example of safe male energy (for sexually abused women); provides support when needing objectivity; avoid during pregnancy because it can stimulate menstrual flow; strengthens our connection with the divine.
Rosewood	uplifting; balancing; opening; calming	cell and tissue regenerator; relieves pain; headaches/migraines; immune system stimulant	1st, 4th, 7th	Connects us with Universal Love; heals emotional and physical abuse; promotes open-mindedness and tolerance; calms and relaxes nervous system.

Chart compilation and article collaboration with Robin Spiegel, massage therapist and sound, color, and aromatherapy healer, Rye, New York.

A MULTILEVEL APPROACH TO
DISARMING 15 CHALLENGING
ILLNESSES

The following table is a cross-referenced, multilevel outline that lists 15 common illnesses and provides various vibrational approaches and ways to work with these illnesses and transform them. Each section will list the illness and its supportive psychospiritual-environmental approaches to helping it transform or heal. The table includes several Feng Shui adjustments to apply, health information based on the Chakra Energy System, and recommended colors to wear, eat, and bring into your environment. In addition, it addresses specific essential oils to use, corresponding crystals and semiprecious stones to carry and meditate with, daily affirmations, vibrational sound, and tones to chant and listen to in order to strengthen and support the diseased area of the body while disarming the illness matrix. There is also a section listed on each chart where you are encouraged to do your own personal work regarding the ESPs of your illness.

Many different modalities, holistic and traditional, allopathic and homeopathic, are not listed in this chart or addressed elsewhere in this book. Their omission is not an oversight, nor is it intended to devalue their importance in any way. I choose to focus on the vibrational medicines of Feng Shui Design, the Chakra Energy System, sound, color, crystals, and aromatherapy oils, because they are the medicines in which I am best versed and use regularly as part of my Feng Shui practice and incorporate in my Feng Shui Design and the Chakra Energy System Consultant Training Program. Please note that I am recommending these options to be used in *tandem* with your medical treatment of choice, for these vibrationally sympathetic medicines will work diligently and energetically toward shoring up both your internal environment and your external environment. When these two environments are strengthened, they actually raise the effectiveness of the treatment plan that you are employing, be it Western, Eastern, or otherwise.

Please be sure not to misuse these wonderful healing gifts, and continue to seek and apply the medical treatment of your choice. My theory on the ESPs of Illness states that you *must* address the physical part of your illness, if total and true healing is to occur. So rearrange your furniture, do your cures, meditate, color-breathe, chant, and pray, but be sure to incorporate a medical treatment plan into your approach. Applying both the mundane and transcendental approaches to your illnesses increases your opportunities for getting well and for accelerating your healing process.

Bless every approach that you choose to utilize from the upcoming charts with the Three Secrets Reinforcement Blessing in chapter 9, page 301.

1. ANXIETY DISORDERS

FENG SHUI INTERVENTIONS	
Corresponding gua(s)—augment and make all necessary repairs:	Center/Health Area
Interior and exterior factors to assess; solutions, cures, and adjustments:	Fix all doors (ch. 1, p. 33) Check your electrical systems (ch. 1, p. 35) Take the "clutter challenge" (ch. 4, p. 113) Direct walkways, traffic flow, and rushing ch'i (ch. 1, p. 28) Long, narrow hallways/driveway and fast-moving ch'i (ch. 6, p. 171) Don't have your back to the door (ch. 1, p. 31) Split-view entranceways (ch. 6, p. 172) Brick-wall entranceways (ch. 6, p. 173) Kitchens that share a wall with a bathroom (ch. 6, p. 178) Check lighting, color, and life force (ch. 6, p. 203) Entranceways with contrary doors that open out instead of in (ch. 6, p. 170) Entranceway and bedroom door that opens to small end of the room (ch. 5, p. 155) Bedroom is over a garage (ch. 5, p. 159) Check for high EMFs (ch. 1, p. 37, ch. 5, pp. 137 and 161
Adjustments to make/do/use:	Check for frayed wires, electrical shorts, empty light-bulb sockets. Repair broken appliances. Add a 50-mm crystal on a nine-inch red string to the Center/Health gua in the bedroom.
Interior factors to eliminate/avoid:	All white walls and monochromatic schemes in general. Clear all clutter.

continued

Transcendental Cures/ Meditations:	Inhale-Exhale meditation; Three-Flute Cure (ch. 9, p. 311)

CHAKRA INTERVENTIONS

Corresponding Chakra colors:	Yellow (3rd or Will Center)
Supporting/complementary Chakra color(s):	Indigo (6th or Third Eye Center)
Supporting/parallel Chakra color(s):	Purple (7th or Crown Center)
Color-breathing exercise(s) (9 inhales/exhales each for 27 consecutive days):	Inhale Yellow through the 3rd Chakra or Will Center. Exhale Green out the 4th Chakra or Heart Center.

VIBRATIONAL MEDICINES

Sound/tone to use:	The Note E
Natural crystals to wear and carry:	Agate, Amethyst, Malachite
Pure essential oils to use:	Fennel, Lemon, Marjoram

YOUR PERSONAL WORK

Daily affirmation (9 times each day for 27 consecutive days):	Everything is in perfect order. I trust in the divine plan.
Your own affirmation(s):	
Emotional underpinning(s):	
Spiritual opportunity, growth, and reason for contracting illness:	
Physical challenge(s); care needed to take:	
Your medical/treatment plan(s):	

2. ARTHRITIS

FENG SHUI INTERVENTIONS	
Corresponding gua(s)—augment and make all necessary repairs:	Knowledge (problems with hands) Wealth (problems with hips) Family (problems with knees)
Interior and exterior factors to assess; solutions, cures, and adjustments:	Fix all doors (ch. 1, p. 33) Bedroom door opens to small end of the room (chapter 5, p. 155) Entranceways with contrary doors that open to the small of the room (ch. 6, p. 169) Bathroom in Wealth gua (ch. 6, p. 181) Staircase too close to the front door (ch. 6, p. 194) Structural beam over the bed (ch. 5, p. 143, ch. 6, p. 197) Long and narrow entranceways, foyers, and hallways (ch. 6, p. 171)
Adjustments to make/do/use:	Check all hinges, doors, and doorknobs and make sure they are in good working order. Lubricate all latches and hinges. Add a 50-mm crystal on a nine-inch red string to the Center/Health gua in the bedroom.
Interior factors to eliminate/avoid:	Doors, cabinets, and locks that don't open easily
Transcendental Cures/Meditations:	The Great Sunshine Buddha Meditation (chapter 9 p. 306)

CHAKRA INTERVENTIONS			
Corresponding Chakra color(s):	Hands: Hips: Knees:	Green Orange Red	(4th or Heart Center) (2nd or Social Center) (1st or Survival Center)
Supporting/complementary Chakra color(s):	Hands: Hips: Knees:	Purple Light Blue Green	(7th or Crown Center) (5th or Throat Center) (4th or Heart Center)
Supporting/parallel Chakra color(s):	Hands: Hips: Knees:	White Indigo Light Blue	(8th or Transpersonal Center) (6th or Third Eye Center) (5th or Throat Center)

continued

Color-breathing exercise(s) (9 inhales/exhales each for 27 consecutive days):	Overall Color Breathing (chapter 8, closing chapter meditation, p. 246)	

VIBRATIONAL MEDICINES

Sound/tone to use:	Hands:	The Note F
	Hips:	The Note D
	Knees:	The Note C

Natural crystals to wear and carry:	Hands:	Emeralds, Aventurine
	Hips:	Citrine, Carnelian
	Knees:	Garnet, Black Tourmaline

Pure essential oils to use:	Eucalyptus, Lemon, German Chamomile, Roman Chamomile, Marjoram, Rosemary

YOUR PERSONAL WORK

Daily affirmation (9 times each day for 27 consecutive days):	I release my grip on my fear of living.

Your own affirmation(s):	

Emotional underpinning(s):	

Spiritual opportunity, growth, and reason for contracting illness:	

Physical challenge(s); care needed to take:	

Your medical/treatment plan(s):	

3. CANCER

FENG SHUI INTERVENTIONS	
Corresponding gua(s)—augment make all necessary repairs:	Relationship (breast cancer) Center (lung cancer) Wealth (colon and prostate cancer)
Interior and exterior factors to assess; solutions, cures, and adjustments:	Check EMF levels (ch. 1, p. 37, ch. 5, pp. 137 and 161) Clean all sewers, plumbing, air-conditioning ducts (ch. 1, p. 38) Assess the Three Visceral Cavities for breast cancer (ch. 4, p. 121 and Figs. 11a and 11b) Check if the bedroom is over a garage (ch. 5, p. 159) Check stove location (ch. 6, p. 191) Check EMF levels in the bedroom (ch. 5, pp. 137, 154 and 161) Bathroom over a front door or entryway (ch. 6, p. 180) Bedroom/kitchen; bedroom/bathroom (ch. 5, pp. 150–55)
Adjustments to make/do/use:	Add and raise wattage of all lighting. Check and fix all waterworks and electrical systems. Add a 50-mm crystal on a nine-inch red string to the Center/Health gua in the bedroom
Interior factors to eliminate/avoid:	Excessive use of the color Red
Transcendental Cures/ Meditations:	The Great Sunshine Buddha (ch. 9, p. 306); The Medicine Buddha (Appendix A); Six Ch'i Healing Sounds Meditation (ch. 10, p. 334)
CHAKRA INTERVENTIONS	
Corresponding Chakra color(s):	Breast: Green (4th or Heart Center); Lung: Green (4th or Heart Center); colon/prostate: Red (1st or Survival Center)
Supporting/complementary Chakra color(s):	Breast: Purple (7th or Crown Center); lung: Purple (7th or Crown Center); colon/prostate: Green (4th or Heart Center)
Supporting/parallel Chakra color(s):	Breast: White (8th or Transpersonal Center); lung: White (8th or Transpersonal Center); colon/prostate: Light Blue (5th or Throat Center)

continued 353

Color-breathing exercise(s) (9 inhales/exhales each for 27 consecutive days):	Overall color breathing; breathe in the specific color of the diseased area/Chakra; exhale Green through the Heart Center.

VIBRATIONAL MEDICINES

Sound/tone to use:	Breast: The Note F; lung: The Note F; colon/prostate: The Note C
Natural crystals to wear and carry:	Breast: Pink Tourmaline, Rose Quartz, Sodalite; lung: Green Tourmaline, Aventurine; colon/prostate: Garnet, Black Tourmaline
Pure essential oils to use:	Do not use essential oils at the same time as chemotherapy. Bergamot, Cedarwood, Eucalyptus, Frankincense, Geranium, Lavender, to treat burns from radiation therapy; Rosemary, for regrowth of hair after chemotherapy

YOUR PERSONAL WORK

Daily affirmation (9 times each day for 27 consecutive days):	I release all past resentments, hurts, and anger.
Your own affirmation(s):	
Emotional underpinning(s):	
Spiritual opportunity, growth; and reason for contracting illness:	
Physical challenge(s); care needed to take:	
Your medical/treatment plan(s):	

4. DEPRESSION

FENG SHUI INTERVENTIONS	
Corresponding gua(s)—augment and make all necessary repairs:	Center Career Health Family Children
Interior and exterior factors to assess; solutions, cures, and adjustments:	Repair all leaks (ch. 1, p. 32) Fix all doors (ch. 1, p. 33) Clear all clutter (ch. 1, p. 34; ch. 4, p. 113) Check electrical systems (ch. 1, p. 35) Clean all sewers, plumbing, air-conditioning ducts (ch. 1, p. 38) Low lighting (ch. 1, p. 36, ch. 6, p. 203) Bedroom door opens to small of the room (ch. 5, p. 155) Headboard shares bathroom wall (ch. 5, p. 151) Bedroom is in the basement or below entranceway level (ch. 5, p. 159) Brick wall/split view entranceway (ch. 6, p. 173) Doors are blocked and broken or don't open—and at one time did (ch. 6, p. 201) House is without much color (ch. 6, p. 203, ch. 7, pp. 238–42) Assess your view (ch. 1, p. 27) Proximity to buildings, businesses, or places of worship (ch. 1, p. 24)
Adjustments to make/do/use:	Life-force adjustments: live plants, strong lighting, fish tanks, pets, things that have movement. Add a 50-mm crystal on a nine-inch red string in the Center/Health gua in the bedroom.
Interior factors to eliminate/avoid:	Dark colors, monochromatic schemes, both in your environment and your clothing
Transcendental Cures/ Meditations:	The Great Sunshine Buddha (chapter 9, p. 306); Medicine Buddha (Appendix A); the Six Ch'i Healing Sounds (ch. 10, p. 334); 3 Bamboo Flutes Cure (chapter 9, p. 311)

continued

CHAKRA INTERVENTIONS

Corresponding Chakra color(s):	Orange (2nd or Social Center); Yellow (3rd or Will Center)
Supporting/complementary Chakra color(s):	Light Blue (5th or Throat Center) for 2nd Chakra; Indigo (6th or Third Eye Center) for 3rd Chakra
Supporting/parallel Chakra color(s):	Indigo (6th or Third Eye Center) for 2nd Chakra; Purple (7th or Crown Center) for 3rd Chakra
Color-breathing exercises(s) (9 inhales/exhales each for 27 consecutive days):	Overall color breathing and also inhale Orange through the 2nd Chakra or Social Center, and exhale Light Blue through the 5th Chakra or Throat Center.

VIBRATIONAL MEDICINES

Sound/tone to use:	The Note D (2nd Chakra); The Note E (3rd Chakra)
Natural crystals to wear and carry:	Aventurine, Botswana Agate, Citrine, Clear Quartz, Malachite, Pyrite, Rutilated Quartz
Pure essential oils to use:	Bergamot, Blood Orange, Frankincense, Geranium, Jasmine, Lavender, Lemon, Neroli, Sandalwood, Ylang-ylang

YOUR PERSONAL WORK

Daily affirmation (9 times each day for 27 consecutive days):	It is safe to have all my feelings, thoughts, and fears.
Your own affirmation(s):	
Emotional underpinning(s):	
Spiritual opportunity, growth, and reason for contracting illness:	
Physical challenge(s); care needed to take:	
Medical/treatment plan(s):	

5. EYE AND SIGHT PROBLEMS

FENG SHUI INTERVENTIONS	
Corresponding gua(s)—augment and make all necessary repairs:	Fame
Interior and exterior factors to assess; solutions, cures, and adjustments:	Too much clutter (ch. 1, p. 34, ch. 4, pp. 113–18) Split-view entranceway (ch. 6, p. 172) Bathroom in Fame gua (ch. 6, p. 181) Boot-shaped floor plan (ch. 6, p. 185) Broken or dirty windows, or windows that don't work (ch. 6, p. 202) Attic disrepair (ch. 4, pages 116 and 119–22)
Adjustments to make/do/use:	Physically clean all windows yourself. Repair all broken glass. Keep Fame gua(s) free of clutter. Hang a 40-mm clear crystal in the Fame gua on a 9-inch red string. Add a 50-mm crystal on a nine-inch red string in the Center/Health gua in the bedroom.
Interior factors to eliminate/avoid:	Water elements in the Fame gua
Transcendental Cures/ Meditations:	Shedding the Golden Cicada (ch. 9, p. 304) Single Mirror Cure (ch. 9, p. 311)

CHAKRA INTERVENTIONS

Corresponding Chakra color(s):	Indigo (6th or Third Eye Center)
Supporting/complementary Chakra color(s):	Yellow (3rd or Will Center)
Supporting/parallel Chakra color(s):	Purple (7th or Crown Center)
Color-breathing exercise(s) (9 inhales/exhales each for 27 consecutive days)	Inhale Indigo from the 6th Chakra or Third Eye Center. Exhale Yellow from the 3rd Chakra or Will Center.

VIBRATIONAL MEDICINES

Sound/tone to use:	The Note A
Natural crystals to wear and carry:	Clear Quartz, Lapis Lazuli, Sodalite

continued

Pure essential oils to use:	Never use essential oils directly on the eyes. Chamomile, Fennel, Jasmine, Lemon, Rose

YOUR PERSONAL WORK

Daily affirmation (9 times each day for 27 consecutive days):	I am at peace with seeing all that is true.
Your own affirmation(s):	
Emotional underpinning(s):	
Spiritual opportunity, growth, and reason for contracting illness:	
Physical Challenge(s); care needed to take:	
Your medical/treatment plan(s):	

6. HEADACHES AND MIGRAINES

FENG SHUI INTERVENTIONS	
Corresponding gua(s)—augment and make all necessary repairs:	Helpful People Fame
Interior and exterior factors to assess; solutions, cures, and adjustments:	Fix all doors (ch. 1, p. 33) Clear all clutter (ch. 1, p. 34) Check types of clutter (ch. 4, pp. 113–16) Bedroom is over the garage (ch. 5, p. 159) Small-nosed floor plan (ch. 6, p. 188) Windows and skylights in good working order? (ch. 6, pp. 202–203) Problematic entranceway (ch. 6., pp. 169–74) "Bad bite" doors (ch. 6, pp. 198–99) Blocked doors, or doors that don't open—and at one time did (ch. 6, p. 201) Attic disrepair (ch. 4, pp. 116 and 119–22) Entranceways with contrary doors that open to the small of a room (ch. 6, p. 169)
Adjustments to make/do/use:	Water adjustments: fountains, fish tanks, all moving water. Wind chimes for metal clarity. Flutes on a diagonal over a headboard. Augmenting the Helpful People gua in general. Add a 50-mm crystal on a nine-inch red string in the Center/Health gua in the bedroom.
Interior factors to eliminate/avoid:	Clutter, especially in the attic. Any dirty or broken windowpanes, entranceways that pinch and constrict.
Transcendental Cures/ Meditations:	Sealing the Doors (ch. 9, p. 307) Golden Circada (ch. 9, p. 304) Single Mirror Cure (ch. 9, p. 311)

CHAKRA INTERVENTIONS	
Corresponding Chakra color(s):	Indigo (6th or Third Eye Center) Purple (7th or Crown Center)
Supporting/complementary Chakra color(s):	Yellow (3rd or Will Center) for 6th Chakra Green (4th or Heart Center) for 3rd Chakra
Supporting/parallel Chakra color(s):	Purple (7th or Crown Center) for 6th Chakra White Light (8th or Transpersonal Center) for 3rd Chakra

359

continued

Color-breathing exercise(s) (9 inhales/exhales each for 27 consecutive days):	Overall color breathing Inhale Purple through the 7th Chakra or Crown Center. Exhale Green through the 4th Chakra or Heart Center. Inhale Indigo (6th or Third Eye Center) and Exhale Yellow (3rd or Will Center) for 6th Chakra.

VIBRATIONAL MEDICINES

Sound/tone to use:	The Note A (6th Chakra) The Note E (3rd Chakra)
Natural crystals to wear and carry:	Amethyst, Aventurine, Clear Quartz, Lapis Lazuli, Sodalite
Pure essential oils to use:	Eucalyptus, Lavender, Marjoram, Roman Chamomile, Rosemary, Rosewood

YOUR PERSONAL WORK

Daily affirmation (9 times each day for 27 consecutive days):	There is order in chaos. I trust fully in the divine plan.
Your own affirmation(s):	
Emotional underpinning(s):	
Spiritual opportunity, growth, and reason for contracting illness:	
Physical Challenge(s); care needed to take:	
Your medical/treatment plan(s):	

7. HEART DISEASE

FENG SHUI INTERVENTIONS	
Corresponding gua(s)—augment and make all necessary repairs.	Relationship Fame
Interior and exterior factors to assess; solutions, cures, and adjustments:	Clear all clutter (ch. 1, p. 34) Check types of clutter (ch. 4, pp. 113 and 116) Clean all sewers, plumbing, air-conditioning ducts (ch. 1, p. 38) Long and narrow entranceways, foyers, and hallways (ch. 6, p. 171) Bedroom is at the end of a hallway (ch. 5, p. 156) Kitchen is the first room you see (ch. 6, p. 175) Small-nosed floor plan (ch. 6, pp. 187–88) Stove is immediately visible from the front door/bedroom (ch. 5, pp. 155 and ch. 6, pp. 191–94) Stove is in the Fame gua of the kitchen (ch. 6, pp. 193–94) Three doors in a row (ch. 6, p. 199) Spiral staircase is in the Center gua or Fame gua (ch. 6, p. 195)
Adjustments to make/do/use:	Wood- and green-related adjustments including plants. Add a 50-mm crystal on a nine-inch red string to the Center/Health gua in the bedroom.
Interior factors to eliminate/avoid:	Fireplaces and excessive red in the Fame and Health area. Three doors in a row.
Transcendental Cures/ Meditations:	The Great Sunshine Buddha (ch. 9, p. 306) The Medicine Buddha (Appendix A) The Six Ch'i Healing Sounds (ch. 10, p. 334) Single and Double Mirror Cure (ch. 9, pp. 311–12)

CHAKRA INTERVENTIONS	
Corresponding Chakra color(s):	Green (4th or Heart Center) Yellow (3rd or Will Center)
Supporting/complementary Chakra color(s):	Red (1st or Survival Center) for 4th Chakra Indigo (6th or Third Eye Center) for 3rd Chakra
Supporting/parallel Chakra color(s):	Light Blue (5th or Throat Center) for 4th Chakra Purple (7th or Crown Center) for 3rd Chakra

A MULTILEVEL APPROACH TO DISARMING 15 CHALLENGING ILLNESSES

Color-breathing exercise(s) (9 inhales/exhales each for 27 consecutive days):	Inhale Green through the 4th Chakra or Heart Center. Exhale Green through the 4th Chakra or Heart Center.

VIBRATIONAL MEDICINES

Sound/tone to use:	The Note F (4th Chakra) The Note E (3rd Chakra)
Natural crystals to wear and carry:	Emerald; Pink, Green, and Watermelon Tourmaline; Rhodochrosite
Pure essential oils to use:	Lavender, Marjoram, Neroli, Peppermint, Rose, Rosemary

YOUR PERSONAL WORK

Daily affirmation (9 times each day for 27 consecutive days):	I reconnect with the joy in life.
Your own affirmation(s):	
Emotional underpinning(s):	
Spiritual opportunity, growth, and reason for contracting illness:	
Physical challenge(s); care needed to take:	
Your medical/treatment plan(s):	

8. IMMUNE SYSTEM AND CIRCULATORY PROBLEMS

FENG SHUI INTERVENTIONS	
Corresponding gua(s)—augment and make all necessary repairs:	Health Center Fame Career Wealth
Interior and exterior factors to assess; solutions, cures, and adjustments:	Check all electrical items (ch. 1, pp. 35 and 37) Clear all sewers, plumbing, air-conditioning ducts (ch. 1, p. 38) Low lighting (ch. 1, p. 36, ch. 6, p. 203) Check stove location (ch. 6, p. 191) Take the "clutter challenge" (ch. 4, p. 113) Assess the Three Visceral Cavities (ch. 4, p. 121) Bed crosses bathroom/shares wall with bathroom (ch. 5, pp. 151–53) Bedroom in the basement or below the entranceway (ch. 5, p. 159) High EMFs (ch. 5, pp. 137 and 161)
Adjustments to make/do/use:	Add bright lights, color, and sound. Water elements, such as water fountains, fish tanks, and ponds, as long as the water is clear. Add a 50-mm crystal on a nine-inch red string to the Center/Health gua in the bedroom.
Interior factors to eliminate/avoid:	Stagnant water. Make sure all the plumbing in the house is in good working order. Check for proper air flow. Remove clutter, fix jammed windows, and check all door functioning. Large furniture, blocking ch'i flow.
Transcendental Cures/ Meditations:	The Great Sunshine Buddha (ch. 9, p. 306) The Medicine Buddha (Appendix A) The Six Ch'i Healing Sounds (ch. 10, p. 334)
CHAKRA INTERVENTIONS	
Corresponding Chakra color(s):	Red (1st or Survival Center) Purple (7th or Crown Center) White (8th or Transpersonal Center)

continued 363

Supporting/complementary Chakra color(s):	Green (4th or Heart Center) use for 7th Chakra and for 1st Chakra. There is no complementary color for the 8th Chakra; reinforce it with itself.
Supporting/parallel Chakra color(s):	Light Blue (5th or Throat Center) for 1st Chakra White (8th or Transpersonal Center) for 7th Chakra Green (4th or Heart Center) for 8th Chakra
Color-breathing exercise(s) (9 inhales/exhales each for 27 consecutive days):	Overall color breathing for the 8th Chakra or Transpersonal Center Inhale Red through the 1st Chakra or Survival Center. Exhale Green from the Heart Center or 1st Chakra. Inhale Purple through the 7th Chakra or Crown Center. Exhale Green through the 4th Chakra or Heart Center or the 7th Chakra or Crown Center.

VIBRATIONAL MEDICINES

Sound/tone to use:	The Note F (for the 7th Chakra) The Note High C for the 8th Chakra
Natural crystals to wear and carry:	Emerald, Garnet, Hematite, Pyrite
Pure essential oils to use:	Cinnamon, Eucalyptus, Frankincense, Geranium, Lemon, Rosemary, Rosewood, Tea Tree, Vetiver

YOUR PERSONAL WORK

Daily affirmation (9 times each day for 27 consecutive days):	I am safe and immune to all hurts, angers, fear, and resentments of the past.
Your own affirmation(s):	
Emotional underpinning(s):	
Spiritual opportunity, growth, and reason for contracting illness:	
Physical challenge(s); care needed to take:	
Your medical/treatment plan(s):	

9. INSOMNIA

FENG SHUI INTERVENTIONS	
Corresponding gua(s)—augment and make all necessary repairs:	Center Career Wealth Family Helpful People
Interior and exterior factors to assess; solutions, cures, and adjustments:	Bedroom door is directly opposite the bathroom door (ch. 5, pp. 150–53) Bedroom is over a garage (ch. 5, p. 159)
Adjustments to make/do/use:	Clean the attic/basement. Check EMF levels in the bedroom. Remove all clock radios or TVs from the bedroom. Check door/window alignment. Add a 50-mm crystal on a nine-inch red string to the Center/Health gua in the bedroom.
Interior factors to eliminate/avoid:	Working in the bedroom; a bed that doesn't have a headboard or is not firmly up against a solid wall; sharing a bedroom wall with a kitchen or bathroom. Too many bright colors, especially red.
Transcendental Cures/ Meditations:	Orange Peel Cure (ch. 2, p. 61) Blessed Rice Cure (ch. 9, p. 309) 3 Bamboo Flutes (ch. 9, p. 311) Single Mirror Cure (ch. 9, p. 311)

CHAKRA INTERVENTIONS	
Corresponding Chakra color(s):	Orange (2nd or Social Center) Yellow (3rd or Will Center) Green (4th or Heart Center) Indigo (6th or Third Eye Center)
Supporting/complementary Chakra color(s):	Light Blue (5th or Throat Center) for 2nd Chakra Indigo (6th or Crown Center) for 3rd Chakra Purple (7th or Crown Center) for 4th Chakra Yellow (3rd or Will Center) for 7th Chakra
Supporting/parallel Chakra color(s):	Indigo (6th or Third Eye Center) for 5th Chakra Purple (7th or Crown Center) for 3rd Chakra White (8th or Transpersonal Center) for 4th Chakra Purple (or Crown Center) for 7th Chakra

continued

Color-breathing exercise(s) (9 inhales/exhales each for 27 consecutive days):	Overall color breathing Inhale Orange through the 2nd Chakra or Social Center. Exhale Light Blue through the 5th Chakra or Throat Center; Inhale Yellow through the 3rd Chakra or Will Center; Exhale Purple through the 7th Chakra or Crown Center. Inhale Green through the 4th Chakra or Heart Center and exhale Green through the 7th Chakra or Heart Center. Inhale White Light through the 8th Chakra or Transpersonal Center and exhale White Light through every Chakra.

VIBRATIONAL MEDICINES

Sound/tone to use:	The Note D (2nd Chakra) The Note E (3rd Chakra) The Note F (4th Chakra) The Note B (7th Chakra)
Natural crystals to wear and carry:	Amethyst, Emerald, Carmelian, Tourmaline in Quartz
Pure essential oils to use:	Blood Orange, Lavender, Marjoram, Neroli, Sandalwood

YOUR PERSONAL WORK

Daily affirmation (9 times each day for 27 consecutive days):	My body safely lets go and I rest comfortably as I am watched over at all times by loving angel guides.
Your own affirmation(s):	
Emotional underpinning(s):	
Spiritual opportunity, growth, and reason for contracting illness:	
Physical challenge(s); care needed to take:	
Your medical/treatment plan(s):	

10. LOW ENERGY

FENG SHUI INTERVENTIONS	
Corresponding gua(s)—augment and make all necessary repairs.	Family Career Center Wealth
Interior and exterior factors to assess; solutions, cures, and adjustments:	Repair all leaks (ch. 1, p. 32) Check electrical systems (ch. 1, p. 35) Take the "clutter challenge" (ch. 4, p. 113) Check types of clutter (ch. 4, p. 116) Bedroom door opens to small of the room (ch. 5, p. 155) Bedroom is over the garage (ch. 5, p. 159)
Adjustments to make/do/use:	Increase lighting and wattage, plants, and life force, and use bright colors and wind chimes. Add brass wind chimes over front door. Add a 50-mm crystal on a nine-inch red string in the Center/Health gua in the bedroom. Play stimulating music.
Interior factors to eliminate/avoid:	No colors, dark colors, mirrors that cut off a view of the head, towering furniture, especially in the bedroom.
Transcendental Cures/ Meditations:	The Great Sunshine Buddha (ch. 9, p. 306) The Orange Peel Cure (ch. 2, p. 61) 3 Bamboo Flute Cure (ch. 9, pp. 310–11)

CHAKRA INTERVENTIONS	
Corresponding Chakra color(s):	Yellow (3rd or Will Center) Orange (2nd or Social Center) Red (1st or Survival Center)
Supporting/complementary Chakra color(s):	Indigo (6th or Third Eye) for 3rd Chakra Light Blue (5th or Throat Center) for 2nd Chakra Green (4th or Heart Center) for 1st Chakra
Supporting/parallel Chakra color(s):	Purple (6th or Third Eye) for 3rd Chakra Indigo (6th or Third Eye) for 2nd Center Light Blue (5th or Throat Center) for 1st Chakra

continued

Color-breathing exercise(s) (9 inhales/exhales each for 27 consecutive days):	Overall color breathing Inhale Yellow through the 3rd Chakra or Will Center. Exhale Yellow Through the 3rd Chakra or Will Center. Inhale Orange through the 2nd Chakra or Social Center. Exhale Light Blue through the 5th Chakra or Throat Center.

VIBRATIONAL MEDICINES

Sound/tone to use:	The Note E (3rd Chakra) The Note D (2nd Chakra) The Note C (1st Chakra)
Natural crystals to wear and carry:	Carnelian, Clear Quartz, Aquamarine
Pure essential oils to use:	Bergamot, Cinnamon, Eucalyptus, Peppermint, Rosemary, Rosewood

YOUR PERSONAL WORK

Daily affirmation (9 times each day for 27 consecutive days):	I experience great joy in being present in my life every day.
Your own affirmation(s):	
Emotional underpinning(s):	
Spiritual opportunity, growth, and reason for contracting illness:	
Physical challenge(s); care needed to take:	
Your medical/treatment plan(s):	

11. REPRODUCTIVE, PREGNANCY, AND MENOPAUSAL ISSUES

FENG SHUI INTERVENTIONS	
Corresponding gua(s)—augment and make all necessary repairs:	Family Relationship Center Children
Interior and exterior factors to assess; solutions, cures, and **adjustments:**	Clear all clutter (ch. 1, p. 34) Kitchen/bathroom in center of house (ch. 6, p. 177) Check electrical systems (ch. 1, p. 35) Clean all sewers, plumbing, and air-conditioning units (ch. 1, p. 38) Remove all EMFs from bedroom (ch. 1, p. 37, ch. 5, pp. 137 and 161) Check for long, narrow entranceways, foyers, and hallways (ch. 6, p. 171) Mandarin duck stairs (ch. 6, p. 195) Check for all types of clutter (ch. 4, p. 113) Bedroom door opens to the small of the room (ch. 5, p. 155) Bed crosses door (ch. 5, p. 161, ch. 6, pp. 191–92) Bedroom is at the end of a long hallway (ch. 5, p. 156) Headboard on bathroom/kitchen wall (ch. 5, pp.150–55) Bathroom is at the end of a hallway (ch. 6, p. 182) L-shaped floor plan (ch. 6, p. 183) Small-nosed floor plan (ch. 6, p. 188)
Adjustments to make/do/use:	Increase lighting in bedroom. Clear entranceways; check bed positioning; for pregnancies, keep the environment stable. Add nine stalks of bamboo to the Children area of the bedroom. Add a brass wind chime to the entranceway to the house. Add a 50-mm crystal on a nine-inch red string to the Center/Health gua in the bedroom.
Interior factors to eliminate/avoid:	Avoid construction in the home, clutter under the bed, and sweeping under the bed during pregnancies and trying to conceive.
Transcendental Cures/ Meditations:	The Great Sunshine Buddha (ch. 9, p. 306) The Shedding of the Golden Cicada (ch. 9, p. 304) Orange Peel Cure (ch. 2, p. 61)

continued

CHAKRA INTERVENTIONS

Corresponding Chakra color(s):	Red (1st or Survival Center); Orange (2nd or Social Center)
Supporting/complementary Chakra color(s):	Green (4th or Heart Center) for 1st Chakra Light Blue (5th or Throat Center) for 2nd Chakra
Supporting/parallel Chakra color(s):	Light Blue (5th or Throat Center) for 1st Chakra Indigo (6th or Third Eye Center) for 2nd Chakra
Color-breathing exercise(s) (9 inhales/exhales each for 27 consecutive days):	Inhale Red into the 1st Chakra or Survival Center. Exhale Orange from the 2nd Chakra or Social Center. Overall color breathing. Inhale Orange from the 2nd Chakra or Social Center. Exhale Orange from the 2nd Chakra or Social Center.

VIBRATIONAL MEDICINES

Sound/tone to use:	The Note C (1st Chakra) The Note D (2nd Chakra)
Natural crystals to wear and carry:	Carnelian, Citrine, Smoky Quartz, Pink Tourmaline
Pure essential oils to use:	Bergamot, Fennel, Geranium, Jasmine, Marjoram, Roman Chamomile, Rose, Rosemary, Ylang-ylang

YOUR PERSONAL WORK

Daily affirmation (9 times each day for 27 consecutive days):	My body resonates to divine timing and is always in sync with nature and cocreates with God's higher plan.
Client's own affirmation(s):	
Emotional underpinning(s):	
Spiritual opportunity, growth, and reason for contracting illness:	
Physical challenge(s); care needed to take:	
Your medical/treatment plan(s):	

12. RESPIRATORY PROBLEMS

FENG SHUI INTERVENTIONS	
Corresponding gua(s)—augment and make all necessary repairs:	Children Center/Health Relationship
Interior and exterior factors to assess; solutions, cures, and adjustments:	Front-door blockages; small entranceways, small waiting areas (ch. 6, pp. 169–74) Clear all clutter (ch. 1, p. 34) Take the "clutter challenge" (ch. 4, p. 113) Assess types of clutter (ch. 4, p. 116) Repair all leaks (ch. 1, p. 32) Bedroom door opens to the small of the room (ch. 5, p. 155) Check for long and narrow entranceways, foyers, and hallways (ch. 6, p. 172) Check for split-view/brick wall entranceways (ch. 6, pp. 172–73) Small-nosed floor plan (ch. 6, p. 188) Doors that are locked or broken, or that open out instead of in (ch. 1, p. 33; ch. 6, p. 170) Trees or foliage that block ch'i (ch. 1, p. 27)
Adjustments to make/do/use:	Wind chimes to keep energy moving. Increase lighting. Put mirrors in the Relationship and Children guas. Add a 50-mm crystal on a red string to the Center/Health gua in the bedroom.
Interior factors to eliminate/avoid:	Clutter in entranceways; doors that are jammed; three doors in a row.
Transcendental Cures/ Meditations:	Rice Blessing (ch. 9, p. 309) Six Ch'i Healing Sounds Meditation (ch. 10, p. 334); Double Mirror/Bamboo Pen Holder (ch. 9, p. 312)
CHAKRA INTERVENTIONS	
Corresponding Chakra color(s):	Green (4th or Heart Center) Light Blue (5th or Throat Center)
Supporting/complementary Chakra color(s):	Purple (7th or Crown Center) for 4th Chakra Orange (2nd or Social Center) for 5th Chakra
Supporting/parallel Chakra color(s):	White (8th or Transpersonal Center) for 4th Chakra Indigo (6th or Third Eye Center) for 5th Chakra

continued

| Color-breathing exercise(s) (9 inhales/exhales each for 27 consecutive days): | Inhale Green through the 4th Chakra or Heart Center. Exhale Green out the 4th Chakra or Heart Center. Inhale Yellow through the 3rd Chakra or Will Center. Exhale Green out the 4th Chakra or Heart Center. |

VIBRATIONAL MEDICINES

Sound/tone to use:	The Note F (4th Chakra) The Note G (5th Chakra)
Natural crystals to wear and carry:	Botswana Agate, Garnet, Green Tourmaline, Rose Quartz
Pure essential oils to use:	Eucalyptus, Fennel, Frankincense, Lavender, Lemon, Rosemary, Tea Tree

YOUR PERSONAL WORK

Daily affirmation (9 times each day for 27 consecutive days):	My breath is in perfect timing with the universe and my life's path.
Your own affirmation(s):	
Emotional underpinning(s):	
Spiritual opportunity, growth, and reasons for contracting illness:	
Physical challenge(s); care needed to take:	
Your medical/treatment plan(s):	

13. STOMACH AND INTESTINAL PROBLEMS

FENG SHUI INTERVENTIONS	
Corresponding gua(s)—augment and make all necessary repairs:	Career Center/Health Wealth Relationship
Interior and exterior factors to assess; solutions, cures, and adjustments:	Repair all leaks, particularly for diarrhea and bleeding illnesses (ch. 1, p. 32) Illuminate all dark areas (ch. 1, p. 36, ch. 6, p. 173) Clean all sewers, plumbing, air-conditioning units (ch. 1, p. 38) Assess for three doors in a row (ch. 6, p. 199) Assess the Three Visceral Cavities (ch. 4, p. 121) Bathrooms inside bedrooms (ch. 5, pp. 150–51) Bathroom is the first room you see (ch. 6, p. 175) Kitchen is the first room you see (ch. 6, p. 175)
Adjustments to make/do/use:	Wind chimes, plumbing that is in need of repair. Create hallways and foyers that are open, lit, and colorfully painted. Add a 50-mm crystal on a nine-inch red string to the Center/Health gua in the bedroom.
Interior factors to eliminate/avoid:	Excessive ch'i force, seeing the kitchen upon entering the house, bad stove positioning, kitchen/bathroom in center of the house.
Transcendental Cures/ Meditations:	The Medicine Buddha (Appendix A) The Six Ch'i Healing Sounds Meditation (ch. 10, p. 334) The Great Sunshine Buddha Meditation (ch. 95, p. 306)
CHAKRA INTERVENTIONS	
Corresponding Chakra color(s):	Yellow (3rd or Will Center) Green (4th or Relationship Center)
Supporting/complementary Chakra color(s):	Indigo (6th or Third Eye Center) Red (1st or Survival Center)
Supporting/parallel Chakra color(s):	Purple (7th or Crown Center) Light Blue (5th or Throat Center)

continued

Color-breathing exercise (9 inhales/exhales each for 27 consecutive days):	Inhale Yellow through the 3rd Chakra or Will Center. Exhale Yellow out the 3rd Chakra or Will Center. Inhale Yellow through the 3rd Chakra or Will Center. Exhale Green out the 4th Chakra or Heart Center. Inhale Green through the 4th Chakra or Heart Center. Exhale Red through the 1st Chakra or Survival Center.

VIBRATIONAL MEDICINES

Sound/tone to use:	The Note E
Natural crystals to wear and carry:	Citrine, Malachite, Pyrite
Pure essential oils to use:	Nausea/Vomiting: Fennel, Peppermint Indigestion: Blood Orange, Fennel, Marjoram, Peppermint Constipation: Blood Orange, Fennel, Marjoram

YOUR PERSONAL WORK (PLEASE FILL IN)

Daily affirmation:	I let go of my control and fear, and release myself to trusting in the process of life.
Your own affirmation(s):	
Emotional underpinning(s):	
Spiritual opportunity, and reason for contracting illness:	
Physical Challenge(s); care needed to take:	
Your medical/treatment plan(s):	

14. TEETH, GUMS, AND TMJ

FENG SHUI INTERVENTIONS	
Corresponding gua(s)—augment and make all necessary repairs:	Children
Interior and exterior factors to assess; solutions, cures, and adjustments:	Bad bite doors (ch. 6, p. 198) Entranceways with no physical door (ch. 6, p. 201) Split-view entranceways (ch. 6, p. 172) Brick-wall entranceways (ch. 6, p. 173)
Adjustments to make/do/use:	Pictures with depth of field; mirrors to offset bad-bite doors; wind chimes in the Children gua; entranceways kept clear of clutter; fix water leaks or problems in children's gua. Adjust Helpful People gua. Add a 50-mm crystal to a nine-inch red string in the Center/Health gua in the bedroom.
Interior factors to eliminate/avoid:	Hinges that don't work, bad-bite doors, split-view entranceways, doors that do not work properly
Transcendental Cures/ Meditations:	Sealing the Doors (ch. 9, p. 307) Shedding the Golden Cicada (ch. 9, p. 304) The Great Sunshine Buddha Meditation (ch. 9, p. 306)

CHAKRA INTERVENTIONS	
Corresponding Chakra color(s):	Light Blue (5th or Throat Center)
Supporting/complementary Chakra color(s):	Orange (2nd or Social Center)
Supporting/parallel Chakra color(s):	Indigo (6th or Third Eye Center)
Color-breathing exercise (9 inhales/exhales each for 27 consecutive days):	Inhale Light Blue through the 5th Chakra or Throat Center. Exhale Light Blue out the 5th Chakra or Throat Center. Inhale Light Blue through the 5th Chakra or Throat Center. Exhale Green out the 4th Chakra or Heart Center.

continued

VIBRATIONAL MEDICINES

Sound/tone to use:	The Note G (5th Chakra)
Natural crystals to wear or carry:	Aquamarine, Blue Tourmaline
Pure essential oils to use:	Bergamot, Fennel, Geranium, Neroli, Tea Tree

YOUR PERSONAL WORK

Daily affirmation (9 times each day for 27 consecutive days):	I make all the right decisions for myself with effortless ease.
Your own affirmation(s):	
Emotional underpinning(s):	
Spiritual opportunity, growth, and reason for contracting illness:	
Physical challenge(s); care needed to take:	
Your medical/treatment plan(s):	

15. URINARY TRACT PROBLEMS

FENG SHUI INTERVENTIONS	
Corresponding gua(s)—augment and make necessary repairs:	Family Relationship Center Career
Interior and exterior factors to assess; solutions, cures, and adjustments:	Check types of clutter (ch. 4, p. 116) Assess the Three Visceral Cavities (ch. 4, p. 121) Bathroom inside the bedroom (ch. 5, pp. 150–51) Repair all leaks (ch. 1, p. 32) Bedroom door is directly opposite the bathroom door (ch. 5, p. 152) Check for three doors in a row (ch. 6, p. 199) Bathroom is the first room you see (ch. 6, p. 175) Kitchen contains a bathroom (ch. 6, p. 178) Bathroom is at the end of a long hallway (ch. 6, p. 182) Too many doors in the same area (ch. 6, p. 199)
Adjustments to make/do/use:	Light and crystal adjustments, especially in the Family gua. Add a 50-mm crystal on a nine-inch red string in the Center/Health gua in the bedroom.
Interior factors to eliminate/avoid:	Water-related problems in the bathroom
Transcendental Cures/ Meditations:	Shedding the Golden Cicada (ch. 9, p. 304) The Great Buddhan Meditation (ch. 9, p. 306)

CHAKRA INTERVENTIONS	
Corresponding Chakra color(s):	Orange (2nd or Social Center) Yellow (3rd or Will Center)
Supporting/complementary Chakra color(s):	Light Blue (5th or Throat Center) for 2nd Chakra Indigo (6th or Third Eye Center) for 3rd Chakra
Supporting/parallel Chakra color(s):	Indigo (6th or Third Eye Center) for 2nd Chakra Purple (7th or Crown Center) for 3rd Chakra

continued

Color-breathing exercise (9 inhales/exhales each for 27 consecutive days):	Inhale Orange through the 2nd Chakra or Social Center. Exhale Light Blue out the 5th Chakra or Throat Center. Inhale Yellow through the 3rd Chakra or Will Center. Exhale Green through the 4th Chakra or Heart Center.

VIBRATIONAL MEDICINES

Sound/tone to use:	The Note D (2nd Chakra) The Note C (1st Chakra)
Natural crystals to wear or carry:	Citrine, Garnet
Pure essential oils to use:	Bergamot, Cedarwood, Chamomile, Frankincense, Lavender, Sandalwood, Tea Tree

YOUR PERSONAL WORK

Daily affirmation (9 times each day for 27 consecutive days):	I deal with my anger directly, and release all real or perceived injustices from my body and energy field.
Your own affirmation(s):	
Emotional underpinning(s):	
Spiritual opportunity, growth, and reason for contracting Illness:	
Physical challenge(s); care needed to take:	
Your medical/treatment plan(s):	

CHAPTER CLOSING EXERCISE

Below you will find a blank worksheet for your use in analyzing any other illnesses that weren't directly addressed in the 15 Challenging Illnesses Charts. Let it help assist you with creating a game plan, and a treatment structure for you to do your personal healing work.

ILLNESS CHART WORKSHEET

FENG SHUI INTERVENTIONS
Corresponding gua(s)—augment and make all necessary repairs:
Interior and exterior factors to assess; solutions, cures, and adjustments:
Adjustments to make/do/use:
Interior factors to eliminate/avoid:
Transcendental Cures/Meditations:
CHAKRA INTERVENTIONS
Corresponding Chakra color(s):
Supporting/complementary Chakra color(s):
Supporting/parallel Chakra color(s):
Color-breathing exercise (9 inhales/exhales each for 27 consecutive days):

continued

VIBRATIONAL MEDICINES

Sound/tone to use:

Natural crystals to wear or carry:

Pure essential oils to use:

YOUR PERSONAL WORK

Daily affirmation (9 times each day for 27 consecutive days):

Your own affirmation(s):

Emotional underpinning:

Spiritual opportunity, growth, and reason for contracting illness:

Physical challenge(s); care needed to take:

Your medical/treatment plan(s):

DIVINE INTERVENTIONS

Clients' Stories in Their Own Words

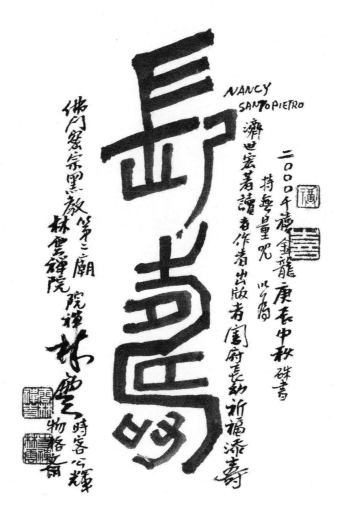

"Longevity."

CALLIGRAPHY BY H. H. PROFESSOR THOMAS LIN YUN RINPOCHE

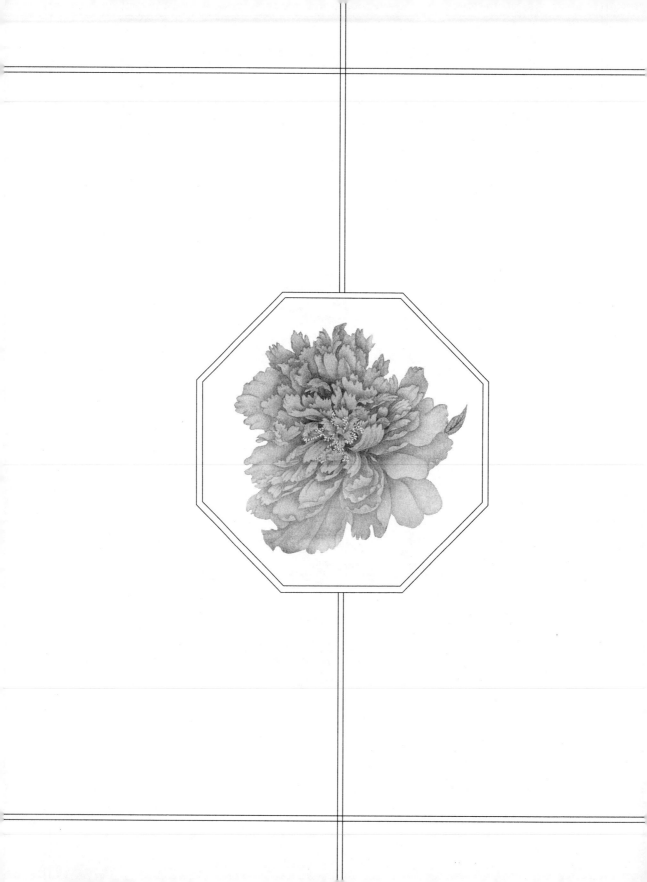

THIS PART OF THE BOOK is very precious to me, and I hope it will become just as important to you. The clients in this chapter *and* throughout this book have selflessly shared their lives, pains, disappointments, and joys to help you learn more about Feng Shui, healing, and the commonalities that we will all encounter. Our lives, our homes, and the everyday things we have to face while on this planet are very private and very close to our hearts. They have been gracious enough to take the time out of their very busy lives to assist me in this last chapter of my book, contributing both their stories, in their own words, and the floor plans of their homes. Understanding the importance of doing service for the higher good of all, from both a spiritual and practical perspective, they have given of themselves so that others can benefit. I thank them, honor them, and, with gratitude, bless their lives and all their generous efforts.

Each of the four stories shared here is an authentic slice of someone's real life. I've chosen these stories because they epitomize strength, courage, and the willingness to show up for life, even in the face of adversity. The only thing that has been changed, outside of some basic editing, is their names, in order to protect their anonymity.

"Fall down seven times, get up eight."

— BUDDHIST PROVERB

THE KITCHEN: A METAPHOR FOR CONSTRUCTING A FAMILY

Dawn and Michael's Story

My husband, Michael, and I moved into our apartment about four and a half years ago. We wanted to make some changes, and eventually it was time to redesign our kitchen. This coincided with our decision to have a baby and start a family. It was a lot to take on at once. In fact, we can remember telling the person we hired to do the kitchen that we might actually have to put this project off. Thinking about the new kitchen was fun at first, and we both got caught up in the excitement. But somewhere along the line, something changed. Michael and I were having trouble conceiving, and began consulting some fertility experts, which was stressful. The person in charge of the kitchen renovation seemed increasingly erratic, and the estimated costs kept mounting. So it didn't seem so much fun anymore. Something was definitely going on. The woman who worked with us in helping our cat deal with an aggression problem suggested that we call Nancy SantoPietro, who did Feng Shui. At first we kept losing her number or forgetting to call. But one day we went out and bought several books about Feng Shui so that we could educate ourselves about it. Once we knew more about the subject, we felt comfortable calling and made an appointment.

When Nancy arrived, she wanted to know what was going on in our lives. Michael and I told her that we were trying to have a baby, and that we were also in the midst of renovating our kitchen. She picked up on a lot of things, including the stress in the house. Then she suggested to us a number of changes that ranged from how to place our furniture to ways of assisting the energy to flow better. Those suggestions helped shift the energy of the entire house. We opened up the entranceway to the apartment, which she said should be clear, because it functioned like a birth canal. We moved some furniture, hung up some crystals, and put some bamboo stalks in various rooms to increase the ch'i.

She also made some specific suggestions and recommended various cures to help us conceive. She wanted us to try making love in different parts of the apartment. She also suggested that we replace the picture behind our bed with one that was more playful and childlike. We adjusted the Family area in our bedroom and created several different altars throughout the house, including one in the baby's room and one in our bedroom. Finally, she had us both take a small circle of paper, write down what we wanted to happen, and put it under the mattress where we slept.

We were impressed with Nancy, and it just seemed natural that she and the kitchen designer should work together, so we set up a meeting. To say it didn't go well was an understatement. Something about the energy exchange between Nancy and the designer made me see him in a new way. He was arrogant and rude, and suddenly some unpleasant personal details began to surface. Still, he had spent a lot of time on the plans and we felt a certain obligation to continue working with him. Over the next several weeks, Michael and I wrestled with what to do.

Finally, the day we were supposed to sign the contract, everything fell apart. It became clear that we needed to take a stand and stop thinking about his needs and start thinking about our own. We needed our house free from all the stress this renovation was creating. There was a major shift when we let the project go. A sense of harmony returned to the apartment. And here's the amazing thing. We were supposed to start the actual renovation in March, and that was when I got pregnant! And something else happened that was also pretty amazing: the bamboo stalks that we placed in the room we were planning to make the baby's room hadn't been doing well. The roots weren't coming in—and some of the bamboo eventually died and had to be replaced. But the minute we decided to put off the renovation, the bamboo stalks took root! We're so grateful, now, that we didn't go ahead with the whole project. We're convinced that having to work together to reach this decision brought us closer and enabled us to conceive, and we know that Feng Shui played a significant role. Having gone through this experience, we are much more aware of energy and how it can affect our lives. When people visit our home, they often say how comfortable it is and how peaceful it seems. This is very pleasing to us.

In December 2000, I gave birth at home to a healthy, beautiful boy. He came into the world in a room that was energetically cleared and surrounded by music and welcoming rose quartz crystals.

Now our goal is to put some final touches on the apartment, in addition to creating a special environment for him that has harmony and balance, and brings with it a lifetime of safety and happiness.

Dawn and Michael's Situation: An Overview

When Dawn called me for a consultation, her original request was that she wanted a consultation because they were ready to begin designing and renovating their kitchen, and wanted my input from a Feng Shui perspective. Shortly into my first meeting with them, Dawn shared with me that they were thinking about having a baby and had been trying to conceive, but hadn't been able to. I checked their floor plan and discovered that their kitchen was located in the Family gua and also partly in the Health gua. That overlap, I quickly realized, was no coincidence; somehow the kitchen was directly tied in to her difficulty with getting pregnant and starting a family. My first instinct as a trained consultant was to recommend that she either delay the kitchen renovations or put off trying to get pregnant; in Black Hat Feng Shui we believe that the stability of the external environment plays a very important role in the ability of a couple not only to conceive, but to maintain a healthy pregnancy throughout the full term.

When any type of renovation or construction is performed in a home, we view that structural change as a form of surgery: just as the house mirrors our life, it also mirrors our body and our health. If every area of the Feng Shui in your home oversees a different area of your body, then wherever the construction is taking place, that corresponding area of the body is having surgery by proxy. Because Dawn wasn't pregnant at the time of my first consultation, I took the opportunity to present to Dawn and Michael the possibility of postponing the renovations until after the baby arrived. They both were pretty set on moving forward with the changes, and were very excited about the proposed designs that the designer created for them. I never felt completely comfortable with their decision, but I agreed to support them and work with them no matter what their final decision was. I was concerned that, given her age (she was in her early forties) and how important this pregnancy was to them, if she did get pregnant while the construction was under way, we would be putting her health and the pregnancy at risk. I enjoyed working with this couple so much that my job then moved beyond a preventive approach to pulling out all the Feng Shui stops, mundane and transcendental, to trying to stabilize the environment—and Dawn and Michael—as much as I could if both things should occur at once. As I started to discuss with Dawn the importance of her kitchen and some of the early memories that she held regarding being in her kitchen, she shared with me some of her deep memories regarding her mother's alcoholism, and some of the traumatic events resulting from her drinking that occurred in the kitchen. With the kitchen overseeing the Family gua, as she entered into the process of changing it and making it more practical and accessible, some of these old memories had to surface if a healing were to occur. Every few weeks Dawn would have a mini-session with me, in which she would update me on the status of the design process. After each of these meetings something would transpire that Dawn would have to assert herself to address. The designer's creative rigidity and recreational drug use provided the catalyst for both Dawn and Michael to reconsider whether he was actually the right person for the job. His talent wasn't in question; this was behind-the-scenes energy that the couple chose not to imbue into the structure of their home, especially as they started to understand the metaphor of the kitchen in their lives. After the budget for the kitchen kept going up and several other problems occurred, they made the bold and courageous decision to stop the renovations and the whole kitchen project for a while. Shortly after they worked through all the realizations, confrontations, and decisions and let go of the project, Dawn became pregnant! The kitchen and the designer served as divine intervention, allowing them as a couple to parent the project and work through fears and decisions they would have to deal with as new parents.

How We Adjusted the Feng Shui of Dawn and Michael's House

One of the main issues Dawn discussed with me in our first session was her inability to focus while in her house. She often felt scattered and unable to complete tasks that she started. Papers would get lost (as my phone number did) and certain areas would become cluttered. So I immediately looked around at her sight line, to see what was in her peripheral view. I first recommended that all the obvious and visible clutter be reorganized and reduced. Her bedroom had two dressers facing the bed, and a smaller table

Fig. 41. Before Adjustments, Floor Plan of Dawn and Michael's Home

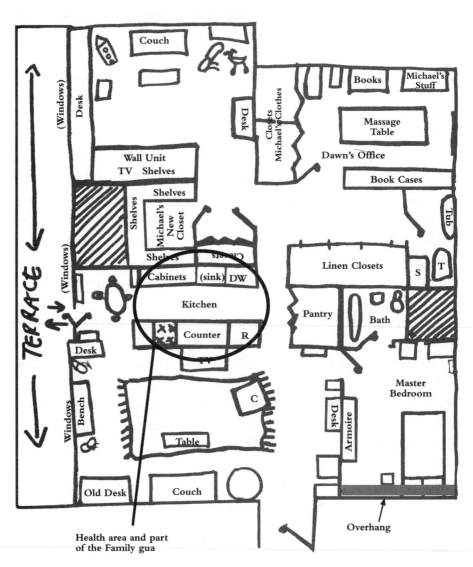

Health area and part of the Family gua

Fig. 42. Dawn and Michael's Home After Adjustments

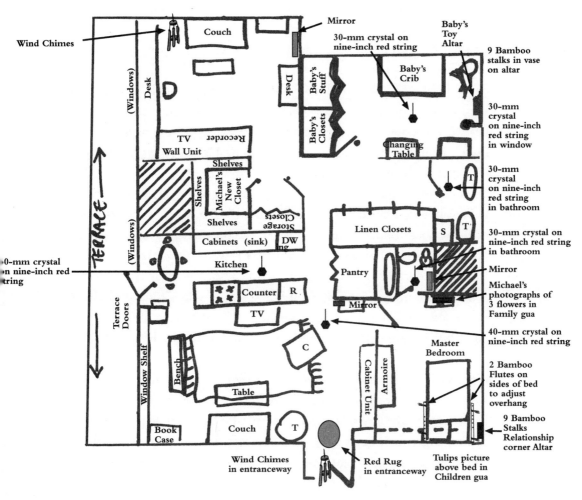

Wind Chimes

Couch

Mirror

30-mm crystal on nine-inch red string

Baby's Toy Altar

9 Bamboo stalks in vase on altar

(Windows)

Desk

Desk

Baby's Stuff

Baby's Crib

30-mm crystal on nine-inch red string in window

TV Wall Unit

Recorder

Baby's Closets

Changing Table

30-mm crystal on nine-inch red string in bathroom

Shelves

Shelves

Michael's New Closet

Shelves

Storage Closets

Linen Closets

S

T

30-mm crystal on nine-inch red string in bathroom

Cabinets (sink)

DW ing

TERRACE

(Windows)

Pantry

Mirror

30-mm crystal on nine-inch red string

Kitchen

Michael's photographs of 3 flowers in Family gua

Counter

R

40-mm crystal on nine-inch red string

TV

Mirror

Terrace Doors

C

Master Bedroom

Window Shelf

Bench

Table

Cabinet Unit

Armoire

2 Bamboo Flutes on sides of bed to adjust overhang

9 Bamboo Stalks Relationship corner Altar

Book Case

Couch

T

Wind Chimes in entranceway

Red Rug in entranceway

Tulips picture above bed in Children gua

that held a VCR and a television. One of the dressers, which had been her mother's, was in the Children section of her overall floor plan. The various furniture pieces were not balanced and were out of order in terms of size, thus creating visual clutter. This pattern was repeated in many of the rooms, especially the room in which Dawn conducted her bodywork practice, and which would eventually become the baby's. The furniture and cabinets were of different sizes and colors; although aesthetically they all worked together, energetically they were causing visual chaos. The energetic patterns reflected some of the confusion around Dawn's pregnancy, and how it would affect her work life and their marriage if a baby came into the picture. Her work space (the baby's room) was in the Relationship gua of the overall apartment. This gua also oversees all mother-related issues.

I suggested that Dawn move some pieces around and also reorganize all the bookcases. The energy patterns were moving in every direction because of the way the books were arranged in the bookcases, with all their various shapes and sizes. This chaos exacerbated Dawn's attention deficit disorder, frustrating her and adding additional and unnecessary stress to her life. In addition, we hung a 50-mm Feng Shui crystal in the center of the room, in the Health area, and created an altar in the Children area of the room, made up of live bamboo plants and nine toys she had around the house. This altar was significant, because it was in creating it that she decided to make the room in her life, work, and relationship for that baby to enter. The hardwood floor in her dining room (the Family area) was replaced, which helped Dawn and Michael to rebuild and restructure their whole foundation. With each change, their life was shifting, and unbeknownst to them, they were working out the pieces that needed to be released through the Feng Shui process, in order for their baby to enter.

In their bedroom, we moved out a litter box that was in the Wealth area and a coat rack in the Relationship area that her brother made when he was a child. We replaced the coat rack with a Relationship altar that eventually housed nine live stalks of bamboo. We added a 40-mm crystal in the center Health area of the room and attached two bamboo flutes, one on either side of the bed's headboard, offsetting the slight overhead beam that extended several inches over their heads. They cleared the metal cases out from under the bed so that the *ling* particles (baby ch'i) that bring life could have access to them while they were trying to conceive. In addition, I recommended no sweeping under the bed during the process of trying to conceive, and I suggested to them a specific pregnancy cure that entailed writing on a circular piece of red paper certain information and placing it under their mattress in their bedroom. The last, but equally important, adjustment in their bedroom was for them to place a picture in the Children section of their bedroom that would represent fertility. Michael is an accomplished photographer, and together they picked out several of his photographs for both the Family section of the bedroom and the Children section, which was located directly on the wall behind their headboard. For the Children section they chose a photograph of a beautiful field of yellow tulips, bursting with light and life force. Behind the picture we placed small mirrors to further open the Children gua, and a beautiful pregnancy ensued. Nine months later, Dawn gave birth at home to a beautiful and healthy baby boy. We welcome him to this world with much love and joy.

AUTISM: A FAMILY'S STORY OF HOPE, COURAGE, AND INSPIRATION

Jane, Mitch, and Mira's Story

This story is one that does not have an ending yet. Feng Shui and its healing benefits have only recently come into our lives. There are things that still need to be worked out, furniture to be moved around, and hopes to be visualized. There are many deep wounds that will eventually have to heal, and sadness that has to be dealt with on a daily basis. But now there is also joy and celebration for the little things that were never noticed before.

Our story goes like this. I woke up one morning to find my life, my husband's life, and my child's life in a state of chaos. Something was happening to my beautiful little girl that neither my body nor my spirit could accept. She was displaying neurological signs of autism, or what we now call pervasive developmental disorder. I was in a constant state of anxiety mixed with depression, and for months I woke up almost every night and never had a good night's sleep. As a practicing speech-language pathologist who was working in early intervention, I knew the seriousness of the disorder and what we could possibly be facing. After several months of praying and making all the necessary calls, I finally put together a team of clinicians to work with my child. Things still did not feel right in our home. Day after day I kept on looking at the faces of these clinicians for reassurance that everything would be okay. It got to the point that I felt so distraught that I began to ask everyone I met if my daughter was going to be all right. It didn't matter who it was—the ice-cream man on the street, a stranger, or someone just passing by. Sometimes I still have those days.

For her first two years, Mira had experienced only happy parents who constantly sang, laughed, cuddled her. Now she was experiencing a different mother who was falling apart, and a father who was constantly worried about how to save the family. She did not seem as happy as she had been.

After three months of therapy, our lives had not changed all that much. I was constantly calling doctors, sending e-mail, reading about diets, and looking for cures. One day I remembered how, when I worked once at a school for children with special needs, in spite of all of their crises, some of the mothers would still manage always to have a smile on their faces. It did not seem to matter how impaired their child was; those children always seemed to do better than the children without that kind of support. I kept on thinking, How could we change things so we could have smiles on our faces again? How could we go back to being a happy family again? I only wanted my daughter to be healthy, and even now we still pray for that.

Then I remembered an old friend who had lost her sister to cancer, and who had introduced me to this design concept called Feng Shui. She said, "If you move things around and make changes in your home, the energy there also changes." I thought about all my past spring cleanings and how they'd made me feel, and a feeling came over me, a freedom that I had never experienced before. Thus my journey into Feng Shui began. One day, while I was chatting with one of Mira's therapists, she shared with me that she had recently experienced the loss of one of her siblings, and that Nancy had worked with her family as part of their healing process. My question, of course, was "Did it help?" Yes, definitely, she said. That night we decided to give Feng Shui a try. I phoned Nancy, and then sent her my biography and floor plans.

A couple of weeks later, Nancy and her associate came to my home. We had no idea what to expect. I thought we would have to get rid of some stuff and buy a few things, but I soon realized that there was much more to it than that. We sat down in the living room, and Nancy asked a couple of questions and proceeded to do a Chakra scan and reading for my whole family. She read our energy like a book; it was a bit scary how accurate her interpretation appeared to be.

She talked about the energy between my husband and me, and how this was affecting my marriage and Mira's healing. She also read Mira's energy and discussed several things about Mira's health, giving us a different perspective on her diagnosis.

Nancy had a good feeling about Mira's healing. She also said that soon people who cared a lot about Mira's healing would be drawn to us. In one month we found a homeopath, a chiropractor with healing hands, and a wonderful doctor who specializes in PDD.

The second time Nancy came to our home, she performed a Transcendental Cure on and around Mira's bed. She explained that quite often things don't change positively at first, and that when you're healing, sometimes you have to go two steps backwards before you can move ahead. This is exactly what happened. For a month we saw Mira's behavior regress. The visualization technique Nancy had given for both Mira and me was becoming difficult for me to do. I was starting to lose hope. Shortly afterward, though, Mira began to regain her lost ground, with even better communication and processing skills.

Healing has definitely occurred, though slowly. Mira is doing better, and looks physically healthier. We have given her a positive affirmation to say every day, which is "I am healthy and strong." We don't really care if she just says it in rote fashion; when she recites it, she usually has a smile on her face, so we know there is some type of understanding. We are beginning to try to do things as a family again. We all went to dinner for the first time in a year, and also lunch at McDonald's (Mira loves the french fries!). We know we have a tough road ahead, but the days that Mira shines with glowing energy and brilliance—those are the days that make me believe we are heading in the right direction.

I have always thought that I was blessed with the ability to pick out a genuine person, a person who has a gift to offer and truly cares. Nancy came into our life for a reason. I have no doubt that she has the ability to help our family.

Mitch and I are continuing to heal Mira and ourselves. I have learned to appreciate where she is right now, and to do my best not to compare her with other children. Although I am often filled with deep sadness and a sense of loss that only another mother could understand, my husband and I believe that Mira will be a happy, healthy, and independent child. We don't know exactly when that will happen, but we feel we are moving closer and closer toward a healing. We know that Nancy will be a big part of that healing, and we are grateful to have her in our lives.

Jane, Mitch, and Mira's Situation: An Overview

When Jane first contacted me, I remember being very struck by the efforts that both she and her husband were making on behalf of getting their child well. She described to me some of the treatment plans they were implementing, and a lot of the obstacles they were facing. After receiving the biography and floor plan, I did some preliminary work, meditating on Mira and the overall dynamics of the family. During my meditation I did a visual scan of Mira's body and Chakra energy system. What I saw was an image of Mira's energy body, very clear on one side and very erratic on the other, with static running up and down the erratic side. At that time I wasn't very sure what the image meant or how I was going to use it, but I committed it to memory and continued making notes on their floor plan.

In the cab ride over to their house, my assistant and I were discussing some of the specifics regarding the floor plan, and I told her about the image that I had in my meditation of Mira's body, then I drew it for her, while still in the back of the cab.

When we first arrived at their house, we sat and talked with the family, and I reviewed their energy. I quickly realized the toll that this whole situation was taking on their marriage, health, and quality of life. This is not an infrequent occurrence with families who are facing illnesses, diseases, and children with special needs. By the time I began to work with this family, the quest for a healing for Mira had become the priority, even though by then it had been at the expense of other needs and aspects of life. This very dedicated couple were now, unknowingly, sacrificing their marriage, their happiness, and the right to live life with any peace of mind.

After I reviewed the situation, I knew I had to begin this very important consultation with regrouping and exhausting the mundane solutions first, then afterward integrate the Transcendental Cures. I knew I had to present to them my take on what was happening, while supporting them in all the ways that they needed to get Mira healed, even if they didn't completely agree with my spiritual theories. My first instinct was to make sure both Jane and Mitch were currently seeing a therapist, because of the amount of strain and pressure that they were both under. When I explored Mitch's energy field, I saw that his solar plexus was very stressed and that his stomach was in knots. He confirmed that that was the part of his body that gave him the most trouble, and that he was under treatment for it. He was also very angry, both at his wife and the overall situation. This was very valuable information because it brought my attention to Jane, and I realized how her intense focus on Mira had resulted in a complete loss of connection to her husband, their marriage, and her own needs. In addition, her tight focus on Mira was energetically shutting Mira down. It seemed to me that she was checking out as a response to being inundated with various therapists, treatment plans, and the burden of having to get well.

I also talked with Jane and Mitch about trying to see this painful situation from a different angle: that Mira had made this choice to be challenged by this developmental condition in this incarnation. This is the hardest talk to have with someone, because when we are in fear and in pain, the last thing we want to hear is that our soul has made a choice to experience this painful situation.

On one level, that suggestion may sound ludicrous, as if I am blaming the person who is sick or has the problem. Nonetheless it becomes very empowering, because the illness or challenge is perceived as something that has a real purpose, and not as something that has come into your life just to haunt you and make you miserable. So my explanation of why Mira was ill helped take some of the burden from her parents for their self-blame, and shifted them out of the victim mind-set also. This small but powerful shift helped them let go, open up to other ways of healing the situation, honor Mira's soul, and, hard as it was, respect her choices. This doesn't mean that we stopped pursuing all methods for getting her well; it just meant going at them from a different perspective. Upon further work with Jane, together we realized that she also was working on some of her own mother/adolescent issues (Throat Chakra) that had been triggered by this very difficult challenge.

While I was working with Mitch and Jane at this session, I was sitting opposite from them on another couch. On the couch next to Jane sat my associate, who at one point looked over at the notes that Jane was taking. On the page was a doodle of Mira. To my associate's surprise, the drawings depicted the same frenetic energy patterns I had drawn in the cab for her on the way here (see Fig. 43a and 43b).

Figs. 43a and 43b. Two Sketches of Mira by Nancy SantoPietro *(top)* and Jane *(bottom)*.

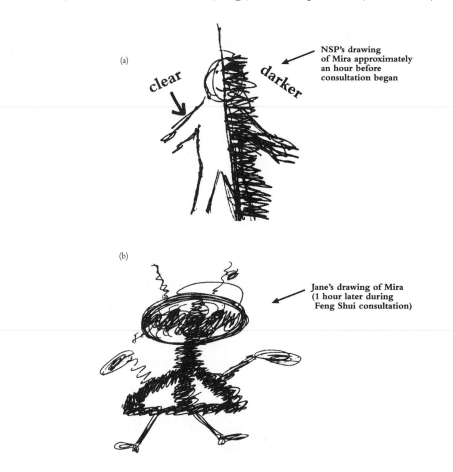

(a)

clear

darker

NSP's drawing of Mira approximately an hour before consultation began

(b)

Jane's drawing of Mira (1 hour later during Feng Shui consultation)

Several weeks after the consultation, I was emptying out a box that held some of my old notepads from my Black Hat Sect classes, and a loose piece of paper fell to the floor. When I picked it up, I saw it was a cure that I'd received several years ago, for children with autism! I hadn't even known that I had it. On the next visit, Jane, Mitch, and I performed the cure for Mira in her room, along with assigning a series of Chakra color/light visualizations for Jane and Mitch to do with each other and with Mira. A month later she had a developmental setback that lasted a few weeks, but then she came back even stronger.

Five months later we had a very big breakthrough. After rethinking the whole treatment process and coming to terms with the reality that it was not working, both parents decided to make a radical move and leave New York City for Long Island. Mira was accepted at a very reputable school for children with special needs, and a team of specialists then stepped in and oversaw Mira's treatment plan, giving her mom and dad a much-deserved break and help. Both Jane and Mitch have committed themselves to simplifying their lives. They are starting to ask for help from family members, they have cut back on programs and treatments for Mira, and they have shifted the focus to helping her, and themselves, enjoy life as it is *now*. This breakthrough on the emotional grid of the illness will now allow for more help, guidance, and healing. The more Jane lets go, the quicker things will shift and a true healing can come through.

How We Adjusted the Feng Shui of Jane, Mitch, and Mira's Home

Jane and Mitch were open and ready to listen to my suggestions, of which there were five. The first was that we had to work toward putting the focus back on their marriage, and on themselves. This gave Mira a little breathing room from the pressure of getting well. The second was that they consolidate Mira's treatment plans, therapists, and numerous appointments. Third, I suggested a meeting with all the various clinicians, and that someone be put in charge of the overall treatment plan. Fourth, I instructed Jane and Mitch not to implement new treatments until there was a new plan, or at least until the things that Mira was working on had had time to prove their effectiveness. The fifth was to make Feng Shui adjustments.

Fig. 44. Before Adjustments, Floor Plans of Jane, Mitch, and Mira's Home

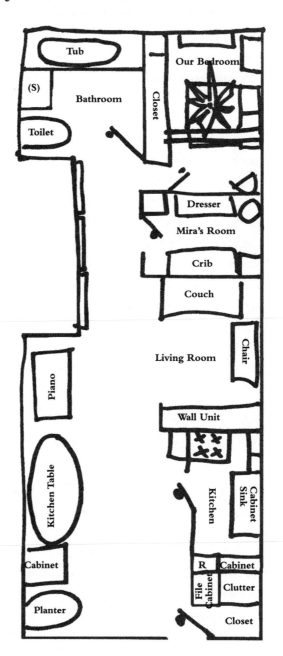

Fig. 45. After Adjustments, Floor Plan of Jane, Mitch, and Mira's Home

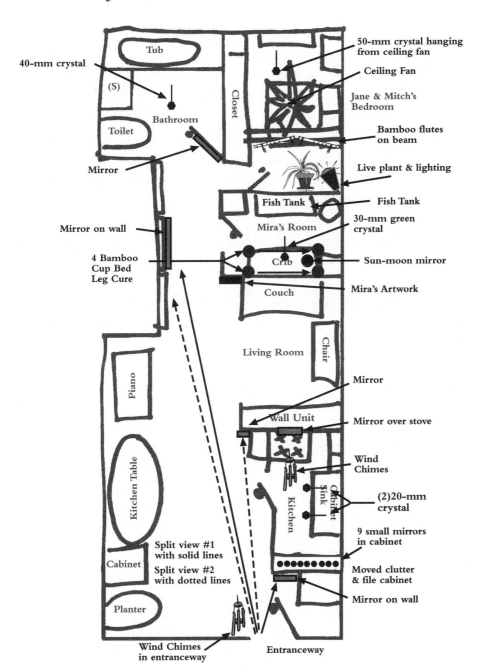

- Tub
- 50-mm crystal hanging from ceiling fan
- 40-mm crystal
- Ceiling Fan
- (S)
- Closet
- Jane & Mitch's Bedroom
- Bathroom
- Toilet
- Bamboo flutes on beam
- Mirror
- Live plant & lighting
- Fish Tank
- Fish Tank
- Mira's Room
- 30-mm green crystal
- Mirror on wall
- Crib
- Sun-moon mirror
- 4 Bamboo Cup Bed Leg Cure
- Mira's Artwork
- Couch
- Living Room
- Chair
- Piano
- Mirror
- Wall Unit
- Mirror over stove
- Wind Chimes
- Kitchen Table
- Kitchen
- Sink
- Cabinet
- (2)20-mm crystal
- 9 small mirrors in cabinet
- Cabinet
- Split view #1 with solid lines
- Split view #2 with dotted lines
- Moved clutter & file cabinet
- Planter
- Mirror on wall
- Wind Chimes in entranceway
- Entranceway

Although I made many recommendations, the ones I deemed most important started at the front door. Upon entering their apartment, I came upon two very serious split views. The first one occurred in the main entranceway, and the second one just a few feet ahead, inches past the kitchen. Both walls jutted out, one more than the other, but nonetheless it was a double split view, creating scattered energy, lack of focus, depression, relationship differences, and a mental split right down the middle. This was the exact image I'd seen when I'd meditated on Mira! The original floor plan did not show a split view, because the drawing's dimensions had been miscalculated. I suggested placing a mirror on each wall of the split views to help the family regain balance, focus, and equilibrium, and so that the two hemispheres of Mira's brain could cooperate and work more efficiently with each other. I had them clear their Helpful People corners, especially the one behind the front door. From that space I had them remove a filing cabinet that was blocking the door from opening fully, thus constricting their flow of Helpful People, which was very important, especially where Mira was concerned.

In the kitchen we augmented the Helpful People corner by placing small mirrors inside the dish closets and adding two 20-mm Feng Shui crystals and lighting under another set of cabinets to augment their Relationship corner. Over their stove I instructed them to place a mirror and hang a brass wind chime on the ceiling in the cook's station to help support and strengthen their finances.

We also adjusted the bathroom, which was sitting in the Wealth area of the overall floor plan, by placing four weights in each corner and hanging a 40-mm crystal on a nine-inch red string in the center of the room.

In Mira's room I had them organize everything in Mira's sight line, and we added her favorite thing to stare at—a small fish tank—in the Family section, directly across from her bed and in her sight line. Jane was also instructed to remove all visual clutter and reduce all busy themes in the room. Because I was told that Mira's blood tests showed a high content of mercury, I checked the location of her room and bed, and found the room to be in the Children gua of the overall floor plan, and her bed in the Children gua of her room. The Children gua in Feng Shui has a corresponding element, and the element of that gua is Metal. Because we did not have another room to place her in, or another area to move the bed to, I suggested that we place a mirror across from the bed in the Family gua, and a mirror in the hallway outside the door, to pull her room and bed symbolically out of the Children gua and away from all that metal. In addition, we hung a 30-mm green crystal over her bed, purchased a new bed that was made out of wood (not metal), and performed a Transcendental Cure specifically for children with brain-related developmental delays, which consisted of wrapping all four legs of her bed frame in a cloth and slipping each leg into a bamboo cup holder with additional mirrors and red string ties. We also placed a sun-moon mirror (Black Hat Sect cure item) on her headboard, directly facing her Crown Chakra, to pull her out of her withdrawn state.

In Jane and Mitch's bedroom I recommended hanging a 50-mm crystal on a nine-inch red string from the ceiling fan located in the center Health gua, and hanging two bamboo flutes on the overhead beam that ran parallel over Jane as she lay in her bed. The other significant adjustments I recommended in their bedroom were to reduce all the clutter and visuals that were overstimulating, and to hang a live plant in their relationship gua, along with some upward lighting to jump-start their Relationship and support all the struggles that they had and will have to face together.

DOUBLE BLESSINGS

David and Lauren's Story

We got married in our late thirties, and knowing that, like any couple, we might face issues with fertility, we decided to try to have children relatively early in our marriage. Our first pregnancy happened more quickly than we had imagined it would, and it ended just as quickly, in a sudden miscarriage. We were devastated, and simply resolved to try again just as soon as we got the medical go-ahead. We did, and once again we had little difficulty conceiving. And once again, as effortlessly and uneventfully as we had conceived, we found ourselves just as swiftly mourning our lost parenthood when another miscarriage ensued. And again we pushed onward, and repeated the cycle. And again. And again. The fifth time, when we made it all the way to twenty-one weeks, we were sure that our dreams were finally going to be realized. And they were not. That time it was no longer just about hopes and dreams. We'd heard her heartbeat, we'd experienced the swelling of the body that meant life was grow-ing inside, and we'd started to count down the weeks until we would be hold-ing our baby in our arms. Instead, again, we cried for days.

We are both firmly grounded in conventional religion. I am a rabbi, and my wife and I are both, at the same time, completely open to the power of alternative avenues to harnessing the healing and edifying powers of the uni-verse. While it would have surprised many in our suburban community to learn that we had decided to employ Feng Shui, we did so with a sense of openness and comfort that what we were doing in no way compromised our religious beliefs, and that it was, in fact, a strong affirmation of our more globally spiritual beliefs. We knew about Feng Shui partly from its increas-ing popularity in Western culture, but mostly because of Nancy, who is a friend of a close friend of ours.

The day we spent with Nancy at our home was intensely meaningful. Of course, we made plans for rearranging furniture, and noted where to hang a crystal in a window and where to plant a small tree by an outside corner of our house. And we talked and wrote and participated in rituals that focused our intentions and our yearnings, and we merged our intentions and ener-gies, and we came away with the strong sense that something inexpressible had substantially shifted. We did everything that Nancy advised us to do, from moving our bed away from the door of our bedroom to placing large rocks along the sides of our driveway. We prayed and we hoped and we focused our energies on becoming parents, the one thing that both of us wanted most.

We became pregnant again, and we held our breath as we got to week twenty-one. Then we breathed a little easier at week twenty-two. And as time went on, we heard heartbeats and saw sonograms, until, a little more than a year after our visit with Nancy, our astonishingly beautiful twins, a son and a daughter, were born.

Of course, we continued to pursue conventional paths of healing and fertility as well, and there is little doubt that we could not have had a suc-cessful pregnancy without the efforts of the physicians who tended to us. But there is equally little doubt in our minds that medicine alone would not have been sufficient. Our children, now four years old, are as beautiful in spirit and soul as they are in body, and we know that all this would not have been, were it not for that special day.

David and Lauren's Situation: An Overview

I knew Lauren through a mutual friend, and I'd heard that they were having a hard time conceiving. I always wanted to help but was waiting for them to be ready and contact me. When Lauren called, she briefly told me the story, and said she was at her wits' end in trying to figure out what kept going wrong. This was an important piece of information that she shared with me regarding her pregnancies. Although some women have a difficult time conceiving, she was able to conceive without any problem, but kept losing the baby. This alerted me that there might be something very obvious in her environment, from a Feng Shui perspective, that was sabotaging her pregnancies and her health.

Prior to going to her home, I reviewed her floor plans very carefully and listened for any information that they might have provided me with subconsciously, as a clue to what may have been going awry. She shared with me a story that seemed almost fictional. Three months into the marriage she'd had her first miscarriage after six weeks. Six months later she was pregnant again, and eight weeks after that she miscarried again. A new doctor discovered that she wasn't producing enough progesterone to hold the baby for the full term of the pregnancy. She was placed on hormonal supplements and got pregnant again, but then, at approximately 20 or so weeks into the pregnancy, she miscarried again. Another doctor, a specialist, detected some structural problem in her uterus. Lauren's exact description was "My uterus looked something like this $\vee$ instead of this $\triangledown$. That little blip acted like a wall that wouldn't allow the baby to grow any further." She had surgery and got pregnant again, and lost the baby yet again. The information and the picture she drew for me of her uterus proved to be key, and very helpful. Although I didn't know what exactly I was looking for, I committed it to memory and then reviewed her floor plans to see if there were any obvious structural concerns regarding her pregnancies and miscarriages.

How We Adjusted the Feng Shui of David and Lauren's Home

First of all, neither David nor Lauren had a lot of Earth in the Five Element charts I drew for them. Earth is a very important element to have and be surrounded by when you are trying to get pregnant, because Earth is where all seeds are planted in order to grow. Without Earth it is hard to hold a pregnancy. One of the first suggestions I made on site was to plant a tree in the somewhat dark and missing Children area outside on their lot. The first floor had a split-view entranceway, with a closet blocking part of the view. I suggested that Lauren mirror the closet door as a cure to open up and balance the view. Other adjustments were made throughout the whole floor for other related issues.

When we went downstairs to the bottom floor, where her bedroom was, the various culprits, from a Feng Shui perspective, became obvious. In addition to the split view upstairs, there was a brick-wall entryway to the downstairs floor. The ch'i was very pinched going downstairs, so I recommended that she mirror the wall at the bottom of the steps to help expand the area and also turn the Bagua around, because, with the current layout, many of those rooms would be outside the Bagua, behind the steps.

Figs. 46a and 46b. Before and After Adjustments, Plans of the First Floor of David and Lauren's Home

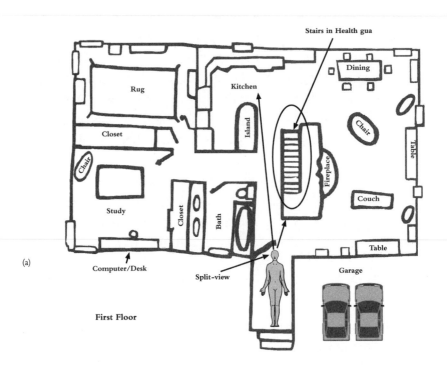

(a)

First Floor

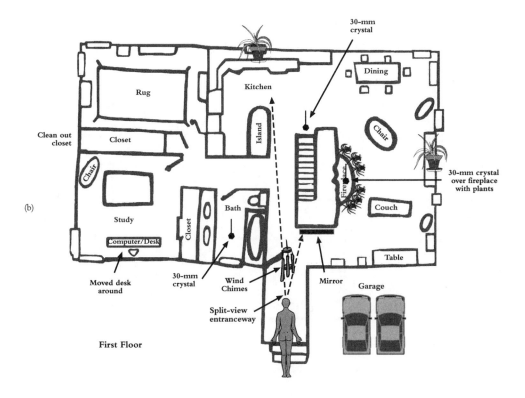

30-mm crystal

Dining

Kitchen

Rug

Island

Chair

Clean out closet

Closet

Chair

30-mm crystal over fireplace with plants

Fireplace

Bath

Closet

Study

Couch

Computer/Desk

Table

Moved desk around

30-mm crystal

Wind Chimes

Mirror

Garage

Split-view entranceway

First Floor

(b)

As we turned left to walk into their bedroom, I noticed that they had a set of "bickering doors"; that is, their closet door and their bedroom door could knock together if you opened them both at the same time. The **V** formation that they made in their open position looked like an exact replica of the shapes and drawings of Lauren's pictures of her uterus! I realized that the opening and closing of those doors created an opening and closing effect energetically on her uterus, fanning it open, then closed, not allowing the baby to hold its place.

As we further explored the bedroom, I immediately noticed two other major problems. The first was that the door opened to the small of the room, facing the closest wall. Remember the importance of entranceways as the "mouths of the ch'i" in Feng Shui. They also oversee the birth canal and uterus, entrance and exits for babies during pregnancy. The entranceway was pinched, and the clashing doors were causing an inconsistent fanning that opened her uterus. I suggested that they take the bedroom door off and rehang it on the opposite side of the frame, so the door, when opened,

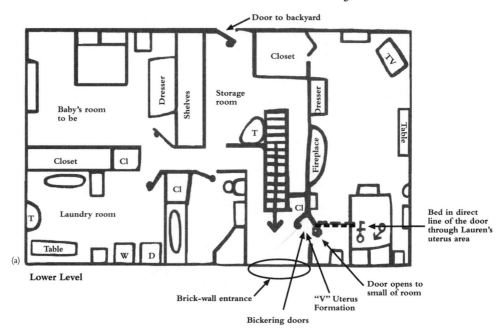

(a)

Door to backyard

Closet

TV

Dresser

Shelves

Storage
room

Baby's room
to be

Dresser

Fireplace

Table

T

Closet

Cl

Cl

Cl

T

Laundry room

Cl

Bed in direct
line of the door
through Lauren's
uterus area

Table

W

D

Lower Level

Brick-wall entrance

Bickering doors

"V" Uterus
Formation

Door opens to
small of room

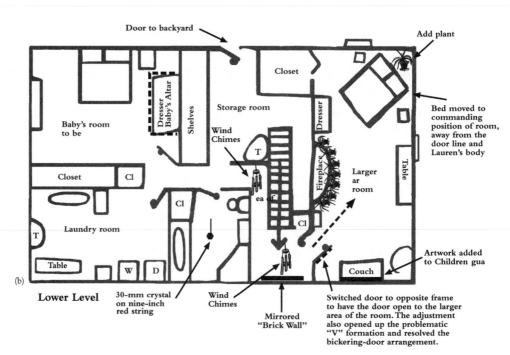

(b)

Door to backyard

Add plant

Closet

Dresser
Baby's Altar

Shelves

Storage room

Dresser

Baby's room
to be

Wind
Chimes

T

Fireplace

Larger
ar
room

Table

Bed moved to
commanding
position of room,
away from the
door line and
Lauren's body

Closet

Cl

Cl

ea of

T

Laundry room

Cl

Table

W

D

Couch

Artwork added
to Children gua

Lower Level

30-mm crystal
on nine-inch
red string

Wind
Chimes

Mirrored
"Brick Wall"

Switched door to opposite frame
to have the door open to the larger
area of the room. The adjustment
also opened up the problematic
"V" formation and resolved the
bickering-door arrangement.

would open to the largest part of the room, thus allowing the ch'i and the baby to flow and grow without restrictions. In addition, this eliminated the "bickering-door" problem, essentially solving two major problems at once.

Their bed was also in a very difficult position, right in the entranceway, in a very stressful position for health. To add a further complication, Lauren slept on the side of the bed closest to the door, with her reproductive organs and uterus crossing the mouth of the ch'i. All these things, along with some of the medical factors, combined to frustrate the couple's wish to start a family. We created altars for the baby, set our intentions in combination with the new proposed layout, created rituals, and said prayers. A year later Lauren gave birth to a beautiful set of healthy twins. Their participation and willingness to join in the process, aggressively make the structural changes, and be open of mind and heart changed their life. As a rabbi and a rabbi's wife, they could have chosen to be closed to other ways of doing and seeing things. Instead, together, we united in our similarities, incorporated our differences, and created a space that welcomed two beautiful little earth angels to the world.

A HOUSE HISTORY AND A SUICIDE ATTEMPT: A PAST TRAUMA REVISITED

Denise's Story

In 1995 my husband and I bought a house. We moved in after doing a lot of work on it. It had a basement apartment that we rented out, which helped pay for some of our mortgage. It was a beautiful studio apartment, and we rented it to a young man in his twenties. He was a good tenant. He had a good job and a nice girlfriend and family. But three months after he moved in, he started to go through a very bad time. His girlfriend left him, and he got laid off from his job, both at the same time. He got very depressed, and eventually tried to kill himself. For several days his lights were out and he never came home, so my husband went down to investigate. To our surprise what we found was the apartment in a total mess, with blood everywhere. It looked as though he had attempted to kill himself in various places, and then left the apartment. The effect was frightening. I was very scared, and it really shook me up badly. My husband and I eventually reached his mother, only to find out that she already knew what had happened. She told us that her son was in a hospital and was being treated. I continued to be very upset by the incident. Even though his mother came over to clean the apartment, I still could not comfortably go downstairs without thinking about the awful thing that had taken place there. Two weeks later the tenant called and wanted his apartment back. Even though I felt sympathy for him and wished him well, I knew I couldn't do that. I told him that without a job he should probably stay with his mother, who could watch over him. He agreed with me. I wished him luck and added that although depression was a terrible thing, he should try to hang in there and get well. After I talked with him, I called his mother to see if she was finished cleaning the apartment. A week later the tenant came over one last time for his belongings and clothes. He never called again. I wasn't able to go downstairs to the basement; I still had very bad feelings whenever I thought about the incident. I called Nancy, who came over to do a space clearing in the apartment. She performed several space-clearing techniques that got all the negative energy out of the apartment. As I watched her perform the clearing ritual, I was very relieved, I felt so much better. I was happy and able once again to go down to the apartment and not feel fear. Finally I was ready to rent the apartment again, being very careful whom I rented it to. I interviewed about ten people, and finally found a very nice man who has been wonderful and has been living here happily ever since.

Denise's Situation: An Overview

Denise and her family had a very traumatic experience that energetically permeated not only her home but her family's state of mind. Experiencing a suicide or an attempted suicide would be traumatic for anyone, but for Denise in particular it was devastating. When she was about eighteen years old, her grandmother had committed suicide. As she started to tell her story, I quickly realized that the traumatic loss of her grandmother still remained in her energy field and parts of what happened were left unresolved. Her Chakra energy system still held the vibration of the trauma, and had pulled in this horrible experience so that it could be free of it.

When I first received the call from her she was very upset and told me that she was having a hard time going down to the basement, where the tenant's apartment was; this was the same floor where her washer and dryer were located, and with two small children it was an area she used daily. When we explored her grandmother's suicide, I realized that her excessive panic and physical shakiness were a residual reaction that had never quite left her body in the twenty intervening years.

As we got further into the Feng Shui process, she shared with me a very interesting detail: *the former owner's grandson had committed suicide by gunshot in what was then a bedroom but was now their living room,* the floor right above the room where her tenant had attempted suicide by cutting his wrists. The Predecessor Law in Feng Shui states that the previous tenant's or owner's energy can remain

Figs. 48a and 48b. Before and After Floor Plans of Denise's Home

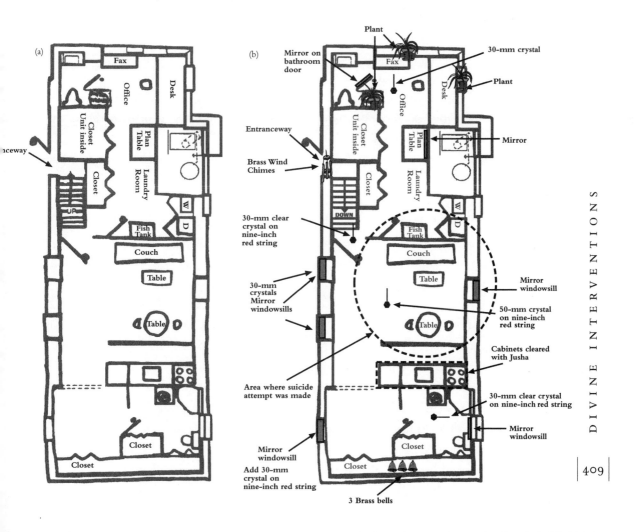

in a space even long after they are gone. It also states that events, especially traumatic ones like domestic violence, suicides, illnesses, and death, can remain energetically in the space, if they are not cleared out or transmuted. The energy field may not only re-create another similar event but also draw in individuals who have similar karmic ties. The owner and her tenant energetically overlapped, and karma occurred. Although on the surface this was a horrifying experience, on a spiritual and emotional level it was a good thing for them both. Denise needed to purge old emotional baggage that was hanging around in her energy field, chipping away at her immunity and eventually making her more susceptible to illness, while the tenant needed to deal with all the emotional losses and fears that he was carrying around with him.

How We Adjusted the Feng Shui of Denise's Home

The main adjustment in a house with this kind of traumatic situation is through space clearing. Although the blood and mess were well cleaned up and gone before I arrived, it wasn't until then that Denise told me some of the other gory details about what had happened. She went on to describe that besides blood being on the floor throughout her tenant's apartment, he'd also written in blood on the kitchen cabinets the words HELP ME. This cry for help really shook her up. The first thing I did was mix a Jusha cure, which contains red cinnabar and alcohol, and had Denise put her finger in the mix and physically go over the now-invisible writing on the kitchen cabinets. Jusha is a very deep red, and when mixed with alcohol it can look very much like blood. As she was symbolically clearing the imprint of the energy, I was doing some very powerful prayers and the Ousting Mudra, releasing all the negative and fearful old energy and also the new energy that had been created. At first Denise was reluctant to do this, but after she'd finished she felt back in control and a bit more distanced from the fear. Then we did the Sealing the Doors cure, and I suggested hanging some crystals in the small basement windows to bring in a "light adjustment" through the rainbows they created in the apartment.

Several months later Denise had another concern that she shared with me. Her youngest daughter wasn't sleeping very well in her room, and exhibited delayed speech patterns and an attention span deficit. When I checked her floor plan again, I quickly realized that her daughter's bedroom

and bed were directly aligned over the area in the basement where the suicide attempt had occurred. The line of energy that ran vertically through
three floors over that spot in the house was very stagnant, and as all ch'i does,
it flowed upward, like smoke. The energy imprint from the first owner's
grandson's suicide, on what was now considered the first floor, spread up to
the child's room on the second floor, and downstairs to the basement apartment, where the tenant had attempted to take his life. We placed a 50-mm
Feng Shui crystal in the Center area of her living room where the original
suicide took place. We space-cleared the whole house with "red jusha rice."
We hung a 30-mm crystal on a nine-inch red string in the center of her
daughter's room, and switched the child's bed to a healthier position, with
her body out of harm's way (the ch'i of the entranceway was too intense).
We added a 30-mm crystal in the center of her other daughter's room, in
the gua that oversees health, and placed plants and other life-force adjustments to bring in life and the positive ch'i force for her home. We also placed

Fig. 49. Denise's Home, Showing the Line of Destructive Predecessor Ch'i Permeating All Three Floors

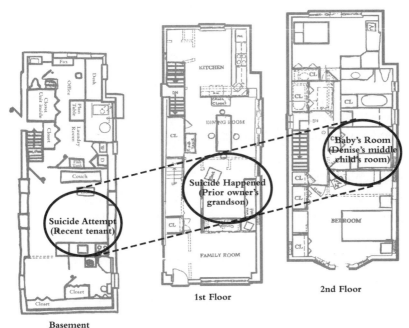

Basement

1st Floor

2nd Floor

a Feng Shui crystal (30- or 40-mm) in her upstairs bathroom, which was located in her Wealth gua. Our last major adjustment was to her side door of entry. This was an area on her floor plan that appeared to be very pinched and tight, with a brick-wall entranceway. There I suggested hanging bells on her door and mirrors on the wall in front of her that was creating a brick-wall entranceway. That kind of entranceway creates a conditioned response of no hope. This was her side door—but it was the tenant's main door, and, confronted as he was with that continual reminder, the no-hope entranceway energetically contributed to his suicide attempt. In addition to her having found a new tenant who is virtually problem-free, her daughter's behavior and speech have improved considerably.

A HERO'S JOURNEY

They say that God never gives you more than you can handle. I only wish that he didn't trust me so much.

— MOTHER TERESA

I've worked with so many different clients and their families over the past two decades, that any of their heartfelt stories could have been told in this book. For obvious reasons they all couldn't be, and some chose not to appear in this, my second book and first book on health.

But during the process of selecting client stories, I came to realize that all of these people (and each of you, the readers) are truly the unsung heroes of this incredible time of great transition and great healing on the planet. The healing is occurring because all of you very courageous souls agreed to come to this planet and help transform various illnesses and life's often-painful challenges. I thank you; we *all* thank you for coming to this often-difficult schoolroom.

Throughout our lives we will be challenged at every turn, with life reminding us constantly to face the challenges and to leave the world in much better shape than when we first arrived. So please do your work here with as much pride, commitment, and integrity as you can muster. Do it quietly. Do it loudly. Paint it. Write it. Live it. Invent it. Challenge it. But, most important . . . love it! For it was *you* who chose to be here, back when we understood and remembered that the gift of life was a privilege and not just a chore.

Thank yourself for being here in spite of having many hurdles to cross, difficulties to face, and bills to pay. Know that you had the perfect spiritual résumé for carrying out the tasks and challenges that were laid before you. Sometimes those challenges come by way of illness.

So, when you are at the end of your day or at the end of your rope, and you find yourself asking, "Why me? Why was I challenged to face this hardship?" remind yourself of the original truth of why you are here: *because God, in his absence, sent you instead!* Then proceed with that understanding in your heart. Draw on it for comfort, draw on it for strength, but, most of all, draw on it for compassion—for yourself as well as for others.

CLOSING STATEMENT

Feng Shui: Complementary Medicine for All Religions and Spiritual Practices

---

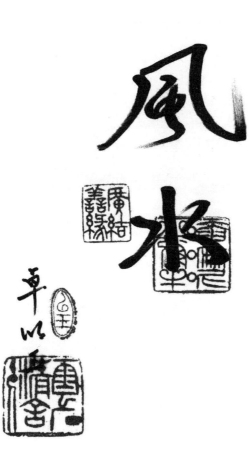

"Feng Shui."
CALLIGRAPHY BY DR. CATHERINE YI-YU CHO WOO

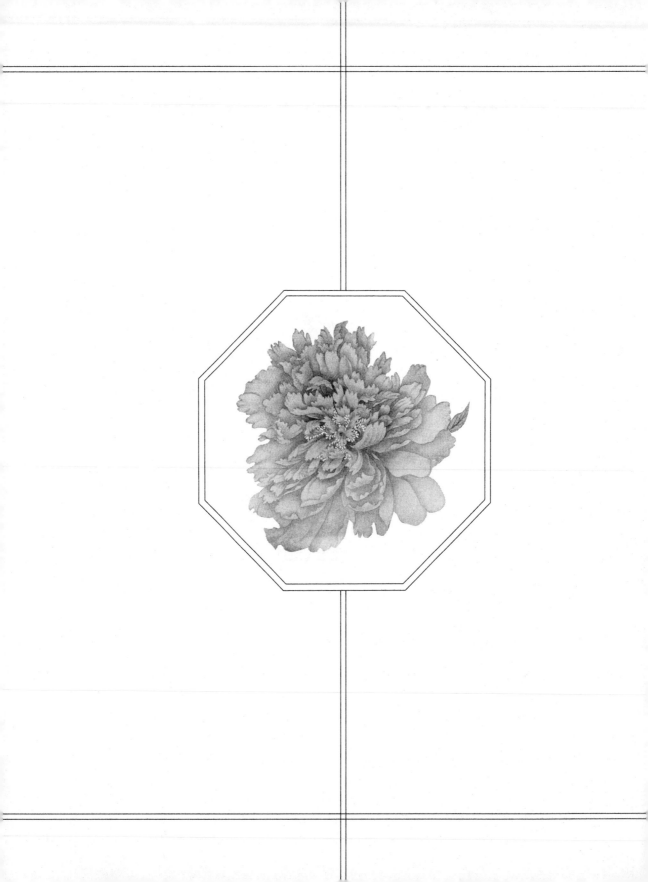

WHEN YOU ARE FACED with an illness, no matter how spiritually evolved you are or how much of the bigger picture you understand, all you really want to do is get well. I have found that no matter what my client's spiritual beliefs were or what religion they practiced, almost everyone eventually turned toward some kind of spiritual practice to help them make sense of their illness and to find comfort and relief from the fears it can elicit, because nothing will render you more helpless and vulnerable than a life-threatening illness.

Although the spiritual roots of the Black Hat Sect School of Feng Shui are firmly planted in the practices of Tibetan Tantric Buddhism, please keep in mind that you *do not* have to be a Buddhist, or even believe in Buddhism, in order to apply its principles to your home, health, or life. At its core, the philosophy of Buddhism is very much like any other honorable spiritual practice whose principles mainly encourage people to do good, help others, and leave the world in a little better shape than that in which they found it. There are so many different spiritual practices, with various beliefs and views on life, but no matter what the philosophical differences, or what language the prayers are spoken in, the one common bond that every evolved group shares is the wisdom of the heart. And the heart knows the truth, no matter what you believe or how you approach it.

I am a third-generation Italian American who was raised Catholic and went to Catholic school. In my early twenties, frustrated and a bit lost, I stopped believing that there was any God worth depending on, never mind praying to on a regular basis. As I began to explore other religions, I had to work very hard on trying to stay open to seeing spirituality and God in a different way than my earlier years of religious training had taught me. I questioned God and totally rebelled against the dogma part of Catholicism.

While growing up, I always felt an innate affinity with all things Eastern, so even without fully understanding Buddhism at the time, I found myself, over the years, gravitating naturally toward it. As I learned more about its principles and beliefs, I soon realized that it very much mirrored many of my own emerging beliefs about life, death, and reincarnation. But like most of the other religions with which I was becoming familiar, I didn't agree totally with all its principles, though I did with most of them. As I was developing spiritually, I began to take bits and pieces from different religions and piece them together in a form that spiritually made sense to me. Over time I became very comfortable with praying to a lot of the great avatars of various religions, including Christ, Buddha, and Krishna. I guess I never believed that God favored just one religion, and that the rest were all there to trip us up in our search for the "correct" one. I also figured that if I prayed to many different spiritual figures, I would raise the percentages in my own behalf, and that when I died, I'd be covered, no matter who was ultimately in charge.

When I first met Professor Lin Yun, eleven years ago, I was very surprised by something he said. Just before he began guiding us through a Black Hat Sect meditation, as his Mandarin words filtered through the translator, he said, "I will be using words or phrases that make reference to Buddha, but please feel free to replace the word 'Buddha' with the name of any religious or spiritual deity, higher power, or aspect of nature you feel connected with or pray to."

I was so touched by that simple act of compassion and understanding that I knew instantly I had found my teacher and mentor. As I've studied with him over the years, I have developed an incredibly deep love and esteem for him. Time after time I have come to appreciate how eloquently he teaches us all, in very humble ways, to dwell on the commonalities of all people, while at the same time respecting our differences. To me this is a sign of a wise teacher and a great spiritual leader. It truly has been my honor and privilege to study all these years with him.

When I first started studying Feng Shui, I didn't want to have to convert to Buddhism, give up my other spiritual beliefs, or adhere to restrictive dogma. But I soon learned that practicing Feng Shui, or getting a Feng Shui consultation, had nothing to do with becoming a Buddhist, any more than one needs to be a practicing Buddhist in order to get a shiatsu massage or an acupuncture treatment, or to eat an egg roll in one's local Chinese restaurant!

So, if all the mudras and mantras have left you in a conflict about working with Black Hat Feng Shui, please know that from a Black Hat perspective, there are *no conflicts* with any other religious beliefs. And although Feng Shui originated in the East, it is not just Chinese. The bottom line is that energy flow (ch'i) impacts on the health and lives of *all humankind*. Energy itself is genderless, without ethnicity, and doesn't have a set of spiritual beliefs or principles to enforce on anyone. The aspects of life that are not neutral, such as religion, politics, and personal opinions, are created by human beings, not by the unbiased elements of nature, or from the all-encompassing universal flow of energy. Good Feng Shui Design principles are teachings about energy, harnessing the natural forces of nature and living with its support, and in accordance with the higher plan. This applies to all creatures, all religions, and all living things.

In the end, if you believe in a Divine Plan, a Higher Self, God, Krishna, Christ, Buddha, Allah, or the Messiah, then those are the Higher Powers that ultimately co-create with you and make the final decisions as to whether your illness will heal, if you will become pregnant, or hit that big lottery next week. But Feng Shui, when used appropriately and not as a magic bullet, can help raise those percentages and reduce the environmental factors, stresses, and obstacles that may be contributing to your particular life situation or health issue. God always helps those who help themselves. Feng Shui, and its application to your home and life, is just another way of helping yourself.

Remember, *everything* that exists is part of God's plan, even the resurrection of this 4,000-year-old design system called Feng Shui. It has been divinely sent to us now to help us heal, transform, and create happy, healthy, and abundant lives. This is our birthright. This is what our Higher Power wants for us, and not one *Om Ma Ni Pad Me Hum* less.

Sickness is a difficult schoolroom, but it is nonetheless one of the journeys that our soul chooses to take as a path to our truth, enlightenment, and inner sense of wholeness. If you embrace your illness and use it correctly, you will be rewarded with insights, personal growth, and spiritual epiphanies beyond your imagination, for in doing this courageous act, you are honoring and loving the parts of yourself that long to be heard, healed, and transformed. By opening up to the underlying teachings that your illness brings, you will consequently discover your own true nature and be closer to God and Spirit in ways that you could never have imagined.

Deep inside of us exists a very special and unique inner space I call our "Sacred Heart Room." It is there, in that place of awareness, that no matter how sick you are or how far away from yourself you have grown, you will always, always recognize Truth. It is the inner voice that you must constantly seek, because at the center of that voice is the voice of your own soul, waiting patiently to remind you who you are and what you came here to do. Anything not in alignment (or exactly in alignment) with your soul's original purpose for incarnating will be revealed—and sometimes it's through the schoolroom of illness.

Keep in mind that, in the end, every experience, every person in your life, every hardship or illness that you might have had to face, was never about the other person or situation; *it was only and always about you, your life, and your relationship with the Divine.* Nothing more, nothing less.

Anyway
by Mother Teresa

People are often unreasonable, illogical and self-centered;
Forgive them anyway

If you are kind, people may accuse you of selfish, ulterior motives;
Be kind anyway

If you are successful, you will win some false friends and some true enemies;
Succeed anyway

If you are honest and frank, people may cheat you;
Be honest and frank anyway

What you spend years building, someone could destroy overnight;
Build anyway

If you find serenity and happiness, others may be jealous;
Be happy anyway

The good you do today, people will often forget tomorrow;
Do good anyway

Give the world the best you have, and it may never be enough;
Give the world the best you have anyway

You see, in the final analysis, it was always between you and God;
And it was never between you and them, anyway.

Appendix A

MEDICINE BUDDHA
(YAO SHI FU)

IN THE BLACK HAT SECT SCHOOL OF FENG SHUI there are more than a hundred deities, Transcendental Cures, and mantras that we use for different needs and in different situations. Some are used frequently, such as *Om Ma Ni Pad Me Hum,* while others are passed down orally and taught to the student only during very auspicious times. It is those particular cures and mantras that will ultimately have the most impact on your life and produce the highest results, because of the karmic nature of how and when you received them. It is not uncommon, when you are studying Feng Shui, to receive certain cures or teachings over and over again. But not until you connect with them one day on a deeper level, or until that "I got it!" lightbulb goes off in your mind, do you realize that at that specific time you are actually in need of that particular cure for your own life situation, or for someone else. You are *now,* as you read this book, and especially this appendix, karmically receiving very powerful cures that can assist you with your health and your life. Besides just reading them, try to take them in and activate the good karma that they bring to you by using them to help change your life. Reading about them alone will not do it. In order to really change your health, you also have to commit to taking action, whether that action means getting treatment, interviewing new doctors, reevaluating your life, leaving your job, praying, asking for help, or learning to take the time to meditate and focus on yourself. Sometimes good karma isn't just in the receiving of the cure itself, but also in meeting the individuals who help connect you with the cure.

I've frequently been very blessed to be at the right place, at the right time. The following story gives one good example of this, and of how I turned my good karma around and passed it along to you.

During the first four or five years of my study and practice of Feng Shui, I was still very sick. Although during that time I was given many different cures and remedies for improving my health, there were also many cures I did not receive, and others I didn't connect with or use. When someone receives a very powerful cure, and that cure changes the person's health or life situation, in Black Hat Sect Feng Shui we refer to that as having very good karma or a very good karmic connection.

In May 1996 I had the very good fortune to be introduced to a woman named Dr. Catherine Yi-yu Cho Woo. Dr. Woo is an internationally known and accomplished scholar, painter, poet, composer, Feng Shui expert, and educator who has made major contributions to the understanding of Chinese philosophy, aesthetics, and culture here and abroad. That year, when I was speaking at the First International Conference on Feng Shui, in San Diego, she was present when Professor Lin handed me his foreword for my first book, *Feng Shui: Harmony by Design* (Perigee, December 1996). I was so excited at the time that I didn't even introduce myself formally to her as she graciously helped translate Professor Lin's kind words from Mandarin into English for me. That was our first official karmic meeting. Over the years, and after many other auspicious meetings, our relationship began to blossom and grow. After discovering that we were both born, although at different times, in the Chinese Year of the Dog, we came to refer to each other affectionately as "Big Dog" and "Little Dog."

Several years ago, when Catherine heard that I was beginning to write my second book, she very generously offered me the use of one of her paintings to actually be used in the book itself. To say the least, I was very honored and grateful. When the present book was almost completed, I reminded her of her very kind offer. When she heard that the book's focus was specifically on health-related issues, she immediately said yes, "especially because it was written on health and its objective is to help alleviate people's sufferings."

When I thought about all her very beautiful paintings and how she somehow managed to magically imbue them with incredible life force (ch'i) and colors and calligraphy that seem to "talk," it became difficult to choose the one that was most appropriate. I already had three pieces of her spiritually inspiring artwork framed and hanging in my home, so I decided to choose from among those three, for they were the ones that were closest to my heart. Anticipating a struggle, I was surprised at how quickly I decided. There really wasn't any choice. The beautiful painting titled *Healing Medicine Buddha* (Yao Shi Fu) was the one that simply had to become part of this book on health. This particular painting was on the wall adjacent to my writing desk, in the Helpful People section of my living room. Thus, after asking Dr. Woo for her permission to use this painting, it became the black-and-white copy in Fig. 51.

In addition to offering me this lovely piece of spiritual art, she gave me several cures to do for my own health, incorporating some of the components written in calligraphy and depicted in her painting. The painting was made with acrylic paints on rice paper, and sitting in the middle of all its healing greens, blues, and purples is a pink lotus flower with eight petals, representing to me the eight Chakras. Hand-drawn over the painting is the Medicine Buddha Prayer written nine times in gold calligraphy, and in white, the mantra *Om Ma Ni Pad Me Hum,* 108 auspicious times. Thus she created not only a very beautiful painting, but also one that resonates to the highest vibration for healing. When admirers of her work look at it, each one sees something different; I always see an oversize pink lotus flower sitting on the top of a green-blue mountain, dispensing healing to all who seek its image for healing and help. For those of you who choose to view it, please visit my website. The painting is also available in a beautiful poster appropriate for framing.

After several late-night talks with my "Chinese mother," I began to work with the Medicine Buddha's image, painting, and prayer more closely on a daily basis for my own healing and as an initiation for my work with others who are ill. My very good karma of receiving this guidance from Catherine has now, in turn, become your very good karma, because this appendix on the Medicine Buddha, and the prayer and meditation for health that follow, were not included in the original proposal for this book.

Although I had connected with Medicine Buddha in the past, I have never worked with him and his healing abilities so closely. He revisited with me during a very much needed time, as I was experiencing a setback with my own health. The Medicine Buddha Prayer, along with certain Transcendental Cures, and a long-overdue visit to my doctor, got me back on

APPENDIX A

425

track and helped restore my physical as well as my emotional and spiritual well-being. I was so inspired by my own connection and transition that I decided to include this appendix and pass my blessings on to you.

We receive many blessings every day, but the wisest people are the ones who know how to utilize them. I believe that it is not only the meek who will inherit the Earth, but also the ones who are willing to live their lives awake enough to receive the gifts that are placed before them.

Medicine Buddha Prayer
Yao Shi Fu

Although there are many different Buddhas, each assigned to various intentions or wishes, one of the most significant and important is the Medicine Buddha. The Medicine Buddha is probably the most precious of all Buddhas because none of us can ever afford to get sick, even a little bit. An illness is a disruptive visitor that can alter the quality of your life in an instant. The Medicine Buddha Prayer invokes the help, guidance, and healing energy of Buddha.

Loosely translated, the prayer asks the Medicine Buddha to cleanse you of all past, present, and future karma that may have contributed to your illness. It asks Buddha to clear all of the unhealthy ch'i from your body so that you can heal and/or not get sick. It also asks Buddha to shield you from known and unknown calamities, protect you from disasters, and help you to avoid accidents, misfortunes, and worries. The prayer also requests that this benevolent Buddha help you sail through all your difficulties, keeping you healthy and blessing you with a long, healthy life.

Please know, even if you really don't master how to pronounce the romanization of the prayer properly, that what makes the prayer most effective is your desire to heal, your strong and clear visualization of your getting well, and, most important, as Professor Lin always says, *your sincerity.* Repeat this prayer nine times every morning for 27 days in a row. Have the artwork (depicted on the NSP&A website) of the Medicine Buddha in front of you and look at it often and breathe in its image and its healing abilities, as you do your Medicine Buddha Prayer every morning. Enlist the Medicine Buddha as a Helpful Person in your life, and incorporate his prayer into your daily praying, along with all the other prayers that you say or deities to whom you pray. Draw on him and the following mantra in times of need. Read this prayer from right to left, top to bottom.

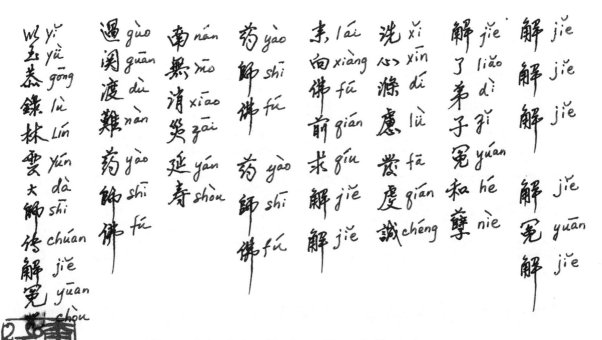

Fig. 50. Medicine Buddha Prayer

CALLIGRAPHY AND ROMANIZATION BY DR. CATHERINE YI-YU CHO WOO

Characters 1–6. Asking Buddha's help to resolve all the grievances.

Characters 7–13. Please resolve your humble disciple's grievances, sins, and past karma.

Characters 14–20. The humble disciple wants to make the most sincere request.

Characters 21–27. Visualize that you are coming forward in front of the Medicine Buddha, asking to be cured.

Characters 28–33. Medicine Buddha, Medicine Buddha.

Characters 34–46. I devote myself to the Medicine Buddha, who can help people get through hardships, prevent misfortunes, and prolong life.

TRANSLATION FOR H. H. PROFESSOR THOMAS LIN YUN

BY LIN-LIN CHENG

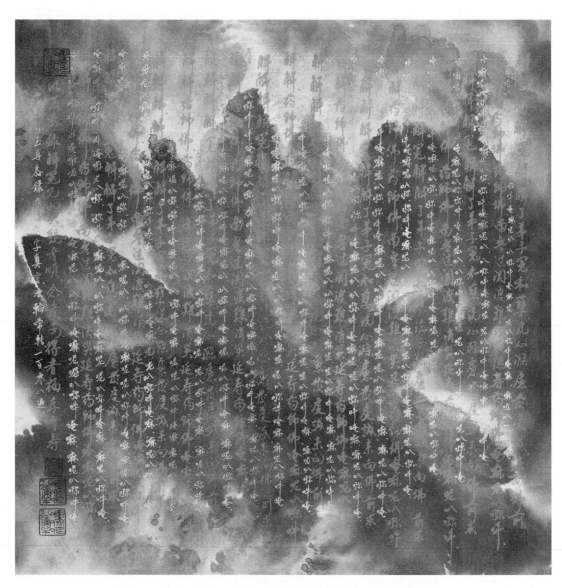

Fig. 51. Healing Medicine Buddha

BY DR. CATHERINE YI-YU CHO WOO

Appendix B

H. H. Grandmaster Professor Thomas Lin Yun Rinpoche's Biography

HIS HOLINESS GRANDMASTER PROFESSOR THOMAS LIN YUN RINPOCHE is the founder and supreme leader of the "contemporary" School of Black Hat Sect Tantric Buddhism, Fourth Stage. He is the world's leading authority on Feng Shui, and an accomplished calligraphy artist, *I Ching* expert, and scholar. In 1986 Professor Lin Yun founded the Yun Lin Temple in Berkeley, California, the first reformist Black Sect Tantric Buddhist temple in the West. In 1994 Professor Lin Yun established the second official temple, Lin Yun Monastery, in Long Island, New York. His inspirational teaching was instrumental in disseminating and popularizing Black Hat Sect Feng Shui throughout the world.

In 1998 His Holiness Lungtok Tenpai Dalai Lama, as one of the five Tantric traditions in Tibet, personally led four high lamas to the United States from India. Their purpose was to conduct enthronement ceremonies, one in Yun Lin Temple in Berkeley, and the other in Lin Yun Monastery in Long Island, to officially present Professor Lin Yun the title His Holiness of Black Sect Tantric Buddhism Fourth Stage. This is the first time in the history of the Tibetan Bon religion that such an honor was bestowed on an individual of Chinese descent.

Over the years, Professor Lin Yun has set up many sanctuary shrines— "Yun Shi Jing She"—all over the world. In addition to promoting Buddhist teachings, Chinese philosophies, and folkloric cultures, Professor Lin Yun's temples and shrines serve to provide blessings and guidance to meet the needs of disciples and people everywhere. His disciples and students come from all nationalities, religions, cultures, and ethnic backgrounds.

For more than three decades Professor Lin Yun has introduced his profound and insightful teachings, especially on Feng Shui, to the West by lecturing at universities, institutions, and religious communities. He has authored many books on Black Hat Sect Feng Shui, the most notable of which are *Interior Design with Feng Shui* and *Living Color,* both coauthored with Sarah Rossbach. Professor Lin Yun has been interviewed on major television networks in the United States, England, Taiwan, Hong Kong, and Southeast Asia. Articles and interviews on Professor Lin Yun and his teachings often appear in newspapers, journals, and magazines throughout the Americas, Europe, and Asia.

DR. CATHERINE YI-YU CHO WOO'S BIOGRAPHY

Dr. Catherine Yi-yu Cho Woo is an internationally known scholar, painter, poet, composer, Feng Shui expert, and educator who has made major contributions to the understanding of Chinese philosophy and aesthetics. Her paintings have been shown throughout Asia and the United States in numerous museums and galleries, including the United Nations, the Sackler Museum at Harvard University, and the National Gallery in Taipei.

Dr. Woo has authored nine books, in Chinese and English, on Chinese literature, art, and culture. She has lectured extensively around the world; her schedule has included such universities as Yale, Harvard, Princeton, MIT, Duke, and UC Berkeley; as well as the United Nations and the National Endowment for the Arts. In 1997 the National Conference of Jews and Christians honored Dr. Woo as Humanitarian of the Year.

As a disciple and devoted student of Grandmaster Lin Yun for the past 25 years, she continues to imbue heart, soul, and radiant life force into all her paintings and creative endeavors.

MEDICINE BUDDHA ARTWORK (SHOWN IN FIG. 51 AND THE NSP&A WEBSITE)

BY DR. CATHERINE YI-YU CHO WOO

The *Medicine Buddha* was painted in 1995 by Dr. Catherine Yi-yu Cho Woo, as she creatively combined the healing colors of green-blue and purple with an eight-petaled pink lotus blossom, representing the opening of one's heart.

Superimposed over the painting, in Mandarin and in gold calligraphy, appears the Medicine Buddha Prayer, nine times. In addition, in white calligraphy is given the powerful Six True Words Mantra, *Om Ma Ni Pad Me Hum,* 108 times (in the dynamic version). Further raising the vibration and healing powers of the painting are the minuscule white dots and lines throughout, representing the ch'i moving out toward people in the direction of all who sincerely come and ask for a healing.

This painting is available as an unframed poster from the Nancy SantoPietro & Associates website, www.fengshui-santopietro.com.

CALLIGRAPHY

CHAPTER 1. *"Opening this book will bring great benefits."* (Calligraphy by H. H. Professor Thomas Lin Yun.)

To be read from right to left, this was written while chanting infinite numbers of mantras in 2000, the Millennium Year of the Golden Dragon, to bestow blessings upon the readers of this book: "May the readers and their family members all receive happiness, wisdom, and safety." The center calligraphy is "Opening this book will bring great benefits." The left was composed by Lin Yun, the "Recluse Scholar Who Emerges with the Dragon,"★ while a visitor at the study of disciple Nancy Wang.

CHAPTER 2. *"Tao."* (Calligraphy by H. H. Professor Thomas Lin Yun.)

To be read from top to bottom. At the top is the Yin-Yang symbol, with smaller symbols contained within. According to Professor Lin Yun, there is Yin in Yang, and there is Yang in Yin. Within the Yang that is in Yin, there is another set of Yin-Yang, and the same within the Yin that is in Yang. And so on. The center is the calligraphy of the Chinese character *Tao.* In smaller script is the definition of *Tao* according to Black Sect Tantric Buddhism: "A Yin and a Yang combine as one, thereby following the laws of nature and set

---

★In the Chinese tradition, it is common for scholars to have many names or aliases. In ancient Chinese folklore, tigers and dragons are regarded as mystical creatures, so that when they appear, it is always with some form of natural phenomenon such as whirling winds or puffs of clouds. Since the word *Yun* in Professor Lin Yun's name means "cloud," he has chosen "Recluse Scholar Who Emerges with the Dragon *(Tsong Long Shan Ren)"* as one of his numerous scholarly names.

in motion continuously." Also in small script is the six-syllable mantra *Om Ma Ni Pad Me Hum,* written by Lin Yun while chanting mantras. The bottom is a prayer for world peace and the well-being of mankind and sentient beings from the Six Realms of Cyclical Existence. "May the readers of Nancy SantoPietro's masterpiece receive happiness, auspiciousness, longevity, wisdom, and safety." It was composed by Lin Tsan Yun while a visitor at the study of disciple Patty Cheng. ("Lin Tsan Yun" is another of Professor Lin Yun's scholarly names.)

CHAPTER 3. *"Bagua."* (Calligraphy by Dr. Catherine Yi-yu Cho Woo, written in the Year of the Dragon, 2000, for Nancy SantoPietro.)

This calligraphy is the Chinese character for the Bagua, the eight-sided map that one superimposes over a floor plan to locate the nine life-situation areas.

CHAPTER 4. *"Buddha's Heart; Divine Skills."* (Calligraphy by H. H. Professor Thomas Lin Yun.)

To be read from right to left, this was written while chanting infinite numbers of mantras in the year 2000 on the day of the Mid-Autumn Festival, to bestow blessings upon the readers, author, and publisher of this book: "May they all receive happiness, longevity, and wisdom." The center calligraphy is "Buddha's Heart; Divine Skills." The left was composed by the Master of *Nien-Hsuan* Den, Lin Yun, while a visitor at the study of disciple Mimi Tsai. (As with their own names, it is common for Chinese scholars to have several names for their studies or dens. *Nien Hsuan* Den is one of the names of Professor Lin Yun's study. The term *Nien Hsuan* means to memorialize one's mother.)

CHAPTER 5. *"Calming Heart."* (Calligraphy by H. H. Professor Thomas Lin Yun.)

To be read from right to left. At the top right is the calligraphy of the Chinese characters for "Calming Heart." At the bottom right is the Heart-Calming Mantra *Gate Gate, Para Gate, Para Sam Gate, Bodhi Swaha,* taken from the Heart Sutra. In the Chinese language, the pronunciations for "Calming Heart" and "Heart Sutra" are almost identical. The left column was written with cinnabar while chanting the highest-order mantras on the day of Mid-Autumn Festival, 2000, to bestow blessings upon the readers, author, and publisher of this book: "May they and their family members all receive happiness, wealth, and safety." It was composed by Lin Yun, the Master of *Wei Shr Hsuan,* while a visitor at the study of disciple Christine Chen. (*Wei Shr Hsuan* is another of the names of Professor Lin Yun's study. The term *Wei Shr* means to appraise and enjoy the refined metals and stones used for Chinese engraving and chops. The word *Hsuan* means den or study.)

CHAPTER 6. *"Talisman."* (Calligraphy by H. H. Professor Thomas Lin Yun.)

To be read from right to left. The right column was written on the day of the Mid-Autumn Festival, 2000, after offering incense and chanting mantras, to bestow blessings upon the readers, author, and publisher of this book: "May they and all their family members receive happiness, wealth, good health, and peace." The center calligraphy is "Talisman." From top to bottom are (1) the Divine order by the highest Taoist deity to immediately offer protection, (2) the Five Thunder Protectors Mantra, (3) the Eight Trigrams, or Bagua, (4) the Six-Syllable Mantra, *Om Ma Ni Pad Me Hum,* (5) Tracing of the Nine Star Path. In the right circles, the Talisman will offer protection to the home of a person with auspicious karma. In the left circles, wealth will arrive at the home of a benevolent and kind person. The left was composed by the Master of Yun Shi Jing She, Lin Yun, while a visitor at the study of disciple Crystal Chu. (Yun Shi Jing She is the name of Professor Lin Yun's shrines and sanctuaries all over the world.)

CHAPTER 7. *"The Seven Colors of the Rainbow/Chakras."* (Calligraphy by Dr. Catherine Yi-yu Cho Woo, written in the Year of the Dragon, 2000, for Nancy SantoPietro.)

This calligraphy comprises the seven Chinese characters for the various colors of the rainbow and Chakras. In the left-hand column, from top to bottom the characters read "red," "orange," "yellow," "green," "blue," "indigo," and "violet." In the right-hand column, from top to bottom, the characters read "violet/purple," "indigo," "blue," "green," "yellow," "orange," and "red."

CHAPTER 8. *"Everyone for Me; I for Everyone."* (Calligraphy by H. H. Professor Thomas Lin Yun.)

To be read from right to left, this was written in oracle-bone scripture, in cinnabar, while chanting infinite numbers of mantras in the year 2000, on the day of the Mid-Autumn Festival, to bestow blessings upon the readers, author, and publisher of this book: "May they receive longevity and may all their wishes come true." It was composed by *"Yun Shr* Scholar" Lin Shr, while a visitor at the study of disciple Belle Tao. (*Yun Shr* and *Lin Shr* are two of Grandmaster Professor Lin Yun's scholarly names.)

CHAPTER 9. *"Spiritual Healing Cures Illnesses, Strengthens the Body, Prolongs Longevity, and Increases Wisdom."* (Calligraphy by H. H. Professor Thomas Lin Yun.)

To be read from right to left, the right column bestows blessings upon the readers, author, and publisher of this book: "May they and their family members all receive happiness, good health, and peace." The center column reads, "Spiritual Healing Cures Illnesses, Strengthens the Body, Prolongs Longevity, and Increases Wisdom." The left column was composed while chanting mantras by Lin Yun, while a visitor at the study of disciple Crystal Chu.

CHAPTER 10. *"Zen."* (Calligraphy by H. H. Professor Thomas Lin Yun.)

To be read from right to left:

Bodhidharma came from the West carrying not a single word
All he insisted upon was his devoted meditation
If the teachings of Buddha can only be obtained from words
Lake Tungting will be dipped dry by all the brush pen tips★

★In ancient times, when Bodhidharma, the founder of Zen Buddhism, came to China from India, he carried with him not a single scripture. He meditated deeply and achieved enlightenment through sudden awakening. The Zen school of Buddhism believed in achieving "sudden enlightenment" through constant meditation, rather than "gradual enlightenment" through studying and memorization of Buddhist scriptures and texts. Therefore, the disciples of Bodhidharma believed that if the teachings of Buddha could only be obtained through studying scriptures and texts, then all the water in the great Lake Tungting might still not be enough to ink the brush pens for writing these scriptures.

The left column bestows blessings upon the families of the readers, author, and publisher of this book: Lin Yun composed it while chanting mantras; at the time he was a visitor at the study of disciple Crystal Chu, in September 2000.

CHAPTER 11. *"Longevity."* (Calligraphy by H. H. Professor Thomas Lin Yun.)

To be read from right to left. The right column was written with cinnabar while chanting infinite numbers of mantras, in the year 2000, the Millennium Year of the Golden Dragon, on the day of the Mid-Autumn Festival. It bestows blessings upon the readers, author, and publisher of this book: "May they and their family members receive happiness and longevity." In the center column are the Chinese characters for "Longevity." The left column was composed by Lin Yun, while a visitor at the study of disciple Robert Chiu.

APPENDIX A. *"The Medicine Buddha Prayer."* (Calligraphy by Dr. Catherine Yi-yu Cho Woo, orally transmitted from H. H. Professor Thomas Lin Yun to Dr. Woo and then from Dr. Woo for Nancy SantoPietro.)

To be read from left to right and top to bottom, the calligraphy is "The Medicine Buddha," hand-drawn calligraphy donated by Dr. Catherine Woo, representing the Medicine Buddha Prayer, English translation by Lin-Lin Cheng for Rev. Crystal Chu, CEO of the Yun Lin Temple. The inscription on the last column (farthest left) reads, "This prayer was passed down from H. H. Grandmaster Professor Lin Yun, Rinpoche, respectfully received by Dr. Catherine Yi-yu Cho Woo."

CLOSING STATEMENT. *"Feng Shui."* (Calligraphy by Dr. Catherine Yi-yu Cho Woo, written in the Year of the Dragon, 2000, for Nancy SantoPietro.)

This calligraphy comprises the two Chinese characters for *Feng Shui,* which means "wind and water."

Notes

1. Source: Yun Lin Temple Newsletter.
2. Becker, *Cross Currents*.
3. Gerber, *Vibrational Medicine for the 21st Century*, 502.
4. Miasm is an energetic mass that exists outside the body; although not an illness in and of itself, it holds the potential for an illness to occur.
5. Wright, *Flower Essences*.
6. For more information on EMFs, see Becker, *Cross Currents*.
7. See Berthold-Bond, *Better Basics for the Home*, and Baker, *Prescriptions for a Healthy House*.
8. Ibid.
9. Braden, *Awakening to Zero Point*.
10. Dr. Heather Anne Harder originated the concept of the "Great Awakening" in her book *Perfect Power in Consciousness*.
11. Braden, *Awakening to Zero Point*.
12. Rodegast and Stanton, *Emmanuel's Book*.
13. Ibid.
14. This section on sound and tone healing was cowritten with Robin Spiegel, massage therapist and sound-and-color healer.
15. Sources for this table include Gurudas, Fox, and Ryerson, *Gem Elixirs and Vibrational Healing;* and Lorusso and Glick, *Healing Stones*.
16. This chart was compiled by Robin Spiegel, massage therapist, aromatherapist, and sound-and-color healer. Ms. Spiegel is the owner of Ancient Aromatics, Rye, N.Y. For more information on therapeutic-grade essential oils, see the Nancy SantoPietro & Associates Web site (www.fengshui-santopietro.com).

Selected Bibliography

Baker, Paula, AIA, Erica Elliott, M.D., and John Banta. *Prescriptions for a Healthy House: A Practical Guide for Architects, Builders, and Homeowners*. Santa Fe: Baker-Laporte and Associates, Inc., 1988.

Ballentine, Rudolph, M.D. *Radical Healing: Integrating the World's Great Therapeutic Traditions to Create a New Transformative Medicine*. New York: Crown Publishing Group, 1996.

Beaulieu, John. *Music and Sound in the Healing Arts: An Energy Approach*. Barrytown, N.Y.: Station Hill Press, 1987.

Becker, Robert O. *Cross Currents: The Promise of Electromedicine, the Perils of Electropollution*. New York: Putnam Publishing Group, 1991.

Berthold-Bond, Annie. *Better Basics for the Home: Simple Solutions for Less Toxic Living*. New York: Crown Publishing Group, 1999.

Braden, Gregg. *Awakening to Zero Point*. Bellevue, Wash.: Radio Bookstore Press, 1997.

Chiazzari, Suzy. *Colour Scents: Healing with Colour and Aroma*. Essex, England: The C. W. Daniel Co., Ltd., 1998. Woodstock: Beekman Publishing, Inc., 1998.

Davis, Patricia. *Aromatherapy A–Z*. Essex, England: The C. W. Daniel Co., Ltd., 1988.

———. *Subtle Aromatherapy*. Essex, England: The C. W. Daniel Co., Ltd., 1991.

Gerber, Richard, M.D. *Vibrational Medicine*. Santa Fe: Bear & Co., 1988.

Gurudas, John Fox, and Kevin Ryerson. *Gem Elixirs and Vibrational Healing*. Vol. 2. Boulder, Colo.: Cassandra Press, 1986.

Gurudas, John Fox, and Kevin Ryerson. *Gem Elixirs and Vibrational Healing*. Vol. 1. Boulder, Colo.: Cassandra Press, 1985.

Harder, Heather Anne, M.D. *Many Were Called, Few Were Chosen: The Story of Mother Earth and the Earth Based Volunteers*. Crowns Point, Ill.: Light Publishing, 1994.

———. *Perfect Power in Consciousness: Seeking Truth Through the Subconscious and Superconscious Mind.* Crowns Point, Ill.: Light Publications, 1994.

Hay, Louise L. *You Can Heal Your Life.* Santa Monica: Hay House, 1984.

Kaminski, Patricia, and Richard Katz. *Flower Essence Repertory: A Comprehensive Guide to North American and English Flower Essences for Emotional and Spiritual Well Being.* Nevada, Calif.: Earth-Spirit, Inc., 1996.

Liberman, Jacob. *Healing with Light and Color.* Denver: Universal Light, 1998.

———. *Light: Medicine of the Future.* Santa Fe: Bear & Co., 1992.

Linn, Denise. *Feng Shui for the Soul.* Santa Monica: Hay House, 1999.

Lorusso, Julia, and Joel Glick. *Healing Stones: The Therapeutic Use of Gems and Minerals.* Albuquerque: Brotherhood of Life, 1984.

Pearson, David. *The New Natural House Book: Creating a Healthy, Harmonious and Ecologically Sound Home.* New York: Simon & Schuster/Fireside, 1989.

Rodegast, Pat, and Judith Stanton. *Emmanuel's Book: A Manual for Living Comfortably in the Cosmos.* New York: Bantam Doubleday Dell Publishing Group, 1985.

Roman, Sanaya. *Soul Love: Awakening Your Heart Centers.* Tiburon, Calif.: Starseed Press, 1997.

———. *Spiritual Growth: Being Your Higher Self.* Tiburon, Calif.: Starseed Press, 1989.

Rosanoff, Nancy. *Intuition Workout.* Fairfield, Conn.: Asian Publishing, 1991.

———. *The Complete Idiot's Guide to Making Money Through Intuition.* New York: Alpha Books, 1999.

Rossbach, Sarah, and Lin Yun. *Living Color: Master Lin Yun's Guide to Feng Shui and the Art of Color.* New York/Tokyo/London: Kodansha America, 1994.

SantoPietro, Nancy. *Feng Shui: Harmony by Design.* New York: Perigee, 1996.

Walters, Derek. *The Feng Shui Handbook: A Practical Guide to Chinese Geomancy* (Five Element Theory). London: Thorsone Publishers, 1991.

Worwood, Valerie Ann. *The Fragrant Mind: Aromatherapy for Personality, Mind, Mood and Emotion.* Novato: New World Library, 1996.

Wright, Machaelle Small. *Flower Essences: Reordering Our Approach to Illness and Health.* Perelandra, Va.: Perelandra, 1988.

Index

body
    Bagua correspondence, 111-12
    Chakra sites, 217, 220, 221
    disease surfacing in, 236-37
    as soul's temple, 213-14
    Three Visceral Cavities, 121-22
Body Secret, 301-2, 304
books, 137-38, 315
Braden, Gregg, 256
Buddha of Healing. *See* Medicine Buddha
Buddhism, 295-96, 417, 418-19. *See also*
    Black Hat Sect
buildings, 14-25, 29-30
burning and fire, 317-18

C

calligraphy, 242, 429
cancer, 131-32, 353-54
candles, 62, 97, 101
Career gua, 81, 86, 87, 92, 267
    Chakra and, 217, 222-23
Chakra Color Breathing Meditation, 162,
    246-51
Chakra Energy System, 6-9, 18, 49, 144,
    209-51
    color system, 215, 240-41
    description of, 50-51, 209-10
    ESPs encoding in, 237
    Feng Shui and, 211-12, 216-51, 259-89,
        316
    functions of, 218
    illness treatment, 237-46, 332-34, 350-79
Chakra Psychology, 210
chanting, 97, 316, 333
ch'i (energy flow), 15-16, 257, 419
    adjustment items, 97-101
    altar area, 317
    assessment of, 18-39, 76
    augmenting/raising, 113
    in body vs. home, 77
    Circle of Life chart of, 235
    clearing emotions and, 61-62
    from clutter, 139
    healing, 297-98, 334-38
    healthy vs. unhealthy, 16
    human and environmental fields, 32-33,
        235-38
    illness and, 51-57
    imbalance/balance, 20, 48
    miasms, 64-65
    natural emission of, 28-29
    predecessor law, 109-11

    realigning, 318-19
    rooms that deplete, 175-76
    rooms that enrich, 174-75
    stagnant, 1, 24, 69, 76, 102-4, 118, 317-18
    two systems of, 49-51
    white light and, 214
Children/Creativity gua, 80, 87, 89, 270-72
    Chakra and, 217, 225-26
Chinese medicine, 48, 79, 297-98
Cinnabar (Jusha) Cures, 307-8
Circle of Life, 18-19, 86, 190, 235
circulatory system, 363-64
clothing color, 239
clutter, 34-35, 113-18, 139
co-creation, 262-64, 326
collectibles, 118, 139
color, 97, 98, 214-15
    in bedrooms, 41, 147-49
    healing with, 7, 8, 27, 215, 238, 242-46,
        317
    as life force, 203
    ways to shift illness, 239-46
color-breathing meditations, 162-63, 241-42,
    246-51, 283
columns, 196, 197
Crown Chakra, 217, 227-29, 231, 275-77
crystals, 27, 28, 69, 97, 113, 297, 338-42
    aurora borealis, 46, 144-45
    chart of properties, 339-42

D

daily activity path, 26, 128-29
death and dying, 62, 287, 323-27
depression, 355-56
desk position, 31-32, 191-93, 197
digestive system, 373-74
divine interventions, 383-411
doorknobs, 34, 41
doorways, 198-202
    Bagua position, 78, 86, 89
    bed position, 31-32, 140, 142, 143, 191
    bedroom, 155-58
    bedroom/bathroom, 152-53
    blocked or broken, 201
    closed to ch'i-depleting rooms, 176
    clutter behind, 116-17
    desk position, 191, 193
    excessive, 198-200
    labeling in floor plan, 84
    opening out, 170-71
    without physical door, 201-2
    problem placements, 198-201

Nancy SantoPietro & Associates, Inc.
Feng Shui Services, Consultant Training Programs, and Healing Retreats

SERVICES

MS. SANTOPIETRO and her associates are available to lecture, teach workshops, and provide Feng Shui health and illness consultations for homes, businesses, hospitals, hospices, and health-related facilities in the United States and internationally.

FENG SHUI CONSULTANT TRAINING PROGRAM

MS. SANTOPIETRO'S highly acclaimed Feng Shui Consultant Training Program, The Accelerated Path™, teaches medical personnel, health-care professionals, interior designers, acupuncturists, healers, and laypeople the art of Feng Shui Design and the Chakra Energy System from a psychospiritual-environmental perspective. With its emphasis on home and health/illness diagnosis, this is the only training program that combines Feng Shui and the Chakra Energy System with adjunct healing disciplines, such as psychic development, mediation, color therapy, and personal daily processing and spiritual enhancement.

ACCELERATED HEALING™ PERSONAL HEALING RETREAT WEEKS (VARIOUS INTERNATIONAL LOCATIONS)

FOR INDIVIDUALS WHO SEEK a safe place to retreat and work on healing personal issues or address the ESP underpinnings of their illness, in addition to addressing one's childhood traumas, unprocessed grief, unresolved issues of the heart, life-path challenges, and past-life obstacles—through the use of Feng Shui Design, the Chakra Energy System, meditations, sound, color, crystals, and essential oils, these life-changing weeks offer an eclectic, progressive approach to transforming blocks, issues, and everyday conflicts.

Website Products, Referrals, and Tools for Healing

NANCY SANTOPIETRO & ASSOCIATES, INCORPORATED, offers Ms. SantoPietro's Guided Chakra Meditation Tapes, Health Videos, Feng Shui Crystals, Therapeutic-Grade Aromatherapy Oils, *Medicine Buddha* (Yao Shi Fu) art poster by Dr. Catherine Yi-yu Cho Woo, and product-related referrals.

Contact Information

FOR MORE INFORMATION, see Nancy SantoPietro & Associates, Inc., Web site. For a free information packet or brochures regarding consultations and health-related services, international Chakra and Feng Shui healing retreats, training programs, class schedules, and products, or to join our mailing list, please contact us by mail, phone, or e-mail at the following address:

NANCY SANTOPIETRO & ASSOCIATES, INC.
1684 80th Street
Brooklyn, NY 11214
Phone: 718-256-2640
Fax: 718-232-8054
E-mail: Nsanpietro@aol.com
Website: www.fengshui-santopietro.com

Yun Lin Temple/Lin Yun Monastery/Professor Lin Yun's Teaching Schedule

FOR INFORMATION on Black Hat Sect Feng Shui teachings and Professor Lin Yun's worldwide lecture itinerary and newsletter, contact:

YUN LIN TEMPLE
2959 Russell Street
Berkeley, CA 94705
Phone: 510-841-2347

LIN YUN MONASTERY
175 Old Westbury Road
Old Westbury, NY 11568-1315
Phone: 516-626-0303
Web site: www.yunlintemple.org
E-mail: info@yulintemple.org